Vasculitis and the Nervous System

Editor

DAVID S. YOUNGER

NEUROLOGIC CLINICS

www.neurologic.theclinics.com

Consulting Editor
RANDOLPH W. EVANS

May 2019 • Volume 37 • Number 2

ELSEVIER

1600 John F. Kennedy Boulevard • Suite 1800 • Philadelphia, Pennsylvania, 19103-2899

http://www.theclinics.com

NEUROLOGIC CLINICS Volume 37, Number 2
May 2019 ISSN 0733-8619, ISBN-13: 978-0-323-67860-5

Editor: Stacy Eastman
Developmental Editor: Donald Mumford

Neurologic Clinics (ISSN 0733-8619) is published quarterly by Elsevier Inc., 360 Park Avenue South, New York, NY 10010–1710. Months of issue are February, May, August, and November. Periodicals postage paid at New York, NY, and additional mailing offices. Subscription prices are $323.00 per year for US individuals, $663.00 per year for US institutions, $100.00 per year for US students, $408.00 per year for Canadian individuals, $803.00 per year for Canadian institutions, $427.00 per year for international individuals, $803.00 per year for international institutions, and $210.00 for Canadian and foreign students/residents. To receive student/resident rate, orders must be accompanied by name of affiliated institution, date of term, and the *signature* of program/residency coordinator on institution letterhead. Orders will be billed at individual rate until proof of status is received. Foreign air speed delivery is included in all *Clinics* subscription prices. All prices are subject to change without notice. **POSTMASTER:** Send address changes to *Neurologic Clinics*, Elsevier Health Sciences Division, Subscription Customer Service, 3251 Riverport Lane, Maryland Heights, MO 63043. **Customer Service: Telephone: 1-800-654-2452 (U.S. and Canada); 314-447-8871 (outside U.S. and Canada). Fax: 314-447-8029. E-mail: journalscustomerservice-usa@elsevier.com (for print support); journalsonlinesupport-usa@elsevier.com (for online support).**

Reprints. For copies of 100 or more of articles in this publication, please contact the Commercial Reprints Department, Elsevier Inc., 360 Park Avenue South, New York, New York, 10010-1710; Tel.: +1-212-633-3874; Fax: +1-212-633-3820, and E-mail: reprints@elsevier.com.

Neurologic Clinics is also published in Spanish by Nueva Editorial Interamericana S.A., Mexico City, Mexico.

Neurologic Clinics is covered in *Current Contents/Clinical Medicine, MEDLINE/PubMed (Index Medicus), EMBASE/Excerpta Medica, and PsycINFO, and ISI/BIOMED.*

Contributors

CONSULTING EDITOR

RANDOLPH W. EVANS, MD
Clinical Professor, Department of Neurology, Baylor College of Medicine, Houston, Texas, USA

EDITOR

DAVID S. YOUNGER, MD, MPH, MS
Department of Neurology, Division of Neuro-Epidemiology, New York University School of Medicine, College of Global Public Health, New York University, Department of Health Policy and Management, Doctoral Candidate, School of Public Health, City University of New York, New York, New York, USA

AUTHORS

ANDREW CARLSON
Department of Pathology, Division of Dermatology and Dermatopathology, Albany Medical College, Albany, New York, USA

FRANCISCO DAVID CARMONA, PhD
Departamento de Genética e Instituto de Biotecnología, Universidad de Granada, Granada, Spain

PATRICIA K. COYLE, MD
Department of Neurology, Vice Chair, Clinical Affairs, Director, MS Comprehensive Care Center, Stony Brook University Medical Center, Stony Brook, New York, USA

HUBERT DE BOYSSON, MD
Department of Internal Medicine, Centre Hospitalier Universitaire de Caen, Caen, France

P. JAMES B. DYCK, MD
Professor, Head of the Peripheral Nerve Section and Peripheral Nerve Laboratory, Department of Neurology, Mayo Clinic, Rochester, Minnesota, USA

MIGUEL A. GONZÁLEZ-GAY, MD, PhD
Epidemiology, Genetics and Atherosclerosis Research Group on Systemic Inflammatory Diseases, Rheumatology Division, IDIVAL, School of Medicine, University of Cantabria, Santander, Spain; Cardiovascular Pathophysiology and Genomics Research Unit, School of Physiology, Faculty of Health Sciences, University of the Witwatersrand, Johannesburg, South Africa

LOÏC GUILLEVIN, MD
Vasculitides and Scleroderma, Department of Internal Medicine, Referral Center for Rare Autoimmune and Systemic Diseases, Hôpital Cochin, Université Paris Descartes, Paris, France

KELLY G. GWATHMEY, MD
Assistant Professor, Department of Neurology, Virginia Commonwealth University, Richmond, Virginia, USA

RAQUEL LÓPEZ-MEJÍAS, PhD
Epidemiology, Genetics and Atherosclerosis Research Group on Systemic Inflammatory Diseases, Rheumatology Division, IDIVAL, Santander, Spain

ANA MÁRQUEZ, PhD
Systemic Autoimmune Diseases Unit, Hospital Clínico San Cecilio and Instituto de Investigación Biosanitaria de Granada (ibs.GRANADA), Granada, Spain

JAVIER MARTÍN, MD, PhD
Instituto de Parasitología y Biomedicina "López-Neyra," IPBLN-CSIC, PTS Granada, Granada, Spain

JENNIFER A. TRACY, MD
Assistant Professor, Department of Neurology, Mayo Clinic, Rochester, Minnesota, USA

DAVID S. YOUNGER, MD, MPH, MS
Department of Neurology, Division of Neuro-Epidemiology, New York University School of Medicine, College of Global Public Health, New York University, Department of Health Policy and Management, Doctoral Candidate, School of Public Health, City University of New York, New York, New York, USA

Contents

Vasculitis is defined as inflammation of blood vessel walls for at least some time during the course of the disease, and affects arteries and veins of varying caliber. Two Chapel Hill Consensus Conferences, in 1994 and 2012, provide consensus on nosology and definitions for the commonest forms of vasculitis. The category of single-organ vasculitis, suggesting the limited expression of a systemic vasculitis, includes primary central nervous system vasculitis and nonsystemic peripheral nervous system vasculitis. The historical aspects of systemic and limited forms of vasculitis are reviewed in 11 relevant themes.

The systemic vasculitides are heterogeneous clinicopathologic disorders that share the common feature of vascular inflammation. The resulting disorder can vary depending on involvement of specific organs, caliber of blood vessels, the underlying inflammatory process, and individual host factors. The cumulative result is diminished blood flow, vascular alterations, and eventual occlusion with variable ischemia, necrosis, and tissue damage. An international revised nomenclature system provides the necessary nosology and findings relevant to classify each of the vasculitides. This article is an introduction and overview of the clinical presentation, differential diagnosis, laboratory evaluation, and treatment of systemic and nervous system vasculitides.

The epidemiology of vasculitis has witnessed extraordinary advances in the past decade influenced by the worldwide increased recognition and accurate classification and diagnosis of the vasculitides, and insights brought by genome-wide association studies and online genetic biological repositories that permit researchers to freely access a wide array of genetic and clinical resources that contribute to the understanding of the heritable factors of the systemic vasculitides. This article reviews the current knowledge of the epidemiology of vasculitides in different global regions.

Vasculitides are a heterogeneous group of inflammatory diseases of blood vessels in which genetic variation plays an important role in their susceptibility and clinical spectrum. Because of the use of novel technologies and the increase of the sample size of the study cohorts, the knowledge of the genetic background of vasculitides has considerably expanded during the last years. However, few insights have been obtained regarding the genetics underlying severe clinical phenotypes, such as those related to the nervous system. In this review the authors provide an updated overview of the genetic landscape behind vasculitis predisposition and development of neurologic manifestations.

There has been extraordinary research in the blood-brain barrier. Once considered a static anatomic barrier to the traffic of molecules in and out of the central nervous system when fully developed in adults, the blood-brain barrier is now known to be not only fully functional in development but also vital in cerebrovascular angiogenesis. Blood-brain barrier breakdown has been recognized as an important factor in a variety of primary neurologic diseases; however, such disturbances have yet to be critically analyzed. This article reviews the history, neurodevelopment, ultrastructure, function, and clinicopathologic correlation and relevance to central nervous system vasculitis.

Neuroimaging plays a vital role in the diagnosis of primary and secondary vasculitic disorders. There multiple neuroimaging options available to accurately describe the underlying clinical deficits of involved cases. Noninvasive neuroimaging modalities provide less risk and when interdigitated, form the basis for a more conclusive understanding of the disease process. There are instances in which invasive cerebral angiography may be needed to image the intricate and at times, small involved vessels. Neuroradiologists should be included in the multidisciplinary team of physicians caring for patients with vasculitides and in research to provide more sensitive and safe modalities for accurate diagnosis.

Granulomatous inflammation, the prototypical histopathology of adult and childhood vasculitis, is characterized by inflammation of blood vessels accompanied by giant cells and epithelioid cells in the walls of cerebral vessels ranging from small leptomeningeal veins to large named cerebral arteries. Headache, hemiparesis, mental changes, abnormal cerebrospinal fluid protein content, and pleocytosis are suggestive features that warrant brain and leptomeningeal biopsy to make the diagnosis certain and begin cytotoxic therapy to improve outcome.

The vasculitides are diseases characterized by inflammation of blood vessels and inflammatory leukocytes in vessel walls. There is an increased propensity for ischemic stroke, resulting from compromise of vessel lumina with distal tissue ischemia; and hemorrhagic or nonhemorrhagic stroke, and aneurysmal formation and bleeding, due to loss of vessel integrity.

The vasculitic neuropathies encompass a wide range of disorders characterized by ischemic injury to the vasa nervorum. Patients with vasculitic neuropathies develop progressive, painful sensory or sensorimotor deficits that are typically multifocal or asymmetric. Depending on the underlying etiology, the vasculitis may be confined to the peripheral nervous system; may be one manifestation of a primary systemic vasculitis; or one manifestation of a systemic vasculitis that is secondary to underlying connective tissue disease, drug exposure, viral infection, or paraneoplastic syndrome. This article reviews the classification, clinical presentation, diagnostic approach, etiologies, and treatment of the vasculitic neuropathies.

Giant cell arteritis (GCA) is a chronic, idiopathic, granulomatous vasculitis of medium and large arteries comprising overlapping phenotypes of cranial arteritis and extracranial GCA. Vascular complications are generally due to delay in diagnosis and initiation of effective treatment. Advancements in MRI and MR angiography, computed tomography angiography, 18fluoro-deoxyglucose/PET, and color duplex ultrasonography have led to improved diagnosis. Corticosteroids are the mainstay of therapy in GCA; however, their use is associated with predictable and occasionally serious side effects. Biological agents are effective and safe corticosteroid-sparing agents in treating GCA. This article reviews the epidemiologic, clinicopathologic features, diagnosis, and treatment of GCA.

Polyarteritis nodosa (PAN) is a necrotizing vasculitis affecting medium-sized vessels whose main manifestations are weight loss, fever, peripheral neuropathy, renal, musculoskeletal, gastrointestinal tract and/or cutaneous involvement(s), hypertension and/or cardiac failure. Peripheral neuropathy is one of the most frequent and earliest symptoms, affecting 50%

to 75% of PAN patients. Central nervous system involvement affects only 2% to 10% of PAN patients, often late during the disease course. Treatment relies on combining corticosteroids and an immunosuppressant (mainly cyclophosphamide) in patients with poor prognoses. In patients with hepatitis B virus-related PAN, plasma exchanges and antiviral drugs should be combined with corticosteroids.

Autoimmune encephalitis is a severe inflammatory disorder of the brain with diverse causes and a complex differential diagnosis. Recent advances in the past decade have led to the identification of new syndromes and biological markers of limbic encephalitis, the commonest presentation of autoimmune encephalitis. The successful use of serum and intrathecal antibodies to diagnose affected patients has resulted in few biopsy and postmortem examinations. In those available, there can be variable infiltrating inflammatory T cells with cytotoxic granules in close apposition to neurons, consistent with an inflammatory autoimmune basis, but true vasculitis is rarely seen. The exception is Hashimoto encephalopathy.

There have been significant advances in the understanding of the vasculitides in the past several years, leading to more precise classification and nosology. Ophthalmologic manifestations may be the presenting feature of and a clue to the diagnosis of vasculitis, or develop in the course of the illness owing to a common disease mechanism. Precise diagnosis and prompt treatment prevents short- and long-term ophthalmologic sequela.

The diagnosis of primary central and peripheral nerve vasculitides should be established with certainty if suspected before commencing potent immunosuppressive therapy. The aim of induction therapy is to rapidly control the underlying inflammatory response and stabilize the blood-brain and blood-nerve barriers, followed by maintenance immunosuppression tailored to the likeliest humoral and cell-mediated autoimmune inflammatory vasculitic processes.

Illicit drug abuse is a common differential diagnosis of acquired central nervous system vasculitis even though there are only a handful of histopathologically confirmed patients in the literature from among the many potential classes of abused drugs traditionally implicated in this disease. This article considers the major classes of illicit drugs in those with and without human immunodeficiency virus type-1 infection and acquired immune deficiency syndrome.

NEUROLOGIC CLINICS

RELATED SERIES

Neuroimaging Clinics
Psychiatric Clinics
Child and Adolescent Psychiatric Clinics

THE CLINICS ARE AVAILABLE ONLINE!
Access your subscription at:
www.theclinics.com

Preface

Vasculitis of the Nervous System

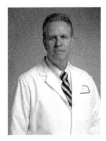

David S. Younger, MD, MPH, MS
Editor

Systemic and nervous system vasculitides are a heterogeneous group of related disorders, each characterized by vascular inflammation such that it has the potential to cause serious morbidity and mortality if unrecognized and therefore untreated. Systemic vasculitis affects all populations and every nationality and walk of life, from childhood to older age. The first issue of "Vasculitis of the Nervous System" published in the *Neurologic Clinics* 30 years ago met the urgent need for a clear, concise, and reliable source of epidemiology, pathogenesis, clinical presentation, laboratory evaluation, and management of these disorders. This updated issue includes many of the original contributors with updated results of translational scientific discoveries, data from clinical trials, and advances in the clinical assessment, pathophysiology, genetic biomarkers, standard of care, and novel therapies of vasculitis.

I am continually inspired at the biennial meetings of The International Vasculitis & ANCA Workshops, which tasks me to summarize their proceedings. This year, the Workshop meets at the University of Pennsylvania in Philadelphia and promises to be an exciting interchange of shared knowledge.

In 2019, I am moving my primary medical school affiliation from New York University to City University of New York (CUNY). I have had the good fortune of interacting with brilliant coauthors, and thought-provoking medical students, neurology trainees, public health doctoral students, and professors at New York University, in the Department of Neurology, Division of Neuro-epidemiology, and the College of Global Public Health; and at City University of New York, where I am a doctoral candidate in Health Policy and Management. Together, we strive to the highest ethical standards in clinical medicine and public health practice and research.

I express thanks to my coauthors, all experts in their individual field of vasculitis, for allowing me to assemble them for the task of producing another monumental issue of "Vasculitis of the Nervous System." I also express my heartfelt appreciation to my wife, Holly, and sons, Adam and Seth, who encourage me to take on projects that promote

Neurol Clin 37 (2019) xi–xii
https://doi.org/10.1016/j.ncl.2019.03.005
0733-8619/19/© 2019 Published by Elsevier Inc.

core values of medicine and humanity, as my patients daily educate me in empathy and humility.

David S. Younger, MD, MPH, MS
Department of Neurology
Division of Neuro-Epidemiology
New York University School of Medicine
College of Global Public Health
New York University
Department of Health Policy and Management
School of Public Health
City University of New York
333 East 34th Street, Suite 1J
New York, NY 10016, USA

E-mail address:
youngd01@nyu.edu

Website:
http://www.davidsyounger.com

Eleven Themes in the History of Systemic and Nervous System Vasculitides

David S. Younger, MD, MPH, MS[a,b,*]

KEYWORDS

- History • Vasculitides • Nervous system

KEY POINTS

- Vasculitis is defined as inflammation of blood vessel walls for at least some time during the course of the disease, and affects arteries and veins of varying caliber.
- Two Chapel Hill Consensus Conferences, 1 in 1994 and the other in 2012, provide consensus on nosology and definitions for the commonest forms of vasculitis.
- The category of single-organ vasculitis, suggesting the limited expression of a systemic vasculitis, includes primary central nervous system vasculitis and nonsystemic peripheral nervous system vasculitis.
- The historical aspects of systemic and limited forms of vasculitis are reviewed in 11 relevant themes.

NOMENCLATURE

Vasculitis is defined as inflammation of blood vessel walls for at least some time during the course of the disease, and affects arteries and veins of varying caliber. Two Chapel Hill Consensus Conferences (CHCCs), one in 1994[1] and the other in 2012,[2] provided consensus on nosology and definitions for the commonest forms of vasculitis. The revised CHCC nomenclature serves as a guide for the categorization of diverse forms of vasculitis based on the vessels involved, and provides a scheme for the neurologic aspects thereof (**Box 1**).

HISTORICAL THEMES

Theme One: The early history of vasculitis is debatable but one fact is clear, the earliest patients with systemic vasculitides had prominent neurologic involvement.

Disclosure Statement: The author has nothing to disclose.
[a] Department of Neurology, Division of Neuro-Epidemiology, New York University School of Medicine, New York, NY 10016, USA; [b] School of Public Health, City University of New York, New York, NY, USA
* 333 East 34th Street, Suite 1J, New York, NY 10016.
E-mail address: youngd01@nyu.edu
Website: http://www.davidsyounger.com

Neurol Clin 37 (2019) 149–170
https://doi.org/10.1016/j.ncl.2019.01.001
0733-8619/19/© 2019 Elsevier Inc. All rights reserved.

neurologic.theclinics.com

Box 1
Childhood and adult vasculitides with nervous system involvement

Large vessel vasculitis
  Giant cell arteritis
  Takayasu arteritis
  Idiopathic aortitis (IgG4)

Medium vessel vasculitis
  Polyarteritis nodosa
  Kawasaki disease

Small vessel vasculitis
  ANCA-associated vasculitis
    Microscopic polyangiitis
    Granulomatosis with polyangiitis (Wegener)
    Eosinophilic granulomatosis with polyangiitis (Churg-Strauss)
  Immune-complex vasculitis
    Cryoglobulinemic vasculitis
    IgA vasculitis (Henoch-Schönlein purpura)
    Hypocomplementemic urticarial vasculitis (IgA vasculitis)

Variable vessel vasculitis
  Behçet disease
  Cogan syndrome

Primary CNS vasculitis

Vasculitis associated with collagen vascular disease
  Systemic lupus erythematosus
  Rheumatoid arthritis

Vasculitis due to substance abuse
  Amphetamines
  Cocaine
  Opioids

Vasculitis and infection
  Bacteria
  Viruses
  Neurosyphilis
  Mycoses
  Parasites
  Human immunodeficiency virus–AIDS

Kussmaul and Maier[3] provided the first complete gross and microscopic description of a patient with leg pains, cramps, and tenderness so prominent that trichinosis was considered in an article entitled, "A Hitherto Undescribed Peculiar Disease of the Arteries Which is Accompanied by Bright's Disease and a Rapidly Progressive General Paralysis of the Muscles." At postmortem examination, there was widespread arteritis that resembled syphilitic periarteritis. The disorder was named periarteritis for the inflammation around blood vessels. In 1908, Longcope[4] described the first American patient with periarteritis, a 35-year-old man with constitutional symptoms and subacute leg pains. Postmortem examination showed widespread necrotizing arteritis and nodules along small-sized and medium-sized vessels of the heart, liver, kidney, pancreas, testicles, brain, nerves, and skeletal muscles, sparing the lungs and spleen. The histologic lesions consisted of mononuclear cell infiltration, necrosis of internal and external elastic lamina of the media, fibrin deposition, aneurysmal dilatation, perivascular inflammation of the adventitia, and intimal proliferation resulting in narrowing of arterial lumina. Kernohan and Woltman[5] summarized the clinical and neuropathologic aspects of adult polyarteritis nodosa (PAN), and Krahulik and colleagues[6] reported the postmortem neurologic findings of fulminant childhood PAN (cPAN). The dominant neurologic picture of both adult PAN and cPAN was a peripheral neuritis that occurred in one-half of patients early in the illness with a predilection for the legs. At postmortem examination, all had arteritic lesions along nutrient arteries of the peripheral nerves, and three-quarters had lesions in arteriae nervorum. The combination of acute and chronic lesions correlated with known exacerbations. Involvement of the central nervous system (CNS) was estimated to occur in 8% of cases, evident by clinically apparent brain infarcts resulting from occlusion of cerebral vessels, which was often insidious in its progression. In PAN, as in the other systemic necrotizing arthritides, the vasculitic lesion proceeded in a characteristic manner, commencing with invasion of the intima, media, and adventitia by polymorphonuclear, plasma cells, eosinophils, and lymphocytes, leading to swelling of the media, and fibrinoid necrosis that clusters around the vasa vasorum, with fragmentation of the internal elastic lamina. There was focal deposition of perivascular connective tissue, vascular necrosis, and denuding of the endothelium, followed by vascular thrombosis, ischemia, aneurysm formation, rupture, and hemorrhage. Healed lesions coexisted with active lesions. Harry Lee Parker conceptualized nerve and muscle biopsy in a discussion of the paper by Kernohan and Woltman[5] commenting, "It occurs to me that in any case in which polyarteritis nodosa may be suspected, it is advisable to take a biopsy from a peripheral nerve, muscle or artery." There are no published series confirming the correlation of the extent of systemic necrotizing arteritis that may be predicted by the singular finding of vasculitis in a cutaneous nerve biopsy specimen. A variant of PAN was recognized in very young children with mucocutaneous lymph node syndrome.[7,8] Although early publications used the term infantile PAN,[9,10] Kawasaki disease (KD) is the preferred term to describe this childhood syndrome with worldwide occurrence, affecting children of all ages and races. Both PAN and KD are prototypical examples of medium vessel vasculitides.

Theme Two: Contemporaneously, small vessel vasculitis (SVV) syndromes were recognized and differentiated from PAN.

First described by Wohlwill[11] in 1923, Davson and colleagues[12] and Wainwright and Davson[13] later described microscopic polyangiitis (MPA) in 34 patients that differed from PAN due to selective involvement of small microscopic arteries, arterioles, capillaries, and venules, including glomerular and pulmonary alveolar capillaries. Fever, arthralgia, purpura, hemoptysis, pulmonary hemorrhage, abdominal pain, and gastrointestinal bleeding likewise preceded the explosive phase of systemic necrotizing vasculitis that affected the kidney and lungs, with rapidly progressive glomerulonephritis and pulmonary capillaritis. Two of 5 deaths were attributed to CNS involvement by vasculitis during periods of disease, respectively at 4 and 8 months; however, that could not be confirmed because postmortem examinations were not performed. The disorder was later reclassified by the CHCC as a necrotizing SVV, with little or no immune-complex deposition that primarily affected the kidney and lungs. Medium-sized arteries might be involved even though the disease was predominantly considered to affect small-sized arteries, arterioles, capillaries, and venules of the 2 organs most affected, with variable systemic necrotizing vasculitis.

The first patient with eosinophilic granulomatosis with polyangiitis (EGPA) was probably Case 1 of Lamb,[14] reported in 1914 under the heading of PAN. That patient, a 26-year-old man with 2 years of worsening asthma, developed fever, palpable purpura, nodular skin lesions, hemoptysis, vomiting, urinary difficulty, and granular urinary casts. He died 1 month later and postmortem examination showed necrotizing arteritis of small arteries, with dense collections of extravascular eosinophils and tissue eosin-ophilia in the heart, stomach, and kidney. Decades later, Churg and Strauss[15] described the clinical and postmortem findings of 13 patients with asthma, fever, and hypereosinophilia, accompanied by eosinophilic exudation, fibrinoid change, and granulomatous proliferation, that constituted the so-called allergic granuloma, that was found within vessels walls and in extravascular connective tissue of major or-gan systems, leading to cardiac, pulmonary, gastrointestinal, skin, peripheral nervous system (PNS), and CNS manifestations. In 1977, Chumbley and colleagues[16] described 30 asthmatic patients from the Mayo Clinic, over the period 1950 to 1974, with necrotizing vasculitis of small arteries and veins, with extravascular granu-lomas and infiltration of vessels, and perivascular tissue with eosinophilia. The lungs, peripheral nerves, and skin were most frequently involved, and renal failure was encountered in only 1 patient. Corticosteroids seemed to confer long-term survival. In 1984, Lanham and colleagues[17] emphasized that the combination of necrotizing vasculitis, tissue infiltration by eosinophils and extravascular granulomas suggested by Churg and Strauss[15] occurred contemporaneously in only a few patients. More-over, such histologic findings could also be encountered in other granulomatous, vas-culitic, and eosinophilic disorders in the absence of clinical asthma, allergic rhinitis, sinusitis, pulmonary infiltrates, and cardiac involvement pathognomonic of EGPA. The investigators described a phasic pattern of EGPA in which allergic disease pre-ceded systemic vasculitis and eosinophilic tissue infiltrates might occur in the absence of peripheral blood eosinophilia. Pulmonary infiltrates and upper respiratory tract and gastrointestinal disease often preceded the vasculitic component of the syndrome, leading to cardiac, cutaneous, nervous system, renal, bone, and muscle involvement. In 1990, the American College of Rheumatology[18] developed criteria for the classifica-tion of EGPA that included ascertainment of 4 or more of the following: asthma, eosin-ophilia of greater than 10%, mononeuropathy or polyneuropathy, nonfixed pulmonary infiltrates on chest radiograph, paranasal sinus abnormality, and extravascular eosin-ophils on tissue biopsy that included an artery, arteriole, or venule. These criteria were inadequate in differentiating the various clinicopathological expressions of SVV and a patient with asthma and paranasal sinusitis could fit the designation of EGPA. The 1994 CHCC[1] characterized EGPA as an eosinophil-rich and granulomatous inflamma-tory process that involved the respiratory tract, with necrotizing vasculitis that affected small-sized to medium-sized vessels, such as capillaries, venules, arterioles, and ar-teries, with associated asthma and eosinophilia.

The syndrome of granulomatosis with polyangiitis (GPA), which included granuloma in the nasopharynx, sinuses, and lower respiratory tract with focal segmental glomer-ulonephritis and disseminated SVV, was described in 1954 by Godman and Churg.[19] Nervous system involvement in GPA was found in up to one-half of patients according to Drachman,[20] who also described a patient with 1 month of headache that awak-ened him from sleep followed by rhinitis, nasal obstruction, epistaxis, mononeurop-athy multiplex, confusion, and hypertension. Active arteritis and necrotizing granuloma were found in the brain, not in peripheral nerves. Two decades later, Fauci and colleagues[21] and Hoffman and colleagues,[22] at the National Institutes of Health (NIH), respectively reported a prospective series of 85 patients with GPA and a retro-spective assessment of 180 patients followed for 6 months to 24 years, describing nervous system involvement in up to 23% of patients. There was a preponderance of mononeuritis multiplex with CNS abnormalities in 8% to 10% of patients. CNS involvement included stroke, cranial nerve abnormalities, and diabetes insipidus. Fauci and colleagues[21] established the efficacy of cyclophosphamide and prednisone in achieving complete remissions in 93% of patients, as well as the tendency of patients to relapse and accrue additive mortality from both disease and treatment; however, alternative immunosuppressive regimens were not equally effective.[22] In a landmark article, Godman and Churg[19] concluded that MPA, EGPA, and GPA were related to one another yet distinct from PAN. This astute conclusion was based mainly on pathologic features and was later substantiated by their common association with antineutrophil cytoplasmic antibody (ANCA) but not so for PAN.

Theme Three: There ensued a renaissance in the understanding of primary systemic vasculitis with convincing clinical evidence to support an important role for ANCA–associated vasculitides (AAVs).

Early observations of ANCA were provided by van der Woude and colleagues[23] in 1985, and Falk and Jennette,[24] followed by progress in the differentiation of these subtypes and understanding of the eponymous manifestations.[25] Proteinase 3 (PR3) is a serine protease found in the azurophilic granules of neutrophils and peroxidase-positive lysosomes of monocytes. Myeloperoxidase (MPO), which constitutes about 5% of the total protein content of the neutrophil cell, is localized to the same cellular compartment as PR3. However, PR3, in contrast to MPO, is also found on the plasma membrane of resting neutrophils and monocytes in many patients. Autoantibodies directed against PR3 and MPO are directed against multiple epitopes. Although sera from different patients may recognize different epitopes, all ANCA recognized restricted epitopes of PR3 involving its catalytic site. The AAV classification seems to better recognize ANCA disease and predict prognosis than other any existing clinical classification systems.[26] However, as with other autoimmune disorders, the etiologic factors and pathogenesis seemed multifactorial, involving the interplay of initiating and predisposing environmental and genetic factors. Important contributing factors to the mediation of vascular and extravascular inflammation included a loss of regulatory T-cell and B-cell function, acute neutrophilic cell injury with release of ANCA-antigens, cytokine priming of neutrophilic cells, subsequent complement activation by fragment crystallizable (Fc) and fragment antigen-binding 2 (Fab2) engagement, and enhancement of complement-dependent cytotoxicity with release of ANCA-antigens into the microenvironment. The ANCA lesion typical of GPA includes both vasculitic and granulomatous features in lung, with focal segmental glomerulonephritis typified pathologically by lysis of glomerular tufts, basement membrane disruption, accumulation of fibrinoid material, thrombosis of glomerular capillary loops, acute tubular necrosis, and cant deposition of immunoglobulin and complement.

There are genetic distinctions between MPO and GPA suggested by the strong association of PR3-ANCA disease with antigenic specificity of HLA-DP and the genes encoding a1-antitrypsin (*SERPINA1*) and PR3 (*PRTN3*), and HLA-DQ for MPO-ANCA.[27] An immunofluorescence technique (IFT) has been standard method for routine determination of ANCA in vasculitis, using ethanol-fixed human neutrophils as substrate. Two main immunofluorescence patterns are distinguished, a cytoplasmic ANCA and perinuclear ANCA. The 1999 "International Consensus Statement on Testing and Reporting anti-neutrophil cytoplasmic antibodies (ANCA)"[28] required laboratories to screen for ANCA by IFT and to confirm the specificity of fluorescent sera by enzyme-linked immunoassay (ELISA) for PR3 and MPO-ANCA. However, conventional ELISA using PR3 immobilized to the surface of the ELISA plate shows great variation in performance and often lacks sensitivity. Capture ELISA is superior in overall diagnostic performance to direct ELISA[29]; however, the sensitivity of capture ELISA may be reduced by the capturing antibodies hiding relevant epitopes. High-sensitivity PR3–ANCA ELISA, which immobilizes PR3 via a bridging molecule to the plastic plate and preserves nearly all epitopes for the binding of ANCA, was superior to direct and capture techniques in GPA.[30]

Theme Four: Hypersensitivity vasculitis leading to cutaneous vasculitis was conceptualized as an immunologic response to antigenic material associated with clinically evident purpura and small vessel inflammation affecting arterioles, capillaries, and postcapillary venules.

Between 1948 and 1952, Zeek[31,32] separated hypersensitivity vasculitis from allergic granulomatous angiitis, rheumatic arteritis, PAN, and giant cell arteritis (GCA). Hemorrhage into the skin or palpable purpura was noted in virtually all patients, resulting from extravasation of erythrocytes, pronounced endothelial swelling, polymorphonuclear, and later mononuclear cell infiltration; followed by fibrosis, necrosis, fibrinoid deposits, and visible polymorphonuclear debris, termed leukocytoclasia. Zeek[33] likened hypersensitivity vasculitis to the anaphylactoid Arthus reaction produced by the experimental injection of horse serum into rabbits.[34] Osler[35] first appreciated the relation of purpuric attacks to cerebral manifestations in the report of a patient with transient hemiparesis and 3 others with potentially fatal cerebral hemorrhages. Gairdner[36] described Henoch-Schönlein purpura (HSP) among 12 patients with anaphylactoid purpura, including 1 child who developed rash, colic, melanotic stools, intussusception, and hematuria, followed by a typical exanthema and convulsion. She died 3 months later and postmortem examination showed scattered cortical hemorrhages associated with cerebral necrotizing arteriolitis. Levitt and Burbank[37] described the clinicopathological findings in 2 previously nonallergic patients with recurrent fatal attacks of HSP after injection of penicillin and ingestion of strawberries, respectively, that included glomerulonephritis alone or with systemic arteriolitis. The finding of IgA deposits in cutaneous blood vessel walls and in glomerular mesangial biopsies of patients with HSP and IgA nephropath[38,39] was circumstantially convincing enough to substitute the term IgA vasculitis for HSP.

Wintrobe and Buell[40] described cryoglobulinemia in a patient with progressive frontal headache, facial pain, Raynaud symptoms, recurrent nosebleeds, exertional dyspnea, palpitation, and changes in the eye grounds due to central vein thrombosis. Postmortem examination showed infiltrating myeloma of the humerus and lumbar vertebra, and splenic enlargement. A unique plasma protein was detected that spontaneously precipitated with cold temperature and solubilized at high temperature and differed from the Bence-Jones proteinuria of other myeloma patients. Lerner and Watson[41] noted the association with purpura and, later, Lerner and Watson[42] described its occurrence in 10% of pathologic sera. Gorevic and colleagues[43] described mixed cutaneous vasculitis in 40 patients, the clinical features of which included palpable purpura in all patients; polyarthralgia in three-quarters; kidney involvement in slightly more than one-half; and deposits of IgG, IgM, and complement, or renal arteritis in a third of patients.

Recurrent attacks of erythematous, urticarial, and hemorrhagic skin lesions that last 24 hours at a time, associated with recurrent attacks of fever, joint swelling, abdominal distress, and low serum complement, indicate hypocomplementemia urticarial vasculitis (HUV) were described by McDuffie and colleagues[44] in 1973; however, small amounts of cryoglobulin were present at 1 time or another in the serum of each patient. When tested by immunodiffusion against purified preparations of rheumatoid factor and human C1q, 2 patients consistently produced bands against the former and 2 others reacted strongly with purified C1q. Skin biopsies showed leukocytoclasia characteristic of necrotizing vasculitis in 1 patient, anaphylactoid purpura in 2 others, and mild nonspecific perivascular infiltration another. Immunofluorescence of skin specimens performed in 3 patients showed fixation of immunoglobulin in the patient with necrotizing vasculitis, whereas in 2 others with a pathologic picture of anaphylactoid purpura or nonspecific dermal infiltrate, immunofluorescence was negative. Renal biopsy in 2 patients showed mild to moderate glomerulonephritis indistinguishable for those seen in other forms of chronic membrane-proliferative glomerulonephritis. The differences from systemic lupus erythematosus (SLE) included more urticarial and purpuric skin lesions, with relatively mild or absent renal and other visceral involvement in the patients with HUV, which was atypical for SLE. Moreover, serum speckled antinuclear and anti-DNA antibodies, and basement membrane immunoglobulin deposits, were absent in those with HUV, also atypical for SLE. An etiopathogenesis related to chronic vascular inflammation, resulting from deposits of immune complexes in small vessel walls seemed likely. Zeiss and colleagues[45] characterized C1q IgG precipitins from HUV sera that precipitated C1q in agarose gel among 4 additional patients. Wisnieski and Naff[46] showed C1q binding activity in IgG from HUV sera, which suggested a relation to SLE but that view was later amended.

Theme Five: The historical account of the category of large vessel vasculitides (LVV) spanned more than a century, with notable advances in the past several years.

Hutchinson[47] provided the first clinical description of temporal arteritis, followed by a pathologic description by Horton and colleagues.[48] Temporal arteritis was named for the site of granulomatous giant cell inflammation and vessel involvement.[49] Those with biopsy-proven temporal arteritis and associated blindness due to vasculitis involvement of ophthalmic and posterior ciliary vessels were classified as having cranial arteritis.[50] The occasional finding of giant cell lesions along the aorta, its branches, and in other medium-sized and large-sized arteries at autopsy in other patients warranted the additional diagnosis of generalized GCA.[51] The pathologic heterogeneity of temporal arteritis was further demonstrated by the finding of intracranial granulomatous arteritic lesions.[52–57] The earliest lesions of GCA consist of vacuolization of smooth muscle cells of the media, with enlargement of mitochondria, infiltration of lymphocytes, plasma cells, and histiocytes. With progression, there is extension of inflammation into the intima and adventitia, leading to segmental fragmentation and necrosis of the elastic lamina, granuloma formation, and proliferation of connective tissue along the vessel wall. This eventuates in vascular thrombosis, intimal proliferation, and fibrosis.

One other LVV, described in the Japanese literature, was change in the central vessels of the retina in the absence of peripheral arterial pulses, typically in women.[58] This pulseless disease, also known as occlusive thromboaortopathy, or Takayasu arteritis, manifested constitutional complaints of malaise, fever, stiffness of the shoulders, nausea, vomiting, night sweats, anorexia, weight loss, and irregularity of menstrual periods weeks to months before the local signs of vasculitis were recognized in up to two-thirds of patients. It is the commonest large vessel vasculitis among Asian women.

Theme Six: One other form of inflammatory aortic disease, or aortitis, came to light in the surgical literature with equally broad and far-reaching implications for concepts of autoimmunity.

In 1972, Walker and colleagues[59] noted that 10% of 217 patients presenting with abdominal aneurysms at Manchester Royal Infirmary between 1958 and 1969 for resection showed excessive thickening of aneurysm walls and perianeurysmal adhesions at operation. Subsequent histologic examination of the walls of the aneurysms showed extensive active chronic inflammatory changes, including plasma-cell infiltration. The clinical features of patients with inflammatory aneurysms differed from those with atherosclerotic disease owing to generally younger age by a decade, lower incidence of rupture, lack of claudication of intermittent the limbs and presence of peripheral pulses, less likelihood of unusual presenting features, elevated erythrocyte sedimentation rate, and lack of calcification on preoperative abdominal radiographs.

In 1985, Pennell and colleagues[60] reported inflammatory aortic or iliac aneurysms in 4.5% of 2816 patients undergoing repair for abdominal aortic aneurysm from 1955 to 1985. Ultrasound and computed tomography imaging suggested the diagnosis in 13.5% and 50% of patients, respectively; the former showing a sonolucent halo with clear definition of the aortic wall posterior to the thickened anterior and lateral aortic walls. In 2000, Rojo-Leyva and colleagues[61] noted idiopathic aortitis in 43% of 1204 aortic specimens gathered over a period of 20 years. In 96% of the patients with idiopathic aortitis and aneurysm formation, aortitis was present only in the thoracic aorta. In 2001, Hamano and colleagues[62] noted a high concentrations of IgG4 associated with sclerosing pancreatitis characterized by obstructive jaundice, infrequent attacks of abdominal pain, irregular narrowing of the pancreatic duct, sonolucent swelling of the parenchyma, lymphoplasmacytic infiltration, fibrosis, and a favorable response to corticosteroid treatment. One year later, Hamano and colleagues[63] noted the association of sclerosing pancreatitis with raised concentrations of IgG4 among those with concomitant hydronephrosis that caused ureteral masses, which were later diagnosed as retroperitoneal fibrosis (RPF). Histologic examination of ureteral and pancreatic tissues revealed abundant tissue infiltration by IgG4-bearing plasma cells. In the same year, 2008, 3 important observations were made. First, Sakata and colleagues[64] concluded that inflammatory abdominal aortic aneurysm (IAAA) was related to IgG4 sclerosing disease. Second, Kasashima and colleagues[65] concluded that IAAA was an IgG4–related disease (RD) together with RPF. Third, Ito and colleagues[66] described a patient with IAAA, hydronephrosis caused by RPF, and high levels of IgG4, in whom treatment with corticosteroids led to clinical improvement and reduction in IgG4 levels. Histologic inspection of the aortic wall specimen showed lymphoplasmacytic infiltration. Immunohistochemical analysis of the tissue showed IgG4-positive plasma cells. The findings suggested that IAAA had an etiopathogenesis similar to autoimmune pancreatitis and that some cases of IAAA and RPF may be aortic and periaortic lesions of an IgG4-RD. One year later, in 2009, Khosroshahi and colleagues[67] described thoracic aortitis due to IgG4-RD with marked elevation of the serum IgG4 levels, with progression to autoimmune pancreatitis. Stone and colleagues[68] described IgG4-related thoracic aortitis with a media-predominant pattern of aortic wall infiltration and marked elevation of serum IgG4 levels, unequivocally linking IgG4-RD with thoracic lymphoplasmacytic aortitis.

Theme Seven: Two forms of variable vessel vasculitides: Behçet disease (BD) and Cogan syndrome (CS), were recognized with very different clinical presentations and systemic involvement.

Adamantiades[69] recognized the disorder of relapsing aphthous ulcers of the mouth, eye, and genitalia, the clinicopathological details of which were later described in detail by Behçet[70,71] in 2 Turkish patients. Nervous system involvement of a 28-year-old Yemenite, with relapsing oral, genital, and oral eruptions over 4 years, was accompanied by severe headache, memory loss, dizziness, lethargy, fatal seizures, and coma. Postmortem examination showed perivascular inflammatory cell infiltration of the meninges, brain, central retinal artery, and optic nerve, with necrotic cerebral lesions. Encephalomyelopathy was detailed at postmortem examination in 2 Australian patients with BD.[72] One presented with hemiparesis, whereas the other patient presented with pseudobulbar affect, vertical gaze palsy, nystagmus, and spastic paraplegias. Postmortem examination showed widespread lesions in cortical and brainstem white matter and hypothalamus, corresponding to small blood vessels, including arterioles and veins that showed perivascular mononuclear cell infiltration. The first well-documented American patient with nervous system involvement of BD was described by Wolf and colleagues.[73] She was a 22-year-old woman with a

5-year history of recurrent oral and genital ulceration, and a 2-year course of progressive visual loss, headache, hemiparesis, ataxia, tremor, dysarthria, cranial nerve palsy, cerebellar and corticospinal tract disease, and mental deterioration, which responded to prednisone therapy. Mogan and Baumgartner[74] described a 26-year-old man with recurrent pain, spasm, redness of the left eye with photophobia, excessive tearing, and marked conjunctival injection, followed by severe attack of dizziness, tinnitus, vertigo, nausea, vomiting, ringing in the ears, profuse perspiration, and deafness. A diagnosis of recurrent interstitial keratitis (IK) and explosive Menière disease was made. In retrospect, he was probably the first reported patient with CS of nonsyphilitic IK.

Vestibuloauditory symptoms were later described by Cogan.[75] Haynes and colleagues[76] set forth diagnostic criteria for typical CS according to the definitions established in a review of 30 patients seen at the National Eye Institute of the NIH by Cogan[75,77] and Norton and Cogan.[78] Symptoms of IK developed abruptly and gradually resolved, associated with photophobia, lacrimation, and eye pain, which may be unilateral or bilateral. Such symptoms tend to recur periodically for years before becoming quiescent. Vestibuloauditory dysfunction was manifested by sudden onset of Menière-like attacks of nausea, vomiting, tinnitus, vertigo, and (frequently) progressive hearing loss that characteristically occurred before or after the onset of IK. However, within 1 to 6 months of the onset of eye symptoms, auditory symptoms progressed to deafness over a period of 1 to 3 months, certainly no longer than 2 years. Cody and Williams[79] provided a description of atypical CS if another significant inflammatory eye lesion in addition to or instead of IK, such as scleritis, episcleritis, retinal artery occlusion, choroiditis, retinal hemorrhage, papilledema, exophthalmos, or tendonitis. Haynes and colleagues[76] defined acute CS as the presence of acute eye disease within 2 weeks of hearing loss, whereas inactive CS was applied to patients without active eye disease or vestibuloauditory dysfunction of greater than 2 weeks before the study. With less than 100 reported patients with this rare childhood and young adult disorder, most reported patients with typical CS appeared as single case reports or patient series, often without pathologic confirmation or evidence of systemic vasculitis in a biopsy or at postmortem examination.

Theme Eight: The concept and clinicopathologic expression of diverse syndromes associated with isolated or nonsystemic peripheral nerve vasculitis (NPNV) intrigued generations of morphologists who later found compelling evidence for distinctive clinicopathologic syndromes associated with inflammatory damage of peripheral nerve microvessels, termed microvasculitis (MV).

The very concept of NPNV, which presumes that the necrotizing vasculitis process is widespread within the PNS and not elsewhere in the body, may yet be called into question for 3 reasons. First, there are reports of equally silent lesions in medium-sized muscular arteries in patients with clinically isolated vasculitic neuropathy.[80] Vasculitis in muscle tissue is included in the definition of nonsystemic vasculitic neuropathy (NSVN),[81] supporting use of the term PNS vasculitis (PNSV) over NPNV. Second, the varied long-term follow-up in cases series ranged from 6 months to 22 years.[82] Third, the presence of only 2 proposed cases from clinicopathologic series have been used as examples of isolated PNSV, both with foci of vasculitis outside the PNS in a visceral organ[5] or the temporal artery,[83] making them anomalous examples of systemic vasculitis, at best.

Contemporaneously, investigators studied patients with inflammatory plexopathy or diabetic neuropathy, elucidating clinicopathologic syndromes characterized by MV in a cutaneous nerve biopsy in peripheral nerve microvessels with a diameter less than 70 μm[81] but with ischemic consequences for the peripheral nerves. Historically, in 1968, Raff and colleagues[84] documented infarctive lesions in a newly diagnosed noninsulin-dependent diabetic, with mononeuritis multiplex and acute asymmetrical leg pain and weakness. Postmortem examination showed a multitude of unilateral small ischemic infarcts of the proximal major nerve trunks of the leg and lumbosacral plexus. In 1984, Bradley and colleagues[85] delineated the syndrome of painful lumbosacral plexopathy with elevated erythrocyte sedimentation rate among 6 patients, 3 of whom were diabetic, including 1 newly diagnosed, with PV in sural nerve biopsies. Johnson and colleagues[86] noted focal fascicular lesions distributed in proximal lumbosacral plexus trunks of 18 out of 32 samples obtained at autopsy from diabetic patients, a quarter of whom were insulin-dependent, using epoxy-embedded and teased nerve fiber sections. These findings suggested a possible propensity for the spontaneous evolution of lumbosacral plexopathy in patients with diabetic neuropathy. Said and colleagues[87] studied 10 noninsulin-dependent diabetics with painful proximal neuropathy and reported ischemic nerve lesions due to necrotizing vasculitis in 3 biopsies of the intermedius cutaneous nerve of the thigh, and 4 others with isolated mononuclear cell inflammation. In 1996, Younger and colleagues[88] characterized microvascular inflammatory lesions in 12 patients with proximal diabetic neuropathy and stepwise or slowly progressive proximal weakness, wasting, and pain, as well as axonopathy, on electrodiagnostic studies. Six nerves showed epineurial MV (**Fig. 1**) composed of cytotoxic-suppressor T cells with activated endoneurial lymphocytes that expressed immunoreactive cytokines, major histocompatibility class II antigens, and endoneurial and epineurial complement C3d and C5b-9. In addition, the nerve tissue of 2 patients with MV had focal pathologic findings indicating ischemia. Dyck and colleagues[89,90] characterized lumbosacral radiculoplexus neuropathy (LSRPN) with and without diabetes. At present, diabetes has not been considered a factor related to vasculitis[81] but there is consensus support for designating nondiabetic LSRPN as a variant of NSVN.[91]

There has also been support for the role of diabetes in both diabetic LSRPN (DLSRPN) and variant forms of diabetic neuropathy. Younger and colleagues[88] reported the clinicopathologic and immunohistochemical findings of sural nerve biopsy

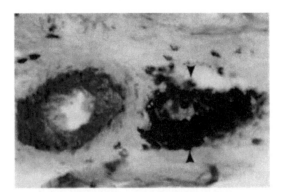

Fig. 1. Peripheral nerve MV in a diabetic. A focal-intense collection of CD3+ T cells efface the wall of a small epineurial blood vessel (*arrowheads*) in a patient with proximal diabetic neuropathy (lumbosacral radiculoplexus neuropathy). In deeper sections (not shown), the same structure stains red in double-labeling with antiactin smooth muscle antigen, a marker for the blood vessel wall (immunoperoxidase, original magnification ×400). (*From* Younger DS, Rosoklija G, Hays AP, Trojaborg W, Latov N. Diabetic peripheral neuropathy: a clinicopathologic and immunohistochemical analysis of sural nerve biopsies. Muscle Nerve 1996;19:722–27; with permission.)

tissues in a cohort of 20 patients with heterogeneous forms of diabetic neuropathy that was continued to a total of 107 patients,[92] of which 3 (3%) showed MV, and 3 (3%) showed necrotizing arteritis (including 2 patients with distal symmetric polyneuropathy and 1 with DLSRPN). The following year, Younger[93] affirmed the existence of DLSRPN in a living case. Despite treatment with 2 g/kg intravenous immunoglobulin for 5 days, followed by 750 mg of intravenous cyclophosphamide and 1000 mg of methylprednisolone intravenously for 3 additional days, the patient died of acute tubular necrosis, increasing lethargy, unresponsiveness, and aspiration pneumonia 4 weeks after admission. General autopsy showed no evidence of systemic or peripheral nerve vasculitis. There was no evidence of systemic vasculitis. Sections of extradural lumbar plexus, sciatic, and femoral nerve tissue showed perivascular epineurial inflammation with infiltration of adjacent endoneurium (**Fig. 2**).

Theme Nine: Diverse clinicopathologic and radiographic syndromes of potentially fatal adult and childhood primary CNS vasculitis have been described; however, none has stood the test of time as well as granulomatous angiitis.

It has been said that efforts to define a disease are attempts to understand the concept of the disease. In no other vasculitis disorder has this been more evident as in granulomatous angiitis of the CNS. No other vasculitis syndrome has captured the attention of so many neurologists and neuropathologists over the decades, and captured the focus of such vigorous debate. In 1922, Harbitz[94] described 2 patients with a previously unrecognized cerebral vasculitis. At age 26 years, a woman noted worsening headaches, mental change, and ataxia, culminating 2 years later in stupor, spastic paraparesis, coma, and death. The other patient, a 46-year-old man, developed hallucinations and confusion, progressing to gait difficulty, stupor, coma, and death in 9 months. At postmortem examination, both had granulomatous vasculitis of the meninges, composed of lymphocytes, multinucleate giant cells, and epithelioid cells, with vessel necrosis and extension into the brain along involved veins and arteries of varying caliber. Over the ensuing quarter century, additional patients reported under the rubric of allergic angiitis and granulomatosis,[95] GCA,[96] and sarcoidosis[97] were described. In 1959, Cravioto and Fegin[98] delineated the clinicopathologic syndrome of granulomatous angiitis, and so named it for the distinctive CNS pathologic findings. For 2 more decades, rare affected patients were identified; however, there was no effective treatment.

Several achievements of the 1980s further transformed the concept of the disorder. In 1983, Cupps and colleagues[99,100] influenced by their advances in the classification, diagnosis, and treatment of systemic vasculitis, advocated cerebral angiography for the diagnosis of isolated CNS angiitis, and prednisone and oral cyclophosphamide therapy for those affected. The angiographic pattern of beading (in 2 patients) or the sausage appearance (in 1 patient) of lesioned vessels, had previously been noted by Hinck and colleagues[101] in a case of giant cell granulomatous angiitis. In 1988, Younger and colleagues[102] analyzed pathologically verified cases of granulomatous angiitis related to herpes zoster virus (HZV) infection, lymphoma, and sarcoidosis, with idiopathic cases. Fever, headache, and mental changes, often leading to focal cerebral signs, with cerebrospinal fluid (CSF) pleocytosis, elevation of the protein content, and normal or nonspecifically abnormal angiographic findings, were found in most patients. In the same year, Calabrese and Mallek[103] reported on so-called primary angiitis of the CNS (PACNS)[103] and isolated angiitis of the CNS (IACNS),[99] emphasizing the restricted nature of the vasculitis, rather than the granulomatous histology, even though antemortem leptomeningeal biopsy of Case 5 of Calabrese and Mallek[103] showed granulomatous SVV affecting meningeal veins (**Fig. 3**) with proliferation of epithelioid cells along vascular walls, sparing the cortex. Cerebral angiography

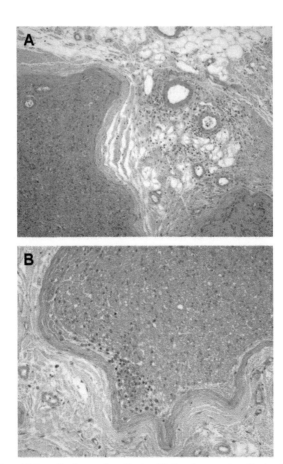

Fig. 2. Postmortem histopathology of patient with lumbosacral radiculoplexus neuropathy. (*A*) Transverse section of the left sciatic nerve shows perivascular chronic inflammation surrounding small blood vessels of the epineurium. (*B*) Transverse section of the left femoral nerve in addition shows perivascular chronic inflammation in the subperineurial area. Inflammatory cells infiltrate the adjacent endoneurium (paraffin, hematoxylin-eosin, original magnification ×200). (*From* Hughes T, Ture-Ozdemir F, Alibaz-Oner F, et al. Epigenome-wide scan identifies a treatment-responsive pattern of altered DNA methylation among cytoskeletal remodeling genes in monocytes and CD4+ T cells from patients with Behçet's disease. Arthritis Rheumatol 2014;66:1648–58; with permission.)

in that patient was negative, showing only tortuosity and some irregularity of the lumen of intracranial vessels without segmental or alternating stenosis and ectasia typical of arteritis. Patients with angiographically negative small-vessel PACNS closely resembled the childhood equivalent, small-vessel (SV)–childhood PACNS (cPACNS),[104] with the difference being that patients with SV-cPACNS are rarely investigated for prototypical granulomatous disease. The prevailing rationale for ignoring the significance of granulomatous disease has been that giant cells and epithelioid cells, usually found at autopsy, were an inconsistent finding in a meningeal and brain biopsy and, therefore, not necessary for antemortem diagnosis.

To illustrate the problem, Younger and colleagues[102] reported that 10 patients with granulomatous angiitis diagnosed antemortem by brain and meningeal biopsy were

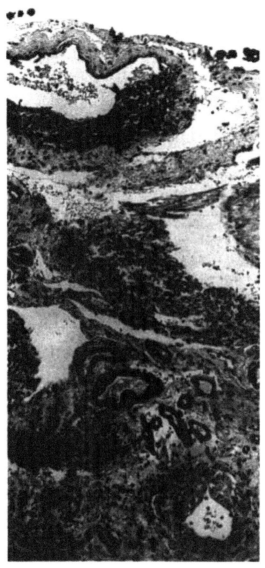

Fig. 3. Section of the leptomeninges (Case #5) showing focal, often eccentric, granuloma-tous Vasculitis predominantly around veins. Note focal proliferation and collection of epithelioid cells (arrowheads) along the vascular walls. (*From* Calabrese HL, Mallek JA. Primary angiitis of the central nervous system: report of 8 new cases, review of the literature, and proposal for diagnostic criteria. Medicine 1988;67:20–39; with permission.)

improved for up to 7 months, whether treated with prednisone, alone (in 3 patients) or with cyclophosphamide (in 3 patients) or azathioprine (in 3 patients); or cyclophospha-mide alone (in 1 patient). Similarly, in a historical survey of 54 pathologically proven cases (**Table 1**),[105] 17 of 94% of untreated patients died, indicating that without ther-apy the disease was usually fatal. Treatment with corticosteroids, alone or in combi-nation with cyclophosphamide, was associated with a considerable reduction in mortality; with the 70% so treated surviving either improved (50%) or clinically

Table 1
Outcome of 54 patients with granulomatous angiitis of the nervous system

Outcome	CS	CS + CYT	CS + AZA	None	Total
Improved	8/0	9/0	1/0	0	18/0
Same	3/0	4/0	0	1/0	8/0
Died	0/6	3/1	0	1/17	4/24

Abbreviations: AZA, azathioprine; CS, corticosteroids; CYT, cyclophosphamide.
Patients diagnosed antemortem in the numerator and postmortem in the denominator.
From Weiss N, Miller F, Cazaubon S, et al. The blood-brain barrier in brain homeostasis and neurological diseases. Biochim Biophys Acta 2009;1788:842–57; with permission.

unchanged. The achievements of the 1980s proved to be the lessons of the 1990s for 2 reasons. First, enthusiasm for the empiric treatment of cerebral vasculitis waned because of the recognition of the unreliability of cerebral angiography in its diagnosis. Several similar patients with beading on cerebral angiography had a benign course without immunosuppressive therapy. Calabrese and colleagues[106] found so-called benign angiopathy of the CNS among young women with the prior diagnosis of PACNS who differed in the onset with a focal cerebral deficit, normal CSF, beading or other previously suggestive features of vasculitis on a cerebral angiogram, lack of progression, and spontaneous resolution. A second factor that lessened interest in empiric therapy with cyclophosphamide for CNS vasculitis, was the recognition of permanent side effects in up to 40% of patients treated with oral cyclophosphamide for GPA. With increasing interest in the etiopathogenic basis of granulomatous angiitis disease, there has been general acceptance for the inclusion of associated disorders; for example, GCA, sarcoidosis, HZV, and lymphoma; and others are emerging.

Commensurate with the refinement in clinical trials methods, the literature reflects a move away from small or single-case series to the experience of larger cohorts of CNS vasculitides, with 1 retrospective series from the Mayo Clinic,[107] a multicenter prospective cohort from the French Vasculitis Study Group, French NeuroVascular Society, and the French Internal Medicine Society,[108] and the PedVas Initiative of AAV (GPA) and PACNS (NIH identifier, NCT02006134). The approach to diagnosis and management of CNS vasculitides in children differs from adults in that suspected cases of cPACNS are first placed into the larger group of inflammatory brain diseases, and then differentiated by angiography and other blood and CSF biomarkers, rarely leptomeningeal and cortical biopsy, to exclude angiography-positive and angiography-negative, brain biopsy-positive mimickers.[109] Notwithstanding, the empiric management of cPACNS with cytotoxic therapy was set back by the early outcome results of the PedVas Initiative, using corticosteroids, cyclophosphamide, methotrexate, or rituximab for remission-induction of childhood GPA,[110] that showed a remission status of 42% and visceral organ damage in 63% of cases so treated.

Theme Ten: Vasculitis due to drug abuse captured the interest of successive generations of investigators.

The earliest reports of misuse of amphetamine sulfate occurred in 1937 when it was used by students to avoid sleep during examination periods.[111] This was followed by reports of death by those who ingested the drug repeatedly as a stimulant for the same purpose[112] in a suicide attempt that resulted in a fatal intracerebral hemorrhage,[113] or accidentally, when dexamphetamine and phenelzine were fatally ingested together decades later.[114] During the Second World War, amphetamine and methamphetamine was used clinically and illicitly but its abuse soared in San Francisco after

1962, wherein it was illegally produced and distributed.[115] By 2009, the United Nations Office on Drugs and Crime estimated that 16 to 51 million persons between the age of 15 and 64 years consumed amphetamine drugs, with more than half using methamphetamine,[116] exceeding the combined consumption of all other drugs of abuse except cannabis.[117] Such drugs agents comprise a large spectrum of agents available in powder, capsule, tablet, and injectable fluid form that can be swallowed, snorted or taken intranasally, smoked, or injected with highly variable purity and dosage equivalence. Histologically confirmed cerebral vasculitis due to amphetamine, methamphetamine, and related agents is exceedingly rare, which is surprising given the number of substances that could cause this disorder if there was a true association.

Theme Eleven: Finally, there has been extraordinary research in the blood–brain barrier (BBB) over the past decade.

Once considered a static anatomic barrier to the traffic of molecules in and out of the CNS when fully developed in adults, and otherwise irrelevant to neuroscience and disease, the BBB is now known to be fully functional in development, and vital in cerebrovascular angiogenesis.[118–122] First postulated as a barrier at the level of the cerebral vessels by Bield and Kraus,[123] and later by Goldman[124] and Lewandowsky,[125] at the turn of the twentieth century, the cellular components and other molecular constituents of the BBB are contained in a neurovascular unit (NVU) protecting the CNS from injury and disease by limiting the passage of toxins, pathogens, and inflammatory effectors of the immune system. In essence, the NVU of the BBB is composed of capillary vascular and neural cells, extracellular matrix components, and a variety of immune cells that mediate local immunity. The schematized and electron microscopic appearance of cerebral capillaries in the BBB shown in **Fig. 4** demonstrate layers of pericytes adherent to the abluminal or parenchymal surface of endothelial cells, together surrounded by a layer of basal lamina composed of proteins and molecules of the extracellular matrix. The endfeet of the neighboring astrocyte processes ensheathe the blood vessels. Monolayers of adjacent endothelial cells that form tight junctions connect adjacent endothelial cells by adhesions of transmembrane occludin, claudin, and junctional associated molecules across the intercellular space, whereas cytoplasmic scaffolding and regulatory proteins, such as zona occludens types 1 and 2 provide linkage to the actin cytoskeleton and initiate several signaling mechanisms via protein–protein interactions. Endothelial BBB cells are also linked by adherens junctions composed of vascular endothelial (VE)-cadherin, which

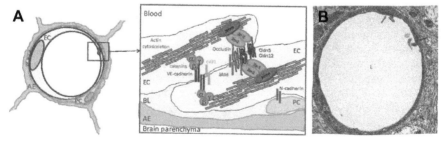

Fig. 4. Human BBB. (*A*) Schematic of a capillary in the human BBB over an endothelial tight junction (*left*). Molecular composition of tight and adherens junctions (*right*). AE, astrocyte endfeet; BL, basal lamina; EC, endothelial cells; PC, pericytes; JAM, junctional associated molecule; VE, vascular endothelial; ZO, zona occludens. (*B*) Electron micrograph of a capillary in the adult murine BBB in which endothelial cells are held together by tight junctions (*red arrows*). (*From* United Nations Office on Drugs and Crime. UNODC 2009 world drug report. Vienne (Austria): United Nations; 2009; with permission.)

mediate cell–cell adhesion interactions, linking adherens junctions to the actin cytoskeleton via catenins. Perivascular and resident macrophages that reside between astrocyte endfeet and the vessel wall act as antigen-presenting cells where novel antigens stimulate naive autoreactive T cells in in the trimolecular complex in the presence of class II main histocompatibility complex molecules, otherwise known as the body's immune playbook. Circulating leukocytes that penetrate the intact BBB via interactions with endothelial cell adhesion molecules that mediate bidirectional crosstalk between immune cells and endothelium for normal surveillance, thereby constituting the extended NVU. Disruption of the BBB is recognized as an important factor in a variety of primary neurologic diseases; however, such disturbances, although common to primary and vasculitis of the CNS, have yet to be critically analyzed but remain a critical element in the search for more effective chemotherapeutic interventions and the establishment of a more favorable metabolic milieu for health and disease in clinically affected patients with vasculitides.

The past several years have witnessed an explosion in the number of genetic and epigenetic association studies respectively termed genome-wide and epigenome-wide association studies (EWAS). Genome-wide association studies investigate the entire genome using single-nucleotide polymorphisms in contrast to specifically testing a small number of specified genetic regions, whereas EWAS analyze the heritable molecular modifications that are independent of the primary DNA sequence. Epigenetic modification occurs at various developmental stages throughout the lifespan and is analyzed by using DNA methylation (DNAm) as a marker for the perturbation that has taken place, whether causally or consequential to the disease phenotype under investigation. The main type of DNAm occurs at cytosines within 5'-cytosine-phosphate-guanine-3' (CpG) dinucleotides, known to be involved in gene expression regulation. Many human diseases, including the vasculitides, arise from genetic and environmental factors and thus the interplay between genes and environment. An EWAS of patients with BD[126] studied 383 CpG sites in blood monocytes, and 125 sites in CD4+ T cells, showing differential methylation between patients and controls. Bioinformatic analysis supported a pattern of aberrant DNAm among genes that regulate cytoskeletal dynamics, suggesting a contribution to BD pathogenesis. Treatment modified these differences with widespread reversal of the direction of DNAm. By studying the epigenome in well-characterized cohorts of vasculitides, it should be possible to discover novel genes and pathways by which genetic factor and environmental exposures influence disease development. Properly performed and with a careful consideration of the characteristics of samples, study design, and key research questions, spurious associations due to confounding and reverse causation can be eliminated from these analyses, leaving the challenge to relate them to accurate epidemiologic data. Genetic research of the vasculitides, integrating multiple phenotypic determinants and biobank data from discrete populations within well-defined geographic boundaries, is the next frontier to uncover novel aspects of disease pathogenesis, and the identification of new targets for monitoring and treatment.

REFERENCES

1. Jennette JC, Falk RJ, Andrassay K, et al. Nomenclature of systemic vasculitides. Proposal of an international conference. Arthritis Rheum 1994;37:187–92.

2. Jennette JC, Falk RJ, Bacon PA, et al. 2012 Revised international chapel hill consensus conference nomenclature of vasculitides. Arthritis Rheum 2013;65: 1–11.

3. Kussmaul A, Maier R. Ueber eine bisher nicht beschriebene eigenthümliche Arterienerkrankung (Periarteritis nodosa), die mit Morbus Brightii und rapid fortschreitender allgemeiner Muskellähmung einhergeht. Deutsches Arch f klin Med 1866;1:484–518.

4. Longcope WT. Periarteritis nodosa with report of a case with autopsy, vol. 1. Philadelphia: Bull Auyer Clin Lab, Pennsylvania Hospital; 1908.

5. Kernohan JW, Woltman HW. Periarteritis nodosa: a clinicopathologic study with special reference to the nervous system. Arch Neurol 1938;39:655–86.

6. Krahulik L, Rosenthal M, Loughlin EH. Periarteritis nodosa (necrotizing panarteritis) in childhood with meningeal involvement. Report of a case with study of pathologic findings. Am J Med Sci 1935;190:308–17.

7. Kawasaki T. MLNS showing particular skin desquamation from the finger and toe in infants. Allergy 1967;16:178–89.

8. Tanaka N, Naoe S, Kawasaki T. Pathological study on autopsy cases of mucocutaneous lymph node syndrome. J Jap Red Cross Cent Hosp 1971;2:85–94.

9. Chamberlain JL, Perry LW. Infantile periarteritis nodosa with coronary and brachial aneurysms: a case diagnosed during life. J Pediatr 1971;78:1039–40.

10. Landing BH, Larson EJ. Are infantile periarteritis nodosa with coronary artery involvement and fatal mucocutaneous lymph node syndrome the same? Comparison of 20 patients from North America with patients from Hawaii and Japan. Pediatrics 1977;59:651–2.

11. Wohlwill F. Uber die mur mikroskopisch erkenbarre form der periarteritis nodosa. Arch Pathol Anat 1923;246:377–411.

12. Davson J, Ball M, Platt R. The kidney in periarteritis nodosa. QJM 1948;17: 175–202.

13. Wainwright J, Davson J. The renal appearance in the microscopic form of periarteritis nodosa. J Pathol Bacteriol 1950;62:189–96.

14. Lamb AR. Periarteritis nodosa-a clinical and pathological review of the disease with a report of two cases. Arch Intern Med 1914;14:481–516.

15. Churg J, Strauss L. Allergic granulomatosis, allergic angiitis, and periarteritis nodosa. Am J Pathol 1951;27:277–301.

16. Chumbley LC, Harrison EG, DeRemee RA. Allergic granulomatosis and angiitis (Churg-Strauss syndrome). Report and analysis of 30 cases. Mayo Clin Proc 1977;52:477–84.

17. Lanham JG, Elkon KB, Pussey CD, et al. Systemic vasculitis with asthma and eosinophilia: a clinical approach to the Churg-Strauss syndrome. Medicine (Baltimore) 1984;63:65–81.

18. Masi AT, Hunder GG, Lie JT, et al. The American College of Rheumatology 1990 criteria for the classification of Churg-Strauss syndrome (Allergic granulomatosis and angiitis). Arthritis Rheum 1990;33:1094–100.

19. Godman GC, Churg J. Wegener's granulomatosis: pathology and review of the literature. Arch Pathol 1954;58:533–53.

20. Drachman DA. Neurological complications of Wegener's granulomatosis. Arch Neurol 1963;8:45–55.

21. Fauci AS, Haynes BF, Katz P, et al. Wegener's granulomatosis: prospective clinical and therapeutic experience with 85 patients over 21 years. Ann Intern Med 1983;98:76–85.

22. Hoffman GS, Kerr GS, Leavitt RY, et al. Wegener granulomatosis: an analysis of 158 patients. Ann Intern Med 1992;116:488–98.

23. van der Woude FJ, Rasmussen N, Lobatto S, et al. Autoantibodies against neutrophils and monocytes: tool for diagnosis and marker of disease activity in Wegener's granulomatosis. Lancet 1985;1:425–9.
24. Falk RJ, Jennette JC. Anti-neutrophil cytoplasmic autoantibodies with specificity for myeloperoxidase in patients with systemic vasculitis and idiopathic necrotizing and crescentic glomerulonephritis. N Engl J Med 1988;318:1651–7.
25. Gadola SD, Gross WL. The renaissance of granulomatous inflammation in AAV. Nat Rev Rheumatol 2012;8:74–6.
26. Lionaki S, Blyth ER, Hogan SL, et al. Classification of anti-neutrophil cytoplasmic autoantibody vasculitides: the role of anti-neutrophil cytoplasmic autoantibody specificity for myeloperoxidase or proteinase 3 in disease recognition and prognosis. Arthritis Rheum 2012;64:3452–62.
27. Lyons PA, Rayner TF, Trivedi S, et al. Genetically distinct subsets within ANCA-associated vasculitis. N Engl J Med 2012;367:214–23.
28. Savige J, Gillis D, Benson E, et al. International consensus statement on testing and reporting of anti-neutrophil cytoplasmic antibodies (ANCA). Am J Clin Pathol 1999;111:507–13.
29. Csernok E, Holle J, Hellmich B, et al. Evaluation of capture ELISA for detection of antineutrophil cytoplasmic antibodies against proteinase-3 in Wegener's granulomatosis: first results from a multicenter study. Rheumatology 2004;43: 174–80.
30. Hellmich B, Csenok E, Fredenhagen G, et al. A novel high sensitivity ELISA for detection of antineutrophil cytoplasm antibodies against proteinase-3. Clin Exp Rheumatol 2007;25(Suppl 44):S1–5.
31. Zeek PM, Smith CC, Weeter JC. Studies on periarteritis nodosa. III. The differentiation between the vascular lesions of periarteritis nodosa and of hypersensitivity. Am J Pathol 1948;24:889–917.
32. Zeek PM. Periarteritis nodosa-a critical review. Am J Clin Pathol 1952;22: 777–90.
33. Zeek PM. Periarteritis nodosa and other forms of necrotizing angiitis. N Engl J Med 1953;248:764–72.
34. Arthus M, Breton M. Lesions cutanées produites par les injections de sérum de cheval chez le lapin anaphylactisé par et pour ce sérum. Compt Rend Soc de Biol 1903;55:1478–80.
35. Osler W. The visceral lesions of purpura and allied conditions. BMJ 1914;1: 517–25.
36. Gairdner D. The Schönlein-Henoch syndrome (anaphylactoid purpura). QJM 1948;17:95–122.
37. Levitt LM, Burbank B. Glomerulonephritis as a complication of the Schonlein-Henoch syndrome. N Engl J Med 1953;248:530–6.
38. Faille-Kuyber EH, Kater L, Kooiker CJ, et al. IgA-deposits in cutaneous blood-vessel walls and mesangium in Henoch-Schonlein syndrome. Lancet 1973;1: 892–3.
39. Conley ME, Cooper MD, Michael AF. Selective deposition of immunoglobulin A1 in immunoglobulin A nephropathy, anaphylactoid purpura nephritis, and systemic lupus erythematosus. J Clin Invest 1980;66:1432–6.
40. Wintrobe MM, Buell MV. Hyperproteinemia associated with multiple myeloma. With report of a case in which an extraordinary hyperproteinemia was associated with thrombosis of the retinal veins and symptoms suggesting Raynauds disease. Bull Johns Hopkins Hosp 1933;52:156–65.

41. Lerner AB, Watson CJ. Studies of cryoglobulins. I. Unusual purpura associated with the presence of a high concentration of cryoglobulin (cold precipitable serum globulin). Am J Med Sci 1947;214:410–5.
42. Lerner AB, Watson CJ. Studies of cryoglobulins. II. The spontaneous precipitation of protein from serum at 5°C in various disease states. Am J Med Sci 1947; 214:416–21.
43. Gorevic PD, Kassab HJ, Levo Y, et al. Mixed cryoglobulinemia: clinical aspects and long-term follow-up of 40 patients. Am J Med 1980;69:287–308.
44. McDuffie FC, Sams WM, Maldonado JE, et al. Hypocomplementemia with cutaneous vasculitis and arthritis. Possible immune complex syndrome. Mayo Clin Proc 1973;48:340–8.
45. Zeiss CR, Burch FX, Marder RJ, et al. A hypocomplementemic vasculitic urticarial syndrome: Report of four new cases and definition of the disease. Am J Med 1980;68:867–75.
46. Wisnieski JJ, Naff GB. Serum IgG antibodies to C1q in hypocomplementemic urticarial vasculitis syndrome. Arthritis Rheum 1989;32:1119–27.
47. Hutchinson J. On a peculiar form of thrombotic arteritis of the aged which is sometimes productive of gangrene. Arch Surg 1890;I:323–9.
48. Horton BT, Magath BT, Brown GE. Arteritis of temporal vessels: report of 7 cases. Mayo Clin Proc 1937;12:548–53.
49. Jennings GH. Arteritis of the temporal vessels. Lancet 1938;1:424–8.
50. Bruce GM. Temporal arteritis as a cause of blindness: review of the literature and report of a case. Trans Am Ophthalmol Soc 1949;47:300–16.
51. Gilmour JR. Giant-cell chronic arteritis. J Pathol Bacteriol 1941;53:263–77.
52. Jellinger K. Giant cell granulomatous angiitis of the central nervous system. J Neurol 1977;215:175–90.
53. Kjeldsen M, Reske-Nielsen E. Pathological changes of the central nervous system in giant cell arteritis. Acta Ophthalmol 1968;46:49–56.
54. McLean C, Gonzalez M, Dowling J. Systemic giant cell arteritis and cerebellar infarction. Stroke 1993;24:899–902.
55. Morrison A, Abitol M. Granulomatous arteritis with myocardial infarction. Ann Intern Med 1955;42:691–700.
56. Ritama V. Temporal arteritis. Ann Med Exp Fenn 1951;40:63–87.
57. Save-Soderbergh J, Malmvall B, Anderson R, et al. Giant cell arteritis as a cause of death. JAMA 1986;255:493–6.
58. Takayasu M. Case with unusual changes of the central vessels in the retina [Japanese]. Acta Soc Ophthal Jap 1908;12:554–5.
59. Walker DI, Bloor K, Williams G, et al. Inflammatory aneurysms of the abdominal aorta. Br J Surg 1972;59:609–14.
60. Pennell RC, Hollier LH, Lie JT, et al. Inflammatory abdominal aortic aneurysms: a thirty year review. J Vasc Surg 1985;2:859–69.
61. Rojo-Leyva F, Ratliff NB, Cosgrove DM, et al. Study of 52 patients with idiopathic aortitis from a cohort of 1,204 surgical cases. Arthritis Rheum 2000;43:901–7.
62. Hamano H, Kawa S, Horiuchi A, et al. High serum IgG4 concentrations in patients with sclerosing pancreatitis. N Engl J Med 2001;344:732–8.
63. Hamano H, Kawa S, Ochi Y, et al. Hydronephrosis associated with retroperitoneal fibrosis and sclerosing pancreatitis. Lancet 2002;359:1403–4.
64. Sakata N, Tashiro T, Uesugi N, et al. IgG4-positive plasma cells in inflammatory abdominal aortic aneurysm: The possibility of an aortic manifestation of IgG4-related sclerosing disease. Am J Surg Pathol 2008;32:553–9.

65. Kasashima S, Zen Y, Kawashima A, et al. Inflammatory abdominal aortic aneurysm: Close relationship to IgG4-releated periaortitis. Am J Surg Pathol 2008;32:197–204.

66. Ito H, Kalzaki Y, Noda Y, et al. IgG4-related inflammatory abdominal aortic aneurysm associated with autoimmune pancreatitis. Pathol Int 2008;58:421–6.

67. Khosroshahi A, Stone JR, Pratt DS, et al. Painless jaundice with serial multiorgan dysfunction. Lancet 2009;373:1494.

68. Stone JH, Khosroshahi A, Hilgenberg A, et al. IgG4-related systemic disease and lymphoplasmacytic aortitis. Arthritis Rheum 2009;60:3139–45.

69. Adamantiades B. Sur un cas d'iritis a hypopion recidivant. Ann D'Ocul 1931;168:271–8.

70. Behçet H. Ueber rezidivierende, aphthöse, durch ein virus verursachte Geschwüre am Mund, am Auge und an den Genitalien. Dermat Wchnschr 1937;105:1152–7.

71. Behçet H, Matteson EL. On relapsing, aphthous ulcers of the mouth, eye and genitalia caused by a virus. 1937. Clin Exp Rheumatol 2010;28(Suppl 60):S2–5.

72. McMenemey WH, Lawrence BJ. Encephalomyelopathy in Behcet's disease. Report of necropsy findings in two cases. Lancet 1957;2:353–8.

73. Wolf SM, Schotland DL, Phillips LL. Involvement of nervous system in Behçet's syndrome. Arch Neurol 1965;12:315–25.

74. Mogan RF, Baumgartner CJ. Meniere's disease complicated by recurrent interstitial keratitis: Excellent results following cervical ganglionectomy. West J Surg 1934;42:628.

75. Cogan DG. Syndrome of nonsyphilitic interstitial keratitis and vestibuloauditory symptoms. Arch Ophthal 1945;33:144–9.

76. Haynes BF, Kaiser-Kupfer MI, Mason P, et al. Cogan's syndrome: Studies in thirteen patients, long-term follow-up, and a review of the literature. Medicine 1980;59:426–41.

77. Cogan DG. Nonsyphilitic interstitial keratitis with vestibuloauditory symptoms. Report of four additional cases. Arch Ophthalmol 1949;42:42–9.

78. Norton EWD, Cogan DG. Syndrome of nonsyphilitic interstitial keratitis and vestibuloauditory symptoms. A long-term follow-up. Arch Ophthalmol 1959;61:695–7.

79. Cody DTR, Williams HL. Cogan's syndrome. Laryngoscope 1960;70:447–78.

80. Said G, Lacroix C, Fujimura H, et al. The peripheral neuropathy of necrotizing arteritis: a clinicopathologic study. Ann Neurol 1988;23:461–5.

81. Collins MP, Dyck PJ, Gronseth GS, et al. Peripheral Nerve Society Guideline on the classification, diagnosis, investigation, and immunosuppressive therapy of non-systemic vasculitic neuropathy: executive summary. J Peripher Nerv Syst 2010;15:176–84.

82. Dyck PJ, Benstead TJ, Conn DL, et al. Nonsystemic vasculitic neuropathy. Brain 1987;110:843–53.

83. Torvik A, Berntzen AE. Necrotizing vasculitis without visceral involvement. Postmortem examination of three cases with affection of skeletal muscles and peripheral nerves. Acta Med Scand 1968;184:69–77.

84. Raff MC, Sangalang V, Asbury AK. Ischemic mononeuropathy multiplex associated with diabetes mellitus. Arch Neurol 1968;18:487–99.

85. Bradley WB, Chad D, Verghese JP, et al. Painful lumbosacral plexopathy with elevated erythrocyte sedimentation rate: a treatable inflammatory syndrome. Ann Neurol 1984;15:457–64.

86. Johnson PC, Doll SC, Cromey DW. Pathogenesis of diabetic neuropathy. Ann Neurol 1986;19:450–7.
87. Said G, Goulon-Goeau C, Lacroix C, et al. Nerve biopsy findings in different patterns of proximal diabetic neuropathy. Ann Neurol 1994;35:559–69.
88. Younger DS, Rosoklija G, Hays AP, et al. Diabetic peripheral neuropathy: a clinicopathologic and immunohistochemical analysis of sural nerve biopsies. Muscle Nerve 1996;19:722–7.
89. Dyck PJ, Norell JE, Dyck PJ. Non-diabetic lumbosacral radiculoplexus neuropathy: natural history, outcome and comparison with the diabetic variety. Brain 2001;124:1197–207.
90. Dyck PJB, Windebank AJ. Diabetic and nondiabetic lumbosacral radiculoplexus neuropathies: new insights into pathophysiology and treatment. Muscle Nerve 2002;25:477–91.
91. Collins MP, Hadden RD. The nonsystemic vasculitic neuropathies. Nat Rev Neurol 2017;13:302–16.
92. Younger DS. Diabetic neuropathy: a clinical and neuropathological study of 107 patients. Neurol Res Int 2010;2010:140379.
93. Younger DS. Diabetic lumbosacral radiculoplexus neuropathy: a postmortem studied patient and review of the literature. J Neurol 2011;258:1364–7.
94. Harbitz F. Unknown forms of arteritis with special reference to their relation to syphilitic arteritis and periarteritis nodosa. Am J Med Sci 1922;163:250–72.
95. Neuman W, Wolf A. Noninfectious granulomatous angiitis involving the central nervous system. Trans Am Neurol Assoc 1952;77:114–7.
96. McCormack H, Neuberger K. Giant cell arteritis involving small meningeal and intracerebral vessels. J Neuropathol Exp Neurol 1958;17:471–8.
97. Meyer J, Foley J, Campagna-Pinto D. Granulomatous angiitis of the meninges in sarcoidosis. Arch Neurol 1953;69:587–600.
98. Cravioto H, Fegin I. Noninfectious granulomatous angiitis with a predilection for the nervous system. Neurology 1959;9:599–607.
99. Cupps TR, Moore PM, Fauci AS. Isolated angiitis of the central nervous system. Prospective diagnostic and therapeutic experience. Am J Med 1983;74:97–105.
100. Cupps T, Fauci A. Central nervous system vasculitis. Major Probl Intern Med 1981;21:123–32.
101. Hinck V, Carter C, Rippey C. Giant cell (cranial) arteritis. A case with angiographic abnormalities. Am J Roentgenol Radium Ther Nucl Med 1964;92:769–75.
102. Younger DS, Hays AP, Brust JCM, et al. Granulomatous angiitis of the brain. An inflammatory reaction of diverse etiology. Arch Neurol 1988;45:514–8.
103. Calabrese HL, Mallek JA. Primary angiitis of the central nervous system: report of 8 new cases, review of the literature, and proposal for diagnostic criteria. Medicine 1988;67:20–39.
104. Benseler SM, deVeber G, Hawkins C, et al. Angiography-negative primary central nervous system vasculitis in children. Arthritis Rheum 2005;52:2159–67.
105. Younger DS, Calabrese LH, Hays AP. Granulomatous angiitis of the nervouse system. Neurol Clin 1997;15:821–34.
106. Calabrese LH, Graff LA, Furlan AJ. Benign angiopathy: a distinct subset of angiographically defined primary angiitis of the central nervous system. J Rheumatol 1993;20:2046.
107. Salvarani C, Brown RD Jr, Christianson TJH, et al. Adult primary central nervous system vasculitis: treatment and course. Arthritis Rheum 2015;67:1637–45.

108. De Boysson H, Arquizan C, Touze E, et al. Treatment and long-term outcomes of primary central nervous system vasculitis. Stroke 2018;49:1946–52.
109. Twilt M, Benseler SM. Central nervous system vasculitis in adults and children. Handb Clin Neurol 2016;133:283–300.
110. Morishita KA, Moorthy LN, Lubieniecka JM, et al. Early outcomes in children with antineutrophil cytoplasmic antibody-associated vasculitis. Arthritis Rheum 2017; 69:1470–9.
111. Editorial: Benzedrine sulfate "pep pills". JAMA 1937;108(23):1973–4.
112. Smith L. Collapse with death following the use of amphetamine sulfate. JAMA 1939;113:1022–3.
113. Gericke O. Suicide by ingestion of amphetamine sulfate. JAMA 1945;128: 1098–9.
114. Lloyd JT, Walker DR. Death after combined dexamphetamine and phenelzine. BMJ 1965;2:168–9.
115. Anglin MD, Burke C, Perrochet B, et al. History of the methamphetamine problem. J Psychoactive Drugs 2000;32:137–41.
116. United Nations Office on Drugs and Crime. UNODC 2009 world drug report. Vienne (Austria): United Nations; 2009.
117. United Nations Office on Drugs and Crime. World drug report 2000. New York: United Nations; 2000.
118. Daneman R. The blood-brain barrier in health and disease. Ann Neurol 2012;72: 648–72.
119. Benarroch EE. Blood-brain barrier. Neurology 2012;78:1268–76.
120. Hawkins BR, Davis TP. The blood-brain barrier/Neurovascular unit in health and disease. Pharmacol Rev 2005;57:173–85.
121. Weiss N, Miller F, Cazaubon S, et al. The blood-brain barrier in brain homeostasis and neurological diseases. Biochim Biophys Acta 2009;1788:842–57.
122. Neuwelt EA, Bauer B, Fahlke C, et al. Engaging neuroscience to advance translational research in brain barrier biology. Nat Rev Neurosci 2011;12:169–82.
123. Bield A, Kraus B. Über eine bisher unbekannte toxische Wirkung der Gallensauren auf das Zentralnervensystem. Zhl Inn Med 1898;19:1185–200.
124. Goldmann EE. Vitalfarbung am Zentral-nervensystem. Abh Preuss Akad Wissensch. Physkol Mathem Klasse 1913;1:1–60.
125. Lewandowsky M. Zür lehre der cerebrospinal flüssigkeit. Z für Klinische Med 1900;40:480–94.
126. Hughes T, Ture-Ozdemir F, Alibaz-Oner F, et al. Epigenome-wide scan identifies a treatment-responsive pattern of altered DNA methylation among cytoskeletal remodeling genes in monocytes and CD4+ T cells from patients with Behçet's disease. Arthritis Rheumatol 2014;66:1648–58.

Overview of the Vasculitides

David S. Younger, MD, MPH, MS[a,b,*]

KEYWORDS

- Primary • Secondary • Vasculitis • Autoimmune • Nervous system

KEY POINTS

- The systemic vasculitides are heterogeneous clinicopathologic disorders that share the common feature of vascular inflammation.
- The 2012 Revised Chapel Hill Consensus Conference serves as a guide for the categorization of diverse forms of vasculitis based on the caliber of the vessels involved.
- The underlying pathophysiology reflects diminished blood flow, vascular alterations, and eventual occlusion with variable ischemia, necrosis, and tissue damage.
- The resulting clinical disorder can vary depending on involvement of specific organs, caliber of blood vessels, the underlying inflammatory process, and individual host factors.
- This article is an introduction and overview of the clinical presentation, differential diagnosis, laboratory evaluation, and treatment of systemic and nervous system vasculitides.

INTRODUCTION

The term vasculitides refers to heterogeneous disorders characterized by vascular inflammation affecting vessels of different sizes from large arteries to capillaries or tiny venules. Vasculitis leads to diminished blood flow or vessel occlusion resulting in ischemia, necrosis, and subsequent tissue damage. Blood vessels themselves can also be damaged in vasculitis, resulting in permanent stenosis, aneurysmal change, or rupture.

CLASSIFICATION AND NOSOLOGY

The 2012 Revised Chapel Hill Consensus Conference (CHCC)[1] serves as a guide for the categorization of diverse forms of vasculitis based on the caliber of the vessels involved (**Boxes 1** and **2**). Large vessel vasculitis (LVV), including giant cell arteritis (GCA) and Takayasu arteritis (TAK), affects the aorta, its major branches, and analogous veins. Medium vessel vasculitis (MVV), inclusive of polyarteritis

Disclosure Statement: The author has nothing to disclose.
[a] Department of Neurology, Division of Neuro-Epidemiology, New York University School of Medicine, New York, New York 10016, USA; [b] School of Public Health, City University of New York, New York, NY, USA
* 333 East 34th Street, Suite 1J, New York, NY 10016.
E-mail address: youngd01@nyu.edu
Website: http://www.davidsyounger.com

Box 1
Classification of vasculitides

Large vessel vasculitis
  Giant cell arteritis
  Takayasu arteritis

Medium vessel vasculitis
  Polyarteritis nodosa
  Kawasaki disease

Small vessel vasculitis
  Antineutrophil cytoplasmic antibody-associated vasculitis
    Microscopic polyangiitis
    Granulomatosis with polyangiitis (Wegener)
    Eosinophilic granulomatosis with polyangiitis (Churg-Strauss)
  Immune-complex vasculitis
    Cryoglobulinemia
    IgA vasculitis (Henoch-Schönlein)
    Hypocomplementemic urticarial vasculitis (anti-C1q)

Variable vessel vasculitis
  Behçet disease
  Cogan syndrome

Single organ vasculitis
  Primary angiitis of the central nervous system
  Nonsystemic peripheral nerve vasculitis
  Idiopathic aortitis (IgG4)

Vasculitis associated with systemic collagen vascular disease
  Systemic lupus erythematosus
  Rheumatoid arthritis vasculitis

Vasculitis associated with infection
  Acute bacterial meningitis
  Mycobacterial tuberculous
  Spirochete disease
    Neurosyphilis
    Lyme neuroborreliosis
  Varicella zoster virus
  Human immunodeficiency virus type-1/AIDS

nodosa (PAN) and Kawasaki disease (KD), involves main visceral arteries and veins and initial branches. Small vessel vasculitic (SVV) involvement affects intraparenchymal arteries, arterioles, capillaries, veins, and venules, with a disease mechanisms related to antineutrophil cytoplasmic antibody (ANCA) or immune complexes (IC).

The category of ANCA-associated vasculitis (AAV) includes granulomatosis with polyangiitis (GPA) (Wegener granulomatosis [WG type]), eosinophilic granulomatosis with polyangiitis (EGPA) (Churg-Strauss syndrome), and microscopic polyangiitis (MPA) (microscopic polyarteritis), whereas vasculitic disorders associated with IC include immunoglobulin A (IgA) vasculitis (IgAV) (Henoch-Schönlein purpura [HSP]), cryoglobulinemic vasculitis (CV), and hypocomplementemia urticarial vasculitis (HUV) associated with C1q antibodies. Vasculitis without a predominant vessel size and caliber, respectively, from small to large, involving arteries, veins, and capillaries, comprises the category of variable vessel vasculitis (VVV), characteristic of Behçet disease (BD) and Cogan syndrome (CS). Vascular inflammation confined to a single

---

Box 2
Laboratory evaluation of systemic and nervous system vasculitides

Studies in Blood, Urine, and Body Fluids

CBC, chemistry panel, ANA, ANCA by IIF; ANCA ELISA serology specific for PR3 and MPO (in those with IIF ANCA seropositivity, other cytoplasmic fluorescence, and ANA that results in homogeneous or peripheral nuclear fluorescence); ESR, CK, T- and B-cell subset panel, circulating IC, acute and convalescent viral, retroviral, bacterial, fungal, TB, syphilis, and Lyme serology; quantitative immunoglobulins, IFE, C1q, complement proteins, RF, cryoglobulins, anticardiolipin, and aPL, LAC, double-stranded DNA antibodies, and appropriate HLA haplotypes; urinalysis for spot and 24-hour collection for chemical and cellular microscopic analysis; bronchoscopy (in those with lung lesions) for lavage; lumbar cerebrospinal fluid analysis for protein, glucose, cell count, IgG level, oligoclonal bands, cytology, VDRL, bacterial Gram stain and culture; India ink, cryptococcal antigen and fungal culture; acid-fast and TB culture; viral encephalitis panel for real-time analysis of DNA and RNA viruses by real-time PCR; *Borrelia* burgdorferi DNA by PCR, Lyme, and HIV1 serology.

Radiological Studies

Screening color Doppler ultrasonography of the temporal arteries and great vessels, 3-T MRI, and high-field MRA or CTA and DSA (as may be appropriate) of vascular beds and major vessels; [18]FDG body PET-CT, nuclear medicine cerebral perfusion with SPECT.

Histopathologic Studies

Punch skin biopsy of for ENF density and histology using PLP 9.5, with IF of vessel walls and microscopic analysis for leukocytoclasia; bronchoscopy or needle tissue biopsy of lung lesion and endoscopic biopsy of kidney tissue; USG-guided temporal artery biopsy; open sural nerve and soleus muscle or superficial fibular nerve and peroneus muscle tissue biopsies for epineurial and epimysial vasculitic foci; meningeal and/or cortical brain biopsy for vasculitic foci in arteries and veins.

Abbreviations: aPL, antiphospholipid; CBC, complete blood count; CK, creatine kinase; ENF, epidermal nerve fiber; IFE, immunofixation electrophoresis; IIF, indirect immunofluorescence; LAC, lupus anticoagulant; PCR, polymerase chain reaction; PLP 9.5, protein gene product 9.5; RBC, red blood cells; SPECT, single-photon emission CT; T and B, thymus and bone marrow–derived cells; USG, ultrasonography; VDRL, venereal disease research laboratory; WBC, white blood cells.

---

organ system, such as vasculitis restricted to the central nervous system (CNS) and peripheral nervous system (PNS), and IgG4 related aortitis (IgG4-related disease [RD]), are collectively referred to as single organ vasculitides (SOV).

There is a separate category for vasculitis associated with systemic disease notably for connective tissue disorders, such as rheumatoid arthritis vasculitis (RAV) and systemic lupus erythematosus (SLE), and another for vasculitis associated with a probable specific cause, such as substance abuse and infection designated by the specific vasculitic disorder with a prefix to denote the causative agent. The category of SOV involves arteries or veins of any size in a single organ without features to indicate that it is a limited expression of a systemic vasculitis that includes granulomatous angiitis of the brain (GAB) and the interchangeable terms primary angiitis of the central nervous system angiitis (PACNS) and primary central nervous system vasculitis (PCNSV); isolated or nonsystemic peripheral nerve vasculitis (NSPNV), and isolated aortitis (IgG4-RD).

In 2008, the Pediatric Rheumatology European Society and the European League against Rheumatism (EULAR) and the Pediatric Rheumatology International Trials Organization (PRINTO) reported methodology and overall clinical, laboratory, and radiographic characteristics for several childhood systemic vasculitides followed by a final validated classification[2,3] based on vessel size, similar to the CHCC nomenclature.[1]

Insight into effective therapies of systemic vasculitides has been guided by collaborative evidence-based randomized clinical trials (RCT) or observational cohorts by the French Vasculitis Study Group (FVSG) database, United States-Canadian Vasculitis Clinical Research Consortium, European Vasculitis Study Society, the EULAR, The French Vasculitis Cohort of Patients with Primary Vasculitis of the Central Nervous System, Diagnostic and Classification Criteria in Vasculitis Study (DCVAS), the Pediatric Vasculitis Initiative (PedVas), , and the Web-based network BrainWorks.

Despite disparities in vessel involvement and end-organ damage, it is possible to reach a presumptive diagnosis of primary and secondary vasculitides in most patients based on the combination of suggestive symptoms and signs, disease-specific serologic studies, and visceral and neurovascular imaging studies, while awaiting the results tissue histopathology.

This article is an overview of primary and secondary vasculitides in adults and children for clinicians treating such patients. Five major challenges encountered in clinical practice are addressed and emphasized. First, clinical, pathologic, and serologic differentiation and diagnosis of the primary vasculitides, including LVV (GCA, TAK), MVV (PAN, KD), SVV (AAV [MPA, GPA, EGPA] and IC-mediated types [IgAV and anti-C1q]), and VVV (BD and CS), all of which share demonstrable histopathologic evidence of systemic vasculitis. Second, recognition of secondary vasculitides associated with underlying primary systemic illness, in which some but not all patients will demonstrate evidence of vasculitis, including CV, RAV, and CNS vasculitis associated with SLE, syphilis, Lyme neuroborreliosis; bacterial meningitis, tuberculosis (TB), varicella zoster virus, human immunodeficiency virus type 1 (HIV1), and AIDS. Third, the identification of the SOV, PCNSA, NSPNV, and IgG4-RD. Fourth, a recommended laboratory approach to the diagnosis of vasculitides. Last, evidence-based treatment options for each of the vasculitides.

DIFFERENTIATION OF PRIMARY VASCULITIDES
Large Vessel Vasculitides

The concepts of GCA and TAK have evolved over a century, with considerable advances in the past decade that have translated into more improved diagnosis and management.

Giant cell arteritis

First named temporal arteritis for the site of granulomatous giant cell inflammation and vessel involvement, those with associated blindness due to vasculitic involvement of ophthalmic and posterior ciliary vessels were subsequently classified as cranial arteritis, and later generalized GCA[4,5] when giant cell lesions were discerned along the aorta, its branches, and in other medium- and large-sized arteries at postmortem examination. There are 5 discriminatory features of GCA, including age greater than 50 years at onset, new localized headache, temporal artery tenderness or decreased temporal artery pulse, erythrocyte sedimentation rate (ESR) greater than 50 mm/h, and biopsy of an artery showing necrotizing arteritis and a predominance of mononuclear cells or granulomatous process with multinucleated giant cells (**Fig. 1**), which collectively serve as useful guideposts in recognizing GCA. If unrecognized and therefore untreated or inadequately treated, there is a high likelihood of large artery

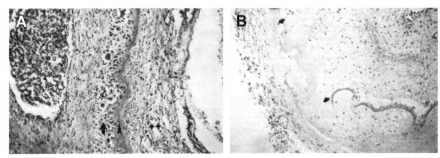

Fig. 1. GCA. (*A*) An early lesion of a large muscular artery, necrosis, inflammation, and giant cell formation (*single arrow*) can be seen immediately adjacent to the internal elastic lamina (*arrowhead*), which is undergoing degenerative changes, and there is some intimal proliferation (*double arrows*) (stain, hematoxylin and eosin, original magnification ×100). (*B*) This more advanced lesion has complete segmental destruction of the internal elastic lamina and virtually the entire media (*arrows*). Marked intimal proliferation has nearly occluded the lumen, and few inflammatory cells remain (stain, hematoxylin and eosin, original magnification ×50). (*From* Younger DS. Vasculitis of the Nervous System. In: Younger DS, editor. Motor Disorders. Third edition. Brookfield, CT: Rothstein Publishing; 2015. p. 235–80; with permission.)

complication. Nuenninghoff and coworkers[6] reported patients with large-artery complications representing 27% of 168 patients in a GCA cohort at the Mayo Clinic between 1950 and 1999 that included aortic aneurysm or dissection in 18%, large artery stenosis in 13%, cervical artery stenosis in 9%, and subclavian, axillary, or brachial artery stenosis in 4%. Temporal artery biopsy is the only sure way of establishing the diagnosis; however, false negative findings on the contemplated affected side may be due to inadvertent sampling of a vasculitic-free length of vessel. The pathologic heterogeneity of GCA was further exemplified by the occasional finding of intracranial lesions in several patients who also qualified for that diagnosis[7]; however, PNS involvement in GCA remains exceedingly uncommon.[8]

Takayasu arteritis

Contemporaneously, another LVV was described in the Japanese literature as unusual changes of the central vessels of the retina in the absence of peripheral arterial pulses in women. Patients with so-called pulseless disease, occlusive thromboaortopathy, or TAK,[9] manifest constitutional complaints of malaise, fever, stiffness of the shoulders, nausea, vomiting, night sweats, anorexia, weight loss, and irregularity of menstrual periods weeks to months before the local signs of vasculitis were recognized in up to two-thirds of patients. TAK is the commonest LVV among Asian women.

The noninvasive assessment of LVV includes performance of color-Doppler sonography (CDS), contrast-enhanced high-resolution MRI combined with MR angiography (MRA), and contrast-enhanced computed tomography (CT) combined with computed tomography angiography (CTA) to visualize the vessel wall and the lumen of large vessels. The signs of early inflammation that include vessel wall thickening and mural inflammation, as well as the late complications of stenosis and aneurysms, can be ascertained. PET with ^{18}F-fluorodeoxyglucose (FDG) detects increased FDG uptake by metabolically active cells, including inflammatory cells infiltrating the vessel wall in vasculitis, whereas digital subtraction angiography (DSA) is a useful modality to demonstrate luminal changes. Moreover, such studies can assist the surgeon in centering on an involved segment of vessel.

Since the early reports of a salutary effect of corticosteroids on GCA in 1950,[10] corticosteroids have remained the standard of care because of their ability to reduce disease-related morbidity, mortality, and symptoms that negatively impact on quality of life. However, they are not curative, do not prevent relapses, and are associated with significant toxicity. Disease-related morbidity in GCA, which largely results from cranial ischemic events or LVV, leads to visual loss in up to 20% of patients. The risk factors for GCA-related ischemic events include visual loss, prior ischemic events, marked intimal hyperplasia on temporal artery biopsy, elevated inflammatory markers, older age at diagnosis, hypertension, ischemic heart disease, and absence of systemic manifestations. Although there is no treatment to date that has been found to completely reverse blindness in GCA once it has occurred, there is strong evidence to suggest that once corticosteroids have been started the risk of visual loss is low.[11] For this reason, corticosteroids should be started while the diagnostic evaluation is in progress and continued for up to 1 year before tapering to the lowest maintenance levels.

Ohigashi and colleagues[12] ascertained an improved prognosis among 106 consecutive patients with TAK in those with onset before 1999 compared with those diagnosed after 2000 (4.2% vs 0%) that was attributed to reduction in the time from onset to diagnosis, replacement of DSA (79% vs 9%) with ultrasound (6% vs 34%), CTA (24% vs 77%), MRA (21% vs 57%), and ^{18}F-FDG PET (0% vs 20%); less frequent complications of moderate or severe aortic regurgitation, and not surprisingly, an increase in the use and maximal dose of corticosteroids (70% vs 97%); and the use of first and second-line immunosuppressant agents (7% vs 42%). Surgical treatment of TKA was similar between those with onset before 1999 and after 2000 (22.5% vs 22.8%).

Medium Vessel Vasculitides

Polyarteritis nodosa and Kawasaki disease

Longcope[13] described the first American patient with periarteritis nodosa in 1908. Kernohan and Woltman[14] summarized the clinicopathologic aspects of adult PAN at postmortem examination, whereas Krahulik and colleagues[15] described fulminant childhood polyarteritis nodosa (cPAN). The dominant clinicopathologic syndrome was peripheral neuritis that occurred in one-half of patients early in the illness with a predilection for the legs. The combination of acute and chronic lesions correlated with known exacerbations. Arteritic lesions along nutrient arteries of the peripheral nerves were characterized by invasion of the intima, media, and adventitia by polymorphonuclear, plasma cells, eosinophils, and lymphocytes associated with swelling of the media, fibrinoid necrosis, and fragmentation of the internal elastic lamina (**Fig. 2**). So impressed was Dr Harry Lee Parker by the frequency of arteritic lesions in the PNS that he conceptualized nerve and muscle biopsy as a useful mode for the diagnosis in life during a discussion of the paper by Kernohan and Woltman.[14] Variants of cPAN were contemporaneously recognized in infants and young children under the rubric of mucocutaneous lymph node syndrome, infantile PAN before arrival at the preferred term KD for the childhood syndrome affecting children of all ages and races, with worldwide occurrence.

A retrospective study of 348 adult patients registered in the FVSG[16] who satisfied criteria for the diagnosis of PAN between 1963 and 2005 noted constitutional findings included fever, weight loss, myalgia, and arthralgia at presentation in 93% of patients; PNS included peripheral neuropathy and mononeuritis multiplex in nearly equal proportion in 79%, and cutaneous involvement, notably, purpura, skin nodules, and livedo reticularis in 50% of patients. CNS involvement was noted in only about 5%

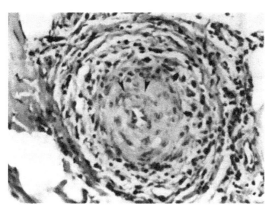

Fig. 2. This small muscular artery from muscle is from a patient with PAN. In the third, or proliferative, phase illustrated here, chronic inflammatory cells replace the neutrophils of the second phase; there is evidence of necrosis of the media (*arrows*), early intimal proliferation (*arrowheads*), and fibrosis. The lumen is almost completely occluded. Ultimately, in the healing phase, this process is replaced by dense, organized connective tissue (stain, hematoxylin and eosin, original magnification ×250). (*From* Younger DS. Vasculitis of the Nervous System. In: Younger DS, editor. Motor Disorders. Third edition. Brookfield, CT: Rothstein Publishing; 2015. p. 235–280; with permission.)

of patients. The classification criteria for cPAN require histologic evidence of necrotizing vasculitis in medium- or small-sized arteries or angiographic abnormalities demonstrating aneurysm formation or vascular occlusions, as a mandatory criterion, plus 2 of 5 features, among them myalgia, skin involvement, hypertension, neuropathy, or abnormal urinalysis or impaired renal function, with disease manifestations ranging from a benign cutaneous form with clinical, laboratory, and molecular characteristics of familial Mediterranean fever to severe disseminated multisystemic disease. Ozen and colleagues[17] studied 110 children with a mean age of 9 years, from 21 pediatric centers worldwide diagnosed with cPAN, dividing them into 4 groups, including systemic PAN (57%), cutaneous PAN (30%), and classic PAN with hepatitis B surface antigen (4.6%).

The FVSG study[16] allowed for a comparison of diagnostic modalities in adult PAN. Only 6 of 47 so tested manifested a positive ANCA finding by immunofluorescent (IF) and enzyme-linked immunosorbent assay (ELISA) techniques, rendering it helpful in support of PAN when negative to differentiate it from AAV, especially MPA. Cutaneous nerve biopsy performed in 129 patients, including 108 with peripheral neuropathy and 21 without peripheral neuropathy, showed typical vasculitic lesions in 83% and 81%, respectively, compared with muscle biopsy that revealed vasculitis in 68% and 60%, respectively. Angiography showed renal and gastrointestinal microaneurysms or stenosis in 66% and 57% of patients, respectively. Patients with hepatitis B virus (HBV)-related PAN had more frequent peripheral neuropathy, abdominal pain, cardiomyopathy, orchitis, and hypertension than those with non-HBV–related PAN, with respective 5-year relapse-free survival rates of 59% and 67% in scheduled therapeutic regimens depending on involvement in clinical trials, or according to the standard of care at the time of diagnosis, among them glucocorticoids and cyclophosphamide.[18,19] The predictors of a poor prognosis were age greater than 65 years, hypertension, and gastrointestinal involvement, and cutaneous manifestations or non-HBV–related PAN had higher rates of relapse. Three positive predictive parameters include HBV antigen and DNA in serum, arteriographic anomalies, and mononeuropathy or polyneuropathy, and 5 negative predictive parameters, including detection of ANCA; asthma, ear, nose and throat signs; glomerulopathy; and cryoglobulinemia, which yielded 70.6% sensitivity for control vasculitides and 92.3% specificity for all controls.

Small Vessel Vasculitides

Antineutrophil cytoplasmic antibody-associated vasculitis

Microscopic polyangiitis Wohlwill,[20] Davson and colleagues,[21] and Wainwright and Davson[22] recognized that fever, arthralgia, purpura, hemoptysis, pulmonary hemorrhage, abdominal pain, and gastrointestinal bleeding preceded the explosive phase of systemic necrotizing vasculitis in some patients with a disorder other than PAN that affected the kidney and lungs, with rapidly progressive glomerulonephritis and pulmonary capillaritis. Such patients with selective involvement of small microscopic arteries, arterioles, capillaries, and venules, including glomerular and pulmonary alveolar capillaries, were deemed to have microscopic PAN. Among 34 such patients described by Savage and colleagues,[23] the clinical symptoms and signs at presentation were constitutional (67%), arthralgia (65%), purpura (44%), hemoptysis in (32%), abdominal pain (32%), mouth ulcers (21%), sensory peripheral neuropathy (18%), and CNS (headache, seizures) (18%). Eighty-five additional patients studied by Guillevin and colleagues[24] with MPA so termed had renal involvement (79%), weight loss (73%), skin involvement (purpura, livedo, nodules, urticarial) (62%), mononeuritis multiplex neuropathy (57%), fever (55%), arthralgia (50%), myalgia (48%), vascular manifestations (hypertension, cardiac failure, pericarditis) (50%), lung involvement (alveolar hemorrhage, pneumonitis, pleurisies) (24%), and CNS involvement (12%). Ahn and colleagues[25] noted perinuclear (p)ANCA or antimyeloperoxidase (MPO) antibody positivity in 69% of Korean MPA patients, compared with 74.5% of positive ANCA in European patients, of whom 87% had a pANCA staining pattern; antibodies to proteinase 3 (PR3) were present in 8% of patients compared with MPO in 61% of those so studied as determined by ELISA. Childhood MPA (cMPA) appears to be very uncommon, and the criteria for diagnosis include 3 of the following features to be present: abnormal urinalysis, granulomatous inflammation on tissue biopsy, nasal sinus inflammation, subglottic, tracheal, or endobronchial stenosis; abnormal chest radiograph or CT scan, and PR3 ANCA or cytoplasmic (c)ANCA staining.[3] Those with cMPA accounted for 4 of the first 32 children in the United States/Canadian ARChiVe registry.[26]

Eosinophilic granulomatosis with polyangiitis EGPA is contemporaneous with the description of MPA, and the first patient with EGPA was probably case 1 of Lamb[27] reported in 1914 also under the heading of PAN. That patient, a 26-year-old man with 2 years of worsening asthma, developed fever, palpable purpura, nodular skin lesions, hemoptysis, vomiting, urinary difficulty, and granular urinary casts. He died 1 month later, and postmortem examination showed necrotizing arteritis of small arteries, with dense collections of extravascular eosinophils and tissue eosinophilia in the heart, stomach, and kidney. Decades later, Churg and Strauss[28] described the clinical and postmortem findings of 13 patients with asthma, fever, and hypereosinophilia, accompanied by eosinophilic exudation, fibrinoid change, and granulomatous proliferation that constituted the so-called allergic granuloma that was found within vessel walls and in extravascular connective tissue of major organ systems, leading to cardiac, pulmonary, gastrointestinal, skin, PNS and CNS manifestations. In 1990, the American College of Rheumatology (ACR)[29] developed criteria for the classification of EGPA that included ascertainment of 4 or more of the following: asthma, eosinophilia of greater than 10%, mononeuropathy or polyneuropathy, nonfixed pulmonary infiltrates on chest radiograph, paranasal sinus abnormality, and extravascular eosinophils on tissue biopsy that included an artery, arteriole, or venule. These criteria were inadequate because a patient with asthma and paranasal sinusitis could fit the designation of EGPA. Among 383 patients enrolled in the FVSG Cohort[30] who satisfied the ACR criteria[29] or the 1994 CHCC definition for EGPA,[31] the mean age at presentation was 50 years without sex predominance. Clinical manifestations at presentation included asthma (91%), peripheral neuropathy (51%), weight loss (49%), ear, nose, and throat signs (48%), nonerosive sinusitis and polyposis (41%), skin lesions (39%), purpuric rash (22%), lung infiltrates (38%), gastrointestinal involvement (23%), renal manifestations (22%), cardiomyopathy (16%), CNS involvement (5%), and cranial nerve involvement (3%). A total of 108 (31%) patients tested positive for ANCA with significantly more frequent ear, nose, and throat, peripheral nerve and renal involvement, but less frequent cardiac manifestations. Small numbers of children have been included in large studies of EGPA sufficient to allow comparisons to adults. Among 133 vasculitic patients in the ARChiVe registry, only 2 were reported to be of the EGPA type.[32]

Granulomatosis with polyangiitis Godman and Churg[33] described the syndrome of GPA that included granuloma in the nasopharynx, sinuses, and lower respiratory tract with focal segmental glomerulonephritis and disseminated small vessel vasculitis. In a landmark article, Godman and Churg[33] concluded that MPA, EGRA, and GPA were related to one another yet distinct from PAN. This astute conclusion was based mainly on pathologic features that were later substantiated by their common association with ANCA, but not so for PAN.[34] Fauci and colleagues[35] and Hoffman and colleagues[36] at the National Institutes of Health (NIH) reported a prospective series of 85 patients with GPA and a retrospective assessment of 180 patients followed for 6 months to 24 years, respectively. The presenting signs included pulmonary infiltrates (71%), sinusitis (67%), arthritis and arthralgia (44%), fever (34%), cough (34%), otitis (25%), and hemoptysis (22%), with an overall predominance of organ system involvement in the lung (94%), paranasal sinuses (91%), kidney (85%), joints (67%), and nasopharynx and nose (64%). Fauci and colleagues[35] established the efficacy of cyclophosphamide and prednisone in achieving complete remissions in 93% of patients as well as the tendency of patients to relapse and accrue additive mortality from both disease and treatment. The characteristic histopathology is a necrotizing granulomatous vasculitis, which may be found in lung and renal biopsy tissue, although the latter is less common. Instead, a focal, segmental glomerulonephritis is often seen. Other inflammatory or vasculitic phenomenon can be encountered, such as leukocytoclastic vasculitis in skin lesions, and acute and chronic inflammation in sinus, retro-orbital, and tracheal tissues. A limited form of GPA without glomerulonephritis was described[37] that is a long-term disease stage or phenotype accounting for about 5% of all patients characterized by destructive and space-consuming lesions associated with relapse rates of 46% and local damage. The 1990 ACR criteria for the classification of GPA,[38] which preceded routine ANCA testing, included the presence of 2 or more from criteria from among 4, including nasal or oral inflammation (painful or painless oral ulcers or purulent or bloody nasal discharge); abnormal chest radiograph (showing nodules, fixed infiltrates, or cavities); urinary sediment (showing microhematuria >5 red blood cells per high-power field, or red cell casts in urinary sediment); and granulomatous inflammation on biopsy tissue (within the wall of an artery or in the perivascular or extravascular area of an artery or arteriole). A proposed classification tree substituted hemoptysis for granulomatous inflammation on a tissue biopsy if the latter was not available. Baseline serum samples for 180 participants in the WG Etanercept Trial Research Group found that when IF, direct, and capture ELISA ANCA testing were performed at baseline, 166 (92%) were seropositive, including 96% with severe disease and 83% with limited disease. Holle and colleagues,[39] who prospectively compared hsPR3-ANCA ELISA with the IFT, noted an excellent performance of hsPR3-ANCA ELISA in identifying GPA and other AAV disorders associated with PR3-ANCA, suggesting that the former be used as screening test.

The past quarter century has witnessed a renaissance in the understanding of primary systemic vasculitis with convincing clinical evidence to support an important role for ANCA in the development of AAV. An AAV classification appears to better recognize ANCA disease and predict prognosis than other any existing clinical classification systems.[40] However, as with other autoimmune disorders, the cause and pathogenesis appear to be multifactorial, involving the interplay of initiating and predisposing environment and genetic factors. Induction with corticosteroids and either cyclophosphamide followed by maintenance with rituximab, or azathioprine is recommended treatment. Among 197 ANCA-positive patients with GPA or MPA in 9 centers participating in the Rituximab in ANCA-Associated Vasculitis-Immune Tolerance Network Research Group multicenter, randomized, double-blind, double-dummy, noninferiority trial[41] of the comparison of rituximab 375 mg per square meter body surface area per week for 4 weeks and cyclophosphamide 2 mg per kilogram of body weight per day controls for severe AAV, was associated with achievement of the primary end point of remission of disease without use of prednisone at 6 months in 67% of study patients compared with 42% of controls. Treatment and efficacy and safety data in children with AAV continue to be largely derived from adult GPA studies; however, as described in ARChiVe, pediatric patients in the United States and Canada are being offered pulse methylprednisolone for 3 to 5 days, followed by oral prednisone, and cyclophosphamide orally or with 1 of 2 intravenous regimens, followed by maintenance therapy, most frequently with methotrexate.

Early outcome results last year for the treatment of childhood AAV, in particular GPA, reported by Morishita and colleagues[42] on behalf of ARChiVe Investigators Network and the Pediatric Vasculitis (PedVas) Initiative were somewhat discouraging. Among 105 children with AAV, mainly GPA, who received corticosteroids, cyclophosphamide, methotrexate, or rituximab for remission-induction, and plasma exchange in conjunction with cyclophosphamide and/or rituximab, 42% achieved remission at 12 months (Pediatric Vasculitis Activity Score of 0, CS dose <0.2 mg/kg/d), 21 (48%) of whom discontinued CS by 12 months; all but 3 remaining on maintenance treatment at 12 months receiving azathioprine, methotrexate, rituximab, mycophenolate mofetil, and cyclophosphamide. However, up to 63% had a Pediatric Vasculitis Damage Index score of 1 or more by 12 months, with the presence of renal, ear, nose, and throat, or pulmonary damage; moreover, 41% of children reported hospitalizations. Thus, a significant proportion of patients were not in remission at 12 months, and more than one-half of the patient cohort experienced damage early in the disease course. The 12-month remission rate of 42% in the cohort was significantly lower than Sacri and colleagues,[43] who reported 73% remission at postinduction and 90% overall remission rate (including secondary remissions after a median time of 6.7 months).

Immune Complex Vasculitis

The foundations for IC-mediated or hypersensitivity vasculitis were conceptualized by Zeek[44,45] between 1948 and 1952, as an immunologic response to antigenic material associated with clinically evident purpura, and small vessel inflammation affecting arterioles, capillaries, and postcapillary venules. It was likened by Zeek[46] to the anaphylactoid Arthus reaction produced by the experimental injection of horse serum into rabbits.[47]

Immunoglobulin A vasculitis (Henoch-Schönlein purpura)

Children with HSP were described by Gairdner[48] with anaphylactoid purpura, including one who developed rash, colic, melanotic stools, intussusception, and hematuria, followed by a typical exanthema and fatal convulsion. Postmortem examination showed scattered cortical hemorrhages associated with cerebral necrotizing arteriolitis. The findings of IgA deposits in cutaneous blood vessel walls and in glomerular mesangial biopsies of patients with HSP and IgA nephropathy[49,50] were circumstantially convincing enough to substitute the term IgAV for HSP. IgAV/HSP is the commonest vasculitis in children. The 1990 ACR criteria[51] for the identification of HSP included age less than or equal to 20 years at disease onset, palpable purpura, acute abdominal pain, and tissue biopsy showing granulocytes in the walls of small arteries or venules. The presence of any 2 or more of these criteria distinguished 85 patients who were diagnosed as having HSP by physicians who submitted cases for the vasculitis criteria compared with 722 patients diagnosed with other forms of vasculitis, arriving at sensitivity of 87.1% and specificity of 87.7%. The addition of gastrointestinal bleeding in a classification tree format increased sensitivity to 89.4% and specificity to 88.1%, respectively.

The EULAR/PRINTO/PReS classification criteria,[3] which recognizes the contribution of IgA deposits, differs in the mandatory finding of purpura with predominance in the legs, and the presence of 1 of the 4 following features: diffuse abdominal pain, arthralgia or arthritis; a biopsy showing predominant IgA deposits; and renal involvement, including proteinuria and hematuria. Derived from the analysis of 827 patients in the database, the calculated sensitivity, specificity for the clinical and laboratory findings in between the consensus panel, and specific definition were 100% and 87%, respectively. Peru and colleagues[52] studied 254 children with IgAV/HSP between 2003 and 2006 with a distribution of skin, joint, gastrointestinal, and renal manifestations of 100%, 66%, 56% and 30%, respectively. The disorder commences with fever and palpable purpura, although early lesions can be urticarial. Arthralgia and abdominal pain precede, accompany, or follow the rash. Melena is common as are signs of peritonitis. Proteinuria and hematuria are of variably severity, and renal pathologic condition may be of a mild glomerulitis to necrotizing or proliferative glomerulonephritis. Ozen and coworkers[3] noted palpable purpura, commonly in crops with lower limb predominance in 89% of patients, arthritis or arthralgia in 78%, diffuse abdominal pain in 60%, proteinuria and hematuria combined in 33%, and IgA deposition in 10% of children. The treatment of IgAV/HSP remains empiric and largely supportive, with conflicting conclusions in retrospective and uncontrolled case series of immune suppression in severe HSP nephritis. Extrarenal manifestations can be managed by symptomatic treatment. A meta-analysis of 15 studies based on a comprehensive review of the literature in the Medline database from 1956 to 2007, and Cochrane Controlled Trials Registry among 15 studies and more than 1300 patients[32] found that early treatment conferred a protective effect on developing persistent renal disease (odds ratio [OR] 0.43) and the likelihood of surgical intervention for abdominal pain (OR 0.75), as well as a statistically significant positive effect on shortening the duration of abdominal symptoms (OR 5.42).

C1q (hypocomplementemic urticarial) vasculitis

McDuffie and colleagues[53] later described several patients with recurrent attacks of erythematous, urticarial, and hemorrhagic skin lesions that lasted 24 hours at a time, associated with recurrent attacks of fever, joint swelling, abdominal distress, and depressed serum complement. When tested by immunodiffusion against purified preparations rheumatoid factor (RF) and human C1q, several patients reacted strongly with purified C1q. Skin biopsies showed leukocytoclasia characteristic of necrotizing vasculitis, anaphylactoid purpura, or mild nonspecific perivascular infiltration. IF of skin specimens showed fixation of immunoglobulin in the patient with necrotizing vasculitis. Renal biopsy showed mild to moderate glomerulonephritis indistinguishable from those seen in other forms of chronic membranoproliferative glomerulonephritis. The differences from SLE included more urticarial and purpuric skin lesions, with relatively mild renal or absent and other visceral involvement in the patients with HUV. An etiopathogenesis related to chronic vascular inflammation resulting from deposits of IC in small vessel walls seemed likely. Zeiss and colleagues[54] characterized C1q IgG precipitins from HUV sera that precipitated C1q in agarose gel among 4 additional patients. Wisnieski and Naff[55] later showed C1q binding activity in IgG from HUV sera. Buck and colleagues[56] recognized the HUV syndrome as the presence of UV with multiorgan involvement, notably arthralgia or arthritis, angioedema, pulmonary, ocular, renal, and pericardial, although anti-C1q antibodies are elevated and the serum low C1q levels are reduced in virtually all children so studied. Antihistamines are the drug of choice with cutaneous lesions to control itching, but they may be insufficient in controlling the formation of IC when given late in the inflammatory cascade. There is yet a consensus on the most effective therapeutic regimen; however, plasmapheresis and intravenous immunoglobulin (IVIG) are alternative immunosuppressant modalities.

Variable Vessel Vasculitis

Behçet disease

Behçet and Matteson[57] described the clinicopathologic findings of a 28-year-old Turkish patient with relapsing oral, genital, and oral eruptions over 4 years, accompanied by severe headache, memory loss, dizziness, lethargy, fatal seizures, and coma. Postmortem examination showed perivascular inflammatory cell infiltration of the meninges, brain, and central retinal artery and optic nerve with necrotic cerebral lesions. The first well-documented American patient with nervous system involvement of BD was described by Wolf and coworkers,[58] namely a 22-year-old woman with a 5-year history of recurrent oral and genital ulceration, and a 2-year course of progressive visual loss, headache, hemiparesis, ataxia, tremor, dysarthria, cranial nerve palsy, cerebellar and corticospinal tract disease, and mental deterioration, which responded to prednisone therapy. The most widely used diagnostic criteria of BD were formulated by the International Study Group[59] that included recurrent oral ulcerations plus any 2 of genital ulceration, typical defined eye lesions, typical skin lesions, or a positive pathergy. Recurrent oral ulcerations were categorized as minor aphthous, major aphthous, and herpetiform ulcerations that recurred at least 3 times in a 12-month period. Recurrent genital ulcerations were defined as aphthous ulceration and scarring. Eye lesions were defined as anterior uveitis, posterior uveitis, or cells in the vitreous on slit-lamp examination, and retinal vasculitis. Compatible skin lesions included erythema nodosum, pseudofolliculitis, papulopustular lesions, and acneiform nodules in postadolescent patients not receiving corticosteroids. A positive pathergy test of cutaneous hypersensitivity was defined as positive when a sterile pustule developed after 24 to 48 hours at the site of a needle prick to the skin.

Although the usual onset of BD is in the third or fourth decade of life, pediatric-onset patients have been described.[60] The neuropathologic findings of BD in brain biopsies and postmortem examination have been remarkably consistent among patients over the past several decades evidencing perivascular cuffing of small meningovascular and parenchymal arteries and veins, rarely medium-sized arteries displaying fibrinoid degeneration and recanalization, and examples of venous thrombosis. Cortical venous sinus thrombosis (CVST) in BD presents with subacute or chronic onset of symptoms of isolated intracranial hypertension accompanied by headache, blurred vision, and diplopia, and underlying necrotizing vasculitis. Venous infarcts occur in up to 63% of those with CVST of other causes, but in only 6% of patients with BD. The inflammatory cell infiltrates are generally composed of lymphocytes, both T- and B cells, macrophages, rarely plasma cells and eosinophils, with reactive astrocytosis and microscopic gliosis in neighboring cerebral, cerebellar, and brainstem white matter. Matsumoto and colleagues[61] noted large vessel lesions in 7 of 8 patients aged 31 to 56 years with BD, including saccular aneurysms of the sinus of Valsalva or aortic arch, thoracic and abdominal aorta, pulmonary, femoral, and iliac arteries, and thrombotic occlusions in the pulmonary vein and superior and inferior vena. Aortitis was noted histologically in 6 of the 8 patients and was active in one, scarred in 6, and intermixed in another. Active aortitis was characterized by intense infiltration of inflammatory cells in the media and adventitia more frequently than in the interim with occasional giant cell formation. Although anticoagulation would not be recommended for BD-related CVST, it might be considered in association with arterial occlusions, with both venous and arterial occlusive episodes, warranting prompt consideration of corticosteroids alone or in association with another immunosuppressant agent.

Cogan syndrome

The first patient with CS of nonsyphilitic interstitial keratitis (IK) was reported by Mogan and Baumgartner,[62] that of a 26-year-old man with recurrent pain, spasm, and redness of the left eye with photophobia, excessive tearing, and marked conjunctival injection, followed by a severe attack of dizziness, tinnitus, vertigo, nausea, vomiting, ringing in the ears, profuse perspiration, and deafness. A diagnosis of recurrent IK and explosive Menière disease was made. Vestibuloauditory symptoms were later described by Cogan.[63] Haynes and colleagues[64] set forth diagnostic criteria for typical CS according to the definitions established in a review of 30 patients seen at the National Eye Institute of the NIH by Cogan. Symptoms of IK develop abruptly and gradually resolve, associated with photophobia, lacrimation, and eye pain, which may be unilateral or bilateral. Such symptoms tend to recur periodically for years before becoming quiescent. Vestibuloauditory dysfunction was manifested by sudden onset of Menière-like attacks of nausea, vomiting, tinnitus, vertigo, and frequently progressive hearing loss that characteristically occurred before or after the onset of IK. However, within 1 to 6 months of the onset of eye symptoms, auditory symptoms progressed to deafness over a period of 1 to 3 months, certainly no longer than 2 years. With less than 100 reported patients with this rare childhood and young adult disorder, most reported patients with typical CS have appeared as single case reports or patient series, often without pathologic confirmation or evidence of systemic vasculitis in a biopsy or at postmortem examination. Early recognition of the diagnosis of childhood CS is important in instituting corticosteroid therapy to preserve hearing especially when hearing loss is a later occurrence. A combination of oral and intravenous corticosteroids may be considered in children who partly but not fully improve. Most patients with CS (58%) so treated with corticosteroids derived a favorable response in both vestibuloauditory and ophthalmologic manifestations, with the remainder demonstrating only ophthalmologic (23%) or vestibuloauditory improvement (19%) alone (100). Other therapies include methotrexate (23%), cyclophosphamide (10%), azathioprine (5%), etanercept (3%), hydroxychloroquine (2%), and IVIG (2%). Surgical cochlear implantation can led to objective and subjective benefits with improved hearing.

RECOGNITION OF SECONDARY VASCULITIDES
Cryoglobulinemic Vasculitis

The presence in the serum of one or more immunoglobulins that precipitate below core body temperatures and redissolve on rewarming is termed cryoglobulinemia. Wintrobe and Buell[65] described the first patient with cryoglobulinemia, that of a 56-year-old woman who presented with progressive frontal headache, left face and eye pain, and right shoulder, neck, and lumbar discomfort after a bout of shingles. These symptoms were followed by Raynaud symptoms, recurrent nosebleeds, exertional dyspnea and palpitation, and changes in the eye ground attributed to central vein thrombosis. Postmortem examination showed infiltrating myeloma of the humerus and lumbar vertebra, and splenic enlargement. A unique plasma protein was detected that spontaneously precipitated with cold temperature and solubilized at high temperature that differed from Bence-Jones proteinuria of other myeloma patients. Brouet and co-workers[66] provided modern classifications of cryoglobulinemia among 86 patients that included type 1, composed of a single monoclonal immunoglobulin, and types II and III as mixed cryoglobulinemia (MC), composed of different immunoglobulins, with a monoclonal component in type II, and polyclonal immunoglobulin in type III. In the absence of well-defined disease, the presence of MC was termed "essential." Since recognition of hepatitis C virus (HCV) infection in patients with MC and the high rate of false-negative serologic tests in type II MC, it became evident that HCV was associated in most patients with MC. CV is characterized by the classical triad of purpura, weakness, and arthralgia, frequent multiple organ involvement, and infrequent late lymphatic and hepatic malignancies. The commonest clinical manifestations of HCV-negative MC vasculitis in the CryoVas survey[67] included purpura (75%), peripheral neuropathy (52%), arthralgia or arthritis (44%), glomerulonephritis (36%), cutaneous ulcers (16%), and cutaneous necrosis (14%). A connective tissue disease was diagnosed in 30% of patients, and B-cell non-Hodgkin lymphoma was noted in 22% of patients, whereas MCV was considered essential in 48% of patients. There was a greater frequency of joint involvement (53% vs 40%), peripheral neuropathy (74% vs 52%), CNS involvement (9% vs 2%) in those with HCV-MC compared with those with HCV-negative MC, with an equal frequency of purpura (71% vs 75%) and renal involvement (34% vs 35%). Cacoub and colleagues[68] noted 5 high prevalent extrahepatic manifestations in chronic HCV infection, including arthralgia (23%), paresthesia (17%), myalgia (15%), pruritus (15%), and sicca syndrome (11%), and a 40% prevalence of cryoglobulins. These findings suggest the possibility of an independent role of HCV infection in the clinicopathologic manifestations of MC and MCV. Among 114 patients, including 18 children and 96 adults, with cryoglobulinemia between 2000 and 2012, children had more frequent prolonged fever (17% vs 3%), petechiae and purpura (27% vs 15%), arthralgia and arthritis (66% vs 16%), and cutaneous involvement (77% vs 50%), than adults.[69] Aggressive optimal therapy for HCV-related CV with PEGylated-interferon-α to improve the pharmacologic properties, and ribavirin with a protease inhibitor in the instance of HCV genotype 1 infection, should be considered induction therapy for CV and administered for 48 weeks for all HCV genotypes.[70] An induction phase of immunosuppression such as rituximab plus antivirals is recommended in patients with more severe HCV-related CV exemplified by worsening renal function, mononeuritis multiplex, extensive skin disease, including ulcers and distal necrosis. Terrier and colleagues[67] showed a greater therapeutic efficacy of rituximab and corticosteroids compared with corticosteroids alone and alkylating agents with cortico-steroids in achieving complete clinical, renal, and immunologic responses and a pred-nisone dosage of less than 10 mg per day at 6 months. However, this regimen was associated with severe infections, particularly when high doses of corticosteroids were used. Plasmapheresis combined with immunosuppression can be useful in fulmi-nant HCV-related CV to engender an immediate effect but should be continued to avoid postpheresis rebound worsening. Rituximab, fludarabine, and cyclophosphamide treatment is effective treatment of refractory CryoVas associated with lymphoma. One-year, 2-year, 5-year, 10-year survival rates of 91%, 89%, 79%, and 65%, respec-tively, have been reported in patients with CV with fatalities related to serious infection and disease flares of CV.

Systemic Lupus Erythematosus

Although distinctly uncommon, 2 collagen-vascular disorders, SLE and rheumatoid arthritis (RA), can be associated with vasculitis of the nervous system. The early con-cepts of the collagen-vascular disorders introduced by Klemperer[71,72] stemmed from the appreciation of fibrinoid necrosis using collagen staining in patients with SLE. As collagen swells and fragments, it dissolves to form a homogeneous hyaline and granular periodic acid–Schiff-positive material. The latter fibrinoid material contains immunoglobulins, antigen-antibody complexes, complement, and fibrinogen. The organ-specific responses to this fibrinoid material, especially of the CNS, lead to recognizable clinical sequela due to vascular and parenchymal damage. The ACR delineated criteria for the diagnosis of SLE.[73] The recognition of neuropsychiatric lupus (NPSLE) was noted in 6.4% of a cohort of 1253 SLE patients defined by the ACR; those with late-onset SLE due to development of disease after age 50 years, had a frequency of NPSLE of 6.6% compared with 36.6% in early-onset disease despite less major organ involvement and more benign course. Once thought to be an important cause of CNS or cerebral lupus, true vasculitis was present in only 12% of postmortem examinations in the series of Johnson and Richardswon,[74] and in 26.7% of late-onset SLE patients compared with 16.6% of those with early-onset SLE. A comparison of the cumulative incidence of clinical manifestations in the 2 latter groups showed that seizures were more common in early-onset patients compared with later-onset patients (6.6% vs 0%), similarly for multiple cerebrovascular attacks (23.3% vs 3.3%), cranial and peripheral neuropathy (6.6% vs 3.3%). Devinsky and col-leagues[75] noted a prevalence of 3.5% of psychiatric involvement that included organic affective, delusional, and hallucinatory syndromes in a cohort of 50 patients with SLE, one-half of whom had CNS lesions. Feinglass and colleagues[76] noted neuropsychi-atric manifestations at onset of SLE among 3% of 140 patients compared with 37% in the course of the illness; however, headache was not specifically tabulated. Cere-bral dysfunction in SLE can be caused by large vessel or small vessel involvement or both. In the series by Feinglass and colleagues,[76] vasculitis was noted overall in 28% of patients as well as in 46% of those with neuropsychiatric involvement compared with 17% of patients lacking neuropsychiatric involvement. Postmortem examination of the CNS in 10 of 19 fatalities showed 2 cases of multiple large and small infarcts, which in one of them, demonstrated inflammatory cells infiltrates in the walls of medium-sized vessels, and perivascular infiltrates around small arterioles. Although active CNS vasculitis was absent in the brain and spinal tissue of all 50 patients re-ported by Devinsky and colleagues,[75] 2 had evidence of inactive healed CNS vascu-litis so suggested by focal disruption of the elastic lamina and mild intimal proliferation of a single medium-sized artery, one of which had active systemic vasculitis of the PAN type, both of which evidenced Libman-Sacks endocarditis and embolic brain infarcts. Focal angiitis of the CNS with cystlike formation around affected blood vessels was noted at postmortem in the patient described by Mintz and Fraga[77] with typical SLE rash, cutaneous vasculitis, and active neuropsychiatric involvement. Trevor and colleagues[78] summarized the literature of large named cerebral vessel occlusions from 1958 to 1965 noting 1 patient with a middle cerebral artery (MCA) stenosis progressing to occlusion and 3 others with angiographic internal carotid artery (ICA) occlusions, adding 3 new patients and suggesting a relation of the occurrence to cerebral arteritis. Two women, one aged 21 and the other aged 42 years, presented with headache followed by focal neurologic symptoms attributed to lesions along the left MCA followed by right ICA occlusions, and a right MCA stenosis progressing to occlusion in 4 months, respectively. A third patient had a left ICA occlusion without mention of headache. Among the 4 literature patients, one had angiographic occlusion of the MCA and 3 others had occlusion of the ICA. Johnson and Richardswon[74] attributed the vasculitic nature of this process histopathologically to cerebral vasculitis mediated by acute inflammation and necrosis. Younger and colleagues[79] reported large named cerebral vessel occlusion attributed to circulating anticardiolipin antibodies in a young man in whom a vasculitic mechanism was not evoked. IC-mediated vasculitis probably affecting small vessels is thought to account for much of the damage in CNS lupus in light of the paucity of cerebral vasculitis evident in the form of inflammatory infiltrates in vessel walls at postmortem examination. In those with discrete vascular infarcts, there is a known association with the presence of circulating pathogenic antibodies, which predisposes some individuals to a high risk of stroke due to both small and large vessel occlusion.

Rheumatoid Arthritis Vasculitis

A joint working group from the ACR and the EULAR published the 2010 classification criteria for RA.[80] Extra-articular RA (ExRA) occurrence is associated with increased comorbidity and mortality.[81] Criteria for severe ExRA were proposed in 2004.[82] Active RA with high disease activity is associated with increased risk of severe ExRA manifestations. Major cutaneous vasculitis and vasculitis involving other organs are 2 such ExRA occurrences. The diagnosis of RAV has generally been ascertained according to the criteria of Scott and Bacon[82] according to the presence of one or more of the following: (1) mononeuritis multiplex; (2) peripheral gangrene; (3) biopsy evidence of acute necrotizing arteritis plus fever and weight loss; and (4) deep cutaneous ulcers or active ExRA disease if associated with typical digital infarcts or biopsy evidence of vasculitis.

The markers of RA severity, including RA positivity, erosion and joint destructive changes (21% among those in the 1985–1994 cohort, compared with 29% in 1995–2007), use of methotrexate, other disease-modifying antirheumatic drugs, and systemic corticosteroids, were significantly associated with ExRA development between 1995 and 2007. Vollerstein and colleagues[83] studied 52 patients with RAV at the Mayo Clinic from 1974 to 1981, who developed clinical vasculitis evidenced by classic ischemic skin lesions, mononeuritis multiplex, or a positive tissue biopsy in comparison to population controls. The initial manifestation of vasculitis was seen in skin (26 patients), nerve (20 patients) or both (3 patients), and mononeuritis multiplex presented in one (2 patients), 2 (9 patients), 3 (5 patients) or 4 nerves (4 patients). More than 90% of tissue biopsy specimens revealed vascular necrosis and inflammation. At diagnosis, 80% of patients began therapy with aspirin and other nonsteroidal anti-inflammatory drugs; however, three-fourths continued or began corticosteroid therapy. Sixteen of the original 52 patients eventually received cytotoxic immunosuppressive therapy. Compared with the general population, those with RAV had decreased survival that was immediately evident and continued for 6 years. The survival of RAV was not different from classic RA.

The factors that predicted decreased survival in RAV include older age, failure to receive previous nonsteroidal anti-inflammatory drugs, previous administration of cytotoxic immunosuppressive agents, a higher dose of corticosteroids at diagnosis, decision to continue or initiate corticosteroids, and abnormal urinary sediment. Puéchal and colleagues[84] found vasculitic involvement of vasa nervorum of both small- and medium-sized arteries indistinguishable from PAN in 64% of patients, with a mortality ranging from 28% to 44% according to the length of follow-up. Epineurial and perineurial vasculitis was observed with the same frequency among those with primary sensory neuropathy as others with predominant motor involvement, 67% versus 64%, respectively. A greater extent of the neuropathy and motor involvement tended to predict decreased survival; however, mononeuritis multiplex was not associated with a poor 5-year survival rate (57%) than was distal symmetric sensory or sensorimotor neuropathy (55%). Scott and Bacon[82] reported that 5 patients (24%) died in the group receiving methylprednisolone and cyclophosphamide; postmortem examination in 4 failed to demonstrate active vasculitis. By comparison, 7 patients (29%) died receiving other treatments, of which one so studied at postmortem examination showed active vasculitis.

Three forms of vasculitis classically occur in RA affecting all calibers of blood vessels from dermal postcapillary venules to the aorta, usually in association with circulating IgM and IgG rheumatoid factor as measured by the latex fixation test, decreased complement levels, and a positive antinuclear antibody (ANA). The first form of vasculitis is a proliferative endarteritis of a few organs, notably the heart, skeletal muscle, and nerves, characterized by inflammatory infiltration of all layers of small arteries and arterioles, with intimal proliferation, necrosis, and thrombosis. The second is fulminant vasculitis indistinguishable from PAN with less severe leukocytosis, myalgia, renal and gastrointestinal involvement, and bowel perforation. The third type takes the form of palpable purpura, arthritis, cryoglobulinemia, and low complement levels.

The literature contains references to RAV with involvement of the CNS at postmortem examination in only 9 patients. Detailed postmortem findings evidencing CNS vasculitis have been reported in only 9 patients[84–91] with accompanying clinical neurologic findings including, delirium, confusion, seizures, hemiparesis, Gerstman-like syndrome, blindness, and peripheral neuropathy. Postmortem examination has shown widespread systemic vasculitis, single major cerebral artery involvement, generalized PAN-like changes in the CNS, isolated CNS vasculitis affecting the temporal lobes and brainstem with diffuse infiltrative thickening of the pia arachnoid, rheumatoid nodular formation, and inflammatory cell infiltration of leptomeningeal vessels in subjacent brain tissue, including the midbrain, medulla, and upper cervical cord, and chronic perivasculitis and transmural chronic inflammatory cell infiltration with severe fibrinoid necrosis of the media of small leptomeningeal vessels and cortical arterioles. Despite development of new and potent drugs for RA, there are no available evidence-based recommendations for treatment of systemic rheumatoid vasculitis. Complete remission of systemic rheumatoid vasculitis occurs in nearly three-fourths treated with rituximab, with a significant decrease in daily prednisone dosage and an acceptable toxicity profile, making it a suitable therapeutic option to induce remission, but maintenance therapy was necessary. Prednisone therapy initially decreases systemic inflammation with a dose dependent on the degree of systemic inflammation and level of organ system involvement. The presence of CNS involvement mandates intravenous corticosteroid therapy and consideration of cytotoxic or biologic agents, including methotrexate, azathioprine, cyclophosphamide, anti–tumor necrosis factor

(TNF) agents and rituximab. Bartolucci and colleagues[92] reported the successful induction of a prompt symptomatic response in 10 patients with systemic vasculitis not responsive to conventional treatment, including 2 with RA and associated vasculitis. Puéchal and colleagues[93] demonstrated evidence of efficacy of adjunctive anti-TNF therapy and corticosteroids for treatment of active refractory systemic RAV with remission achieved in two-thirds of patients, and a significant decrease in prednisone dose, with a higher risk of infection in the most severely ill patients.

IDENTIFICATION OF SINGLE-ORGAN VASCULITIDES
Primary Angiitis of the Central Nervous System

Adult- and childhood-isolated angiitis and vasculitis are prototypical primary vasculitic disorders restricted to the CNS. The diagnosis of PACNS[94] like IACNS[95] originally relied on classic angiographic (**Fig. 3**) or histopathologic features of angiitis within the CNS in the absence of systemic vasculitis or another cause for the observed findings. The typical patient with PACNS presented with headache of gradual onset often accompanied by the signs and symptoms of dementia, while only later developing focal neurologic symptoms and signs. The clinical course might be rapidly progressive over days to weeks, or at times insidiously over many months with seemingly prolonged periods of stabilization. Those with the subset of GAB[96] presented with headache, mental change, and elevated cerebrospinal fluid protein content with or without pleocytosis. Hemiparesis, quadriparesis, and lethargy were associated with a poor prognosis and mandated the need for combined meningeal and brain biopsy to establish the diagnosis with certainty. Granulomatous giant cell and epithelioid cell infiltration in the walls of arteries of various caliber, from named cerebral vessels to small arteries and veins, was noted at postmortem examination (**Fig. 4**).

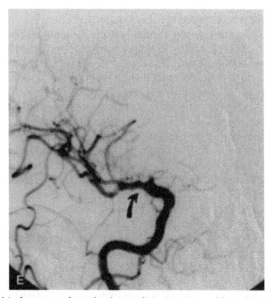

Fig. 3. Radiographic features of cerebral vasculitis. Ectasia and beading in the M1 segment and lack of flow in the A1 segment of the right anterior cerebral artery (*arrow*). (*From* Younger DS. Vasculitis of the Nervous System. In: Younger DS, editor. Motor Disorders. Third edition. Brookfield, CT: Rothstein Publishing; 2015. p. 235–80; with permission.)

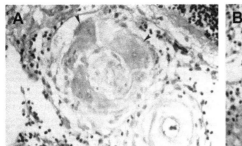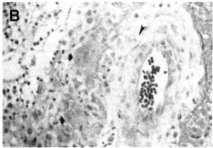

Fig. 4. CNS vasculitis. (*A*) The media and adventitia of this small leptomeningeal artery have been almost completely replaced by multinucleated giant cells (*arrowheads*). There is intimal proliferation with obliteration of the vascular lumen, and a dense, perivascular, mononuclear inflammatory infiltrate can be seen (stain, hematoxylin and eosin, original magnification ×250). (*B*) A somewhat larger leptomeningeal vessel shows necrosis of the media and internal elastic lamina with multinucleated giant cell formation (*arrows*), intimal proliferation (*arrowhead*), and lymphocytic infiltration of the adventitia and neighboring meninges (stain, hematoxylin and eosin, original magnification ×250). (*From* Younger DS. Vasculitis of the Nervous System. In: Younger DS, editor. Motor Disorders. Third edition. Brookfield, CT: Rothstein Publishing; 2015. p. 235–80; with permission.)

The experience of adult PCNSV and GAB was summarized in a single large historical cohort by Younger and colleagues,[97] and 2 observational cohorts, one retrospective from the Mayo Clinic[98] and a multicenter prospective cohort of PACNS from the FVSG, French NeuroVascular Society, and the French Internal Medicine Society[99] have stratified cases of based on clinical, neuroradiographic, and histopathologic laboratory features, offering additional insights into the management of CNS vasculitis.

Awaiting the results of The PedVas Initiative, a Canadian and United Kingdom collaborative study (ARChiVe Investigators Network within the PedVas Initiative [ARChiVe registry], BrainWorks, and DCVAS) of pediatric and adult cases of AAV (GPA) and PACNS (NIH identifier, NCT02006134), there is yet satisfactory prevalence and incidence data or evidence-based guidelines to treat childhood (c)PACNS. The PedVas Initiative has been prospectively collecting clinical and biobank data in January 2013 of registered cases, within 12 months of study entry. The approach to diagnosis and management has been to first differentiate cPACNS and SVcPACNS respectively from angiography-positive, and angiography-negative, brain biopsy-positive mimickers. The approach to adult PACNS and cPACNS has been problematic for several reasons.

First, unlike antemortem pediatric cases of cerebral vasculitis that show angiographic evidence of large named vessel involvement, children with small-vessel (SV)-cPACNS can only be diagnosed conclusively by CNS biopsy tissues that show transmural inflammation of small meningeal and penetrating cortical vessels. Affected patients present with focal symptoms suggesting an association with stroke, but are more likely to develop subacute, nonlocalizing neurologic complaints, such as headache, behavioral changes, seizures, school failure, or cognitive decline. Moreover, childhood strokes may be highly variable in character and distribution.

Second, neuroimaging is far less specific in cPACNS. Noninvasive arterial imaging using CTA and MRA shows typically normal findings even when parenchymal MRI ranges from normal to diffusely abnormal across a wide array of lesion characteristics.

Third, childhood arterial ischemic stroke due to SV-cPACNS may show normal results on conventional angiography. Such cases, referred to as "angiography-negative SV-cPACNS,"[101] are typically unsubstantiated by histopathology even though the categorical term (SV-cPACNS) suggests a corresponding caliber of vessel involvement.

Fourth, despite the similarities to adult forms of PACNS, cPACNS series[100] fails to mention prototypical granulomatouspathologic condition, suggesting a bias of selection, making clinicopathologic comparisons to the adult form and the overall spectrum of CNS vasculitis problematic.

Fifth, awaiting the results of The PedVas Initiative, the approach of cPACNS has largely been to lump such cases into the broader category of IBrainD[102] by systematically excluding "angiography-positive" mimics of cPCANS and "angiography-negative brain biopsy-positive" mimics from true SVcPACNS. Sixth, as the approach to management of SV-cPACNS is patterned after other SVV such as AAV, it becomes difficult to reconcile the disappointing results of the PedVas Initiative[42] that showed a remission status of 42%, and visceral organ damage in 63% of cases following treatment with corticosteroids, cyclophosphamide, methotrexate, or rituximab for remission-induction, and plasma exchange in conjunction with cyclophosphamide and/or rituximab; and azathioprine, methotrexate, rituximab, mycophenolate mofetil, and cyclophosphamide for up to 12 months for remission maintenance.

Idiopathic Aortitis–Immunoglobulin G4-related Disorders

In 1972, an unusual form of inflammatory aortic disease or aortitis came to light in the surgical literature with far-reaching implications for concepts of autoimmunity. Walker and colleagues[103] noted that 10% of 217 patients presenting with abdominal aneurysms at Manchester Royal Infirmary between 1958 and 1969 for resection showed excessive thickening of aneurysm walls and perianeurysmal adhesions at operation. Subsequent histologic examination of the walls of the aneurysms showed extensive active chronic inflammatory changes, including plasma-cell infiltration. The clinical features of patients with inflammatory aneurysms differed from those with atherosclerotic disease due to generally younger age by a decade, lower incidence of rupture, lack of claudication of intermittent the limbs and presence of peripheral pulses, less likelihood of unusual presenting features, elevated ESR, and lack of calcification on preoperative abdominal aortic imaging. Rojo-Leyva and colleagues[104] noted idiopathic aortitis in 43% of 1204 aortic specimens gathered over a period of 20 years. In 96% of the patients with idiopathic aortitis and aneurysm formation, aortitis was present only in the thoracic aorta. In 2001, Hamamo and colleagues[105] noted a high concentrations of IgG4 associated with sclerosing pancreatitis characterized by obstructive jaundice, infrequent attacks of abdominal pain, irregular narrowing of the pancreatic duct, sonolucent swelling of the parenchyma, lymphoplasmacytic infiltration, fibrosis, and a favorable response to corticosteroid treatment. One year later, Hamano and coworkers[106] noted the association of sclerosing pancreatitis with raised concentrations of IgG4 among those with concomitant hydronephrosis that caused ureteral masses later diagnosed as retroperitoneal fibrosis (RPF). Histologic examination of ureteral and pancreatic tissues revealed abundant tissue infiltration by IgG4-bearing plasma cells. In the same year, 2008, three important observations were made. First, Sakata and colleagues[107] concluded that inflammatory abdominal aortic aneurysm (IAAA) was related to IgG4 sclerosing disease. Second, Kasashima and colleagues[108] concluded that IAAA was an IgG-RD together with RPF. Third, Ito and colleagues[109] described a patient with IAAA, hydronephrosis caused by RPF, and high levels of IgG4 in whom treatment with corticosteroids led to clinical improvement and reduction in IgG4 levels. Histologic inspection of the aortic wall specimen showed lymphocytoplasmacytic infiltration. Immunohistochemical analysis of the tissue showed IgG4-positive plasma cells. The findings suggested that IAAA had an etiopathogenesis similar to autoimmune pancreatitis and that some cases of IAAA and RPF may be aortic and periaortic lesions of an IgG4-RD. One year later in 2009,

Khosroshahi and colleagues[110] described thoracic aortitis due to IgG4-RD with marked elevation of the serum IgG4 levels with progression to autoimmune pancreatitis, and Stone and coworkers[111] described IgG4-related thoracic aortitis with a media-predominant pattern of aortic wall infiltration and marked elevation of serum IgG4 levels, unequivocally linking IgG4-RD with thoracic lymphoplasmacytic aortitis. CDS, MR combined with MRA and CTA, which adequately visualize the aortic wall and lumen, combined with FDG PET to detect increased uptake by metabolically active cells, including inflammatory cells infiltrating the vessel wall, are essential in the assessment of the extent and severity of the various forms of aortitis, including IgG4 types. The histopathologic analysis of biopsy specimens has been the cornerstone of the diagnosis of IgG4-RD. A 2012 consensus statement on the pathologic condition of IgG4-RD by Deshpande and colleagues[112] proposed a terminology scheme for the diagnosis of IgG4-RD based on the morphologic appearance and tissue IgG4+ plasma cell counts in biopsy tissue. Three histopathologc features associated with IgG4-RD included a dense lymphoplasmacytic infiltrate, fibrosis arranged at least focally in a storiform pattern, and obliterative phlebitis in morphologic specimens. Most cells were T cell with scattered B cells, and an essential component of plasma cells with occasional eosinophils and macrophages. The level IgG4 antibody, which represents less than 5% of the total IgG in healthy individuals, is tightly regulated and has a unique structure and functional property. It undergoes half antibody exchange in vivo resulting in recombined antibodies composed of 2 different binding specificities. Their production is driven in part by Th2 cytokines that mediate allergic reactions and IgE production. It does not activate complement pathways and has reduced effector function relative to other IgG subtypes. It remains unclear as to whether IgG4 directly mediates the disease process or reflects a protective response induced by anti-inflammatory cytokines, making it simply a valuable biological marker of IgG4-RD.

A Japanese consensus management guideline[113] suggested the initiation of oral prednisolone for induction of remission at a dose of 0.6 mg/kg per day for 2 to 4 weeks, with tapering by 5 mg every 1 to 2 weeks based on clinical manifestations, biochemical blood tests, and repeated imaging, to a maintenance dose of 2.5 to 5 mg per day for up to 3 months. Readministration of corticosteroids is advised for treating relapses. Treatment with azathioprine, mycophenolate mofetil, and methotrexate can be used as corticosteroid-sparing agents or as remission-maintenance drugs after corticosteroid-induced remissions. Patients with recurrent or refractory disease and B-cell depletion may be considered for rituximab.[114]

Nonsystemic Peripheral Nerve Vasculitis

The vasculitic neuropathies are heterogeneous disorders that present in the setting of systemic vasculitis or in the absence thereof where necrotizing arteritis may remain clinically and pathologically restricted to the peripheral nerves as a SOV. The Peripheral Nerve Society[115,116] established respective guidelines for the classification, diagnosis, investigation, and treatment of non-systemic vasculitic neuropathy (NSVN) and vasculitic peripheral neuropathy. Pathologically defined vasculitic neuropathy is defined by active or chronic peripheral nerve and muscle tissue lesions that show cellular invasion of the walls of blood vessels with accompanying acute vascular damage (fibrinoid necrosis, endothelial loss/disruption, internal lamina loss/fragmentation, smooth muscle media loss/fragmentation/separation, acute thrombosis, vascular/perivascular hemorrhage, or leukocytoclasia) or chronic vascular damage (intimal hyperplasia, fibrosis of media, adventitial/periadventitial fibrosis, or chronic thrombosis chronic thrombosis with recanalization), without evidence of another primary disease process that could mimic vasculitis pathologically, such as lymphoma, lymphomatoid granulomatosis, or amyloidosis.

Patients with NSVN lack clinical and laboratory evidence of involvement of other organs (demonstrable by laboratory evidence of PR3-, MPO-ANA, mixed cryoglobulins, anti-Sjögren's antibodies syndrome-related antigen A and B (SSA, SSB), Smith (Sm), ribonuclear protein (RNP), SCL-70, centromere, double-stranded DNA, citrullinated protein (CCP); ESR >100 mm per hour, or tissue biopsy evidence of vasculitis in another organ other than muscle; serologic, polymerase chain reaction or culture evidence of a specific infection associate with vasculitis), and no predisposing factors (other than diabetes) of a connective tissue disease, sarcoidosis, inflammatory bowel disease, active malignancy, HUV, cutaneous PAN, or exposure to drugs likely to cause vasculitis. Inflammation of microvessels less than 40 to 70 μm in diameter without vascular damage is broadly referred to as microscopic vasculitis or microvasculitis (MV).

The management of NPNV has remained uncertain because of the very concept presumes that the vasculitic disease process is widespread within the nerves and not present elsewhere in the body. This assumption has been called into question by 4 lines of evidence.

First, the definition of NPNV allows for the finding of vasculitic lesions in muscle tissue, perhaps making the syndrome more appropriately termed PNS vasculitis. Moreover, the detection of vasculitis in cutaneous nerve and muscle tissue specimens has been incorporated into the FVSG database to establish the diagnosis of systemic vasculitis. Among 129 patients with PAN[16] who underwent nerve biopsy with (108 patients) or without (21 patients) peripheral neuropathy, vasculitic lesions were noted in cutaneous nerve tissue in 83% and 81% of patients, respectively, compared with 68% and 60% of cases where muscle biopsy tissue was examined.

Second, the lack of long-term follow-up in most cases series ranged from 6 months to 22 years.[117]

Third, the report was of only 2 proposed cases, both with foci of vasculitis outside the PNS in a visceral organ[14] or the temporal artery.[118] Patient 1 in the series of pathologically confirmed cases of PAN by Kernohan and Woltman[116] was a 54-year-old man with 5 years of progressive generalized painful peripheral neuropathy that was so severe before death that he was partially paralyzed and unable to speak or swallow. Postmortem examination showed PAN limited to the nerve trunks of the arms and legs. The brain, cranial nerves, and spinal cord were normal except for early acute changes without evidence of vasculitis. Examination of all other organs failed to reveal a single vascular lesion, except one small artery in the capsule of the prostate gland. Torvik and Berntzen[118] described a 76-year-old woman with diffuse fever, pain, and central scotoma of the eye that improved with corticosteroids. A biopsy of the temporal artery and pectoralis muscle disclosed necrotizing arteries of small arteries and arterioles in small adventitial vessels of the temporal artery without frank temporal arteritis. However, postmortem examination showed evidence of healed vasculitis in numerous small arteries and arterioles of muscle and nerve tissue measuring 50 to 200 μm in diameter without vasculitis in visceral organ or the CNS.

Fourth, the inclusion of patients with diabetes according to the 2010 guidelines[115] may be introducing selection bias. Over the years, there has been increasing support for the contribution of autoimmune mechanism in the pathogenesis of diabetic neuropathy. Diabetes itself appears to be caused by autoimmune mechanisms directed at insulin-producing pancreatic beta cells, and a variety of autoantibodies have been detected in patients with type 1 diabetes or insulin-dependent diabetes, including anti-islet cell cytoplasmic antibodies, present in up to 80% of newly diagnosed patients,[119] and glutamic acid decarboxylase antibodies, also present in patients with autoimmune stiff person syndrome.[120] Younger and colleagues[121] reported the clinicopathologic and immunohistochemical findings of sural nerve biopsy tissues in a cohort of 20 patients with heterogeneous forms of diabetic neuropathy. That series was continued to 107 patients,[122] of which 3 (3%) showed MV and 3 (3%) showed necrotizing arteritis. Although diabetes has not been considered a predisposing factor in PNV, the presence or absence of diabetes became a defining feature of patients with lumbosacral radiculoplexus neuropathy (LSRPN).[123,124] In the only postmortem case of LSRPN described by Younger,[125] sural nerve biopsy showed mononuclear inflammatory cells surrounding a small epineurial artery with extension into the vascular wall, with reactive luminal connective tissue suggesting recanalization of a thrombus. An adjacent nerve fascicle showed marked loss of myelinated nerve fibers. The patient was treated for painful LSRPN and peripheral nerve vasculitis according to prevailing standards with 2 g/kg intravenous immunoglobulin for 5 days, followed by 750 mg of intravenous cyclophosphamide and 1000 mg of methylprednisolone intravenously for 3 additional days. Acute tubular necrosis, increasing lethargy, unresponsiveness, and aspiration pneumonia supervened, and the patient expired 4 weeks after admission. General autopsy showed no evidence of systemic or peripheral nerve vasculitis. The brain showed diffuse loss of neurons in all sampled cortical areas, including the cerebellum, consistent with anoxia secondary to cardiac arrest. Sections of extradural lumbar plexus, sciatic, and femoral nerve tissue showed perivascular epineurial inflammation with infiltration of adjacent endoneurium. This case exemplifies the restricted nature of LSRPN as an example of a true NSVN.

There have been far more studies of living cohorts with NSPNV. Kissel and colleagues[126] reported that 4.5% of 350 consecutive nerve biopsies performed at a single institution evidenced peripheral neuropathy secondary to necrotizing angiopathy. Six patients manifested a distal symmetric sensorimotor polyneuropathy, while 10 had a mononeuritis multiplex presentation, 8 of whom had overlapping involvement of peripheral nerves that obscured the picture of mononeuritis. In three-quarters (12 patients), a specific underlying collagen vascular disease was not diagnosed despite extensive clinical, radiologic, and serologic evaluation. Said and colleagues[127] studied 100 patients with necrotizing arteritis in muscle or nerve biopsy tissue that occurred in the context of a connective tissue disorder in 55 patients and in association with a disorder unrelated to connective tissue pathologic condition in 13 others. The commonest complaints at presentation in this cohort were specific cutaneous manifestation of vasculitis, including livedo, cutaneous necrosis, and nodules in one-third. Thirty-two patients had neuropathy only and necrotizing arteritis, the most common complaints of which were spontaneous pain of neurogenic or muscle origin (48%).

Collins and colleagues[128] described 48 patients with NSPNV, 85% of whom had extensive, overlapping involvement of multiple nerves. Peroneal nerve and peroneal muscle tissue biopsy was 58% diagnostically sensitive compared with 47% for sural nerve biopsy for the diagnosis of vasculitis. Combination therapy with corticosteroids and cytotoxic agents was more effective than corticosteroids monotherapy for inducing remission and improving disability, with trends toward reduced relapses and chronic pain. Overall, 10 patients died (21%) over the period of 63 months' follow-up, 5 (10%) of whom were related to the disease or treatment, including 2 patients who succumbed to pulmonary emboli as a result of limited mobility of the legs or myocardial infarction in another, and 2 patients, one of whom had fatal sepsis and another had metastatic bladder cancer as a consequence of cyclophosphamide toxicity.

There are no ongoing observational cohort studies to guide the treatment of NPNV. Recommendations for the treatment of NSPNV[115] include prednisone monotherapy unless there is rapidly progressive neuropathy at the dose of 1 mg/kg per day, with tapering over 1 year to a low dose. Combination therapy using cytotoxic drugs, including cyclophosphamide, methotrexate, and azathioprine, may be used with adjuvant plasma exchange or IVIG. The latter appears to be appropriate, first-line therapeutic modality in NSPNV. Moreover, the benefit of IVIG may be achieved without the risk of potentially fatal cytotoxic side effects. However, there has not been a prospective RCT of IVIG in NSPNV. A variety of mechanisms have been thought to be responsible for the beneficial effects of IVIG in NSPNV and other systemic vasculitides, including neutralization of autoantibodies, inhibition of complement pathways, alteration of Fc receptor expression, and alteration of cytokine profiles. Careful monitoring should be performed to observe desired therapeutic responses and to avoid potentially serious drug side effects.

SUMMARY

In no other disorder have there been so many triumphs as in the diagnosis and treatment of primary systemic vasculitis. Physicians in a variety of subspecialties, including neurology, rheumatology, immunology/allergy, dermatology, and clinical pathology, all working side by side, aided by subspecialities of public health, epidemiology, genetics, and clinical trial specialists, have benefited from the outlook for individual patients and population cohorts around the globe. Nevertheless, it starts with clinical acumen typically of the general practitioner. This article on clinical approach was written with such diverse backgrounds in mind, from generalist to subspecialist, with the hope that it will bring the field up to date and to the present.

REFERENCES

1. Jennette JC, Falk RJ, Bacon PA, et al. 2012 revised international chapel hill consensus conference nomenclature of vasculitides. Arthritis Rheum 2013;65: 1–11.
2. Ruperto N, Ozen S, Pistorio A, et al. EULAR/PINTO/PRES criteria for Henoch-Schönlein purpura, childhood polyarteritis nodosa, childhood Wegener granulomatosis and childhood Takayasu arteritis: Ankara 2008. Part I: overall methodology and clinical characterization. Ann Rheum Dis 2010;69:790–7.
3. Ozen S, Pistorio A, Iusan SM, et al. EULAR/PRINTO/PReS criteria for Henoch-Schönlein purpura, childhood polyarteritis nodosa, childhood Wegener granulomatosis and childhood Takayasu arteritis. Ankara 2008. Part II: final classification. Ann Rheum Dis 2010;69:798–806.
4. Jennings GH. Arteritis of the temporal vessels. Lancet 1938;1:424–8.
5. Gilmour JR. Giant-cell chronic arteritis. J Pathol Bacteriol 1941;53:263–77.
6. Nuenninghoff DM, Hunder GG, Christianson TJH, et al. Incidence and predictors of large-artery complication (aortic aneurysm, aortic dissection, and/or large artery stenosis) in patients with giant cell arteritis. Arthritis Rheum 2003; 48:3522–31.
7. Ritama V. Temporal arteritis. Ann Med Intern Fenn 1951;40:63–87.
8. Save-Soderbergh J, Malmvall B, Anderson R, et al. Giant cell arteritis as a cause of death. JAMA 1986;255:493–6.
9. Nakao K, Ikeda M, Kimata S-I, et al. Takayasu's arteritis: clinical report of eighty-four cases and immunologic studies of seven cases. Circulation 1967; 35:1141–55.

10. Shick RM, Baggenstoss AH, Fuller BF, et al. Effects of cortisone and ACTH on periarteritis nodosa and cranial arteritis. Mayo Clin Proc 1950;25:492–4.

11. Aiello PD, Trautmann JC, McPhee TJ, et al. Visual prognosis in giant cell arteritis. Ophthalmology 1993;100:550–5.

12. Ohigashi H, Haraguchi G, Konishi M, et al. Improved prognosis of Takayasu arteritis over the past decade. Circ J 2012;76:1004–11.

13. Longcope WT. Periarteritis nodosa with report of a case with autopsy, vol. 1. Philadelphia: Bull Auyer Clin Lab Pennsylvania Hospital; 1908.

14. Kernohan JW, Woltman HW. Periarteritis nodosa: a clinicopathologic study with special reference to the nervous system. Arch Neurol 1938;39:655–86.

15. Krahulik L, Rosenthal M, Loughlin EH. Periarteritis nodosa (necrotizing panarteritis) in childhood with meningeal involvement. Report of a case with study of pathologic findings. Am J Med Sci 1935;190:308–17.

16. Pagnoux C, Seror R, Henegar C, et al. Clinical features and outcomes in 348 patients with polyarteritis nodosa. Arthritis Rheum 2010;62:616–26.

17. Ozen S, Anton J, Arisoy N, et al. Juvenile polyarteritis: results of a multicenter survey of 110 children. J Pediatr 2004;145:517–22.

18. Guillevin L, Cohen P, Mahr A, et al, the French Vasculitis Study Group. Treatment of polyarteritis nodosa and microscopic polyangiitis with poor prognosis factors: a prospective trial comparing glucocorticoids and six or twelve cyclophosphamide pulses in sixty-five patients. Arthritis Rheum 2003;49:93–100.

19. Guillevin L, Mahr A, Callard P, et al, for the French Vasculitis Study Group. Hepatitis B virus-associated polyarteritis nodosa: clinical characteristics, outcome, and impact of treatment in 115 patients. Medicine 2005;84:313–22.

20. Wohlwill F. Uber die mur mikroskopisch erkenbarre form der periarteritis nodosa. Arch Pathol Anat 1923;246:377–411.

21. Davson J, Ball M, Platt R. The kidney in periarteritis nodosa. QJM 1948;17:175–202.

22. Wainwright J, Davson J. The renal appearance in the microscopic form of periarteritis nodosa. J Pathol Bacteriol 1950;62:189–96.

23. Savage COS, Winearls CG, Evans DJ, et al. Microscopic polyarteritis: presentation, pathology and prognosis. QJM 1985;220:467–83.

24. Guillevin L, Durand-Gasselin B, Cevallos R, et al. Microscopic polyangiitis. Clinical and laboratory findings in eighty-five patients. Arthritis Rheum 1999;42:421–30.

25. Ahn JK, Hwang J-W, Lee J, et al. Clinical features and outcome of microscopic polyangiitis under a new consensus algorithm of ANCA-associated vasculitides in Korea. Rheumatol Int 2012;32:2979–86.

26. Cabral DA, Uribe AG, Benseler S, et al, for the ARChiVe (A Registry for Childhood Vasculitis: e-entry) Investigators Network. Classification, presentation, and initial treatment of Wegener's granulomatosis in childhood. Arthritis Rheum 2009;60:3413–24.

27. Lamb AR. Periarteritis nodosa-a clinical and pathological review of the disease with a report of two cases. Arch Intern Med 1914;14:481–516.

28. Churg J, Strauss L. Allergic granulomatosis, allergic angiitis, and periarteritis nodosa. Am J Pathol 1951;27:277–301.

29. Masi AT, Hunder GG, Lie JT, et al. The American College of Rheumatology 1990 criteria for the classification of Churg-Strauss syndrome (Allergic granulomatosis and angiitis). Arthritis Rheum 1990;33:1094–100.

30. Comarmond C, Pagnoux C, Khellaf M, et al, for the French Vasculitis Study Group. Eosinophilic granulomatosis with polyangiitis (Churg-Strauss). Arthritis Rheum 2013;65:270–81.
31. Jennette JC, Falk RJ, Andrassay K, et al. Nomenclature of systemic vasculitides. Proposal of an international conference. Arthritis Rheum 1994;37:187–92.
32. O'Neil KM. Progress in pediatric vasculitis. Curr Opin Rheumatol 2009;21: 538–46.
33. Godman GC, Churg J. Wegener's granulomatosis: pathology and review of the literature. Arch Pathol 1954;58:533–53.
34. Guillevin L, Visser H, Noel LH, et al. Antineutrophil cytoplasm antibodies in systemic polyarteritis nodosa with and without hepatitis B virus infection and Churg-Strauss syndrome-62 patients. J Rheumatol 1993;20:1345–9.
35. Fauci AS, Haynes BF, Katz P, et al. Wegener's granulomatosis: Prospective clinical and therapeutic experience with 85 patients over 21 years. Ann Intern Med 1983;98:76–85.
36. Hoffman GS, Kerr GS, Leavitt RY, et al. Wegener granulomatosis: an analysis of 158 patients. Ann Intern Med 1992;116:488–98.
37. Carrington CB, Libow AA. Limited forms of angiitis and granulomatosis of Wegener's type. Am J Med 1966;41:497–527.
38. Leavitt RY, Fauci AS, Bloch DA, et al. The American College of Rheumatology 1990 criteria for the classification of Wegener's granulomatosis. Arthritis Rheum 1990;33:1101–7.
39. Holle JU, Csernok E, Fredenhagen G, et al. Clinical evaluation of hsPR3-ANCA ELISA for detection of antineutrophil cytoplasmic antibodies directed against PR3. Ann Rheum Dis 2010;69:468–9.
40. Lionaki S, Blyth ER, Hogan SL, et al. Classification of anti-neutrophil cytoplasmic autoantibody vasculitides: the role of anti-neutrophil cytoplasmic autoantibody specificity for myeloperoxidase or proteinase 3 in disease recognition and prognosis. Arthritis Rheum 2012;64:3452–62.
41. Miloslavsky EM, Specks U, Merkel P, et al. Clinical outcomes of remission induction therapy for severe antineutrophil cytoplasmic antibody-associated vasculitis. Arthritis Rheum 2013;65:2441–9.
42. Morishita KA, Moorthy LN, Lubieniecka JM, et al. Early outcomes in children with antineutrophil cytoplasmic antibody-associated vasculitis. Arthritis Rheum 2017; 69:1470–9.
43. Sacri AS, Chambaraud T, Ranchin B, et al. Clinical characteristics and outcomes of childhood-onset ANCA-associated vasculitis: a French nationwide study. Nephrol Dial Transplant 2015;30(Suppl 1):i104–12.
44. Zeek PM, Smith CC, Weeter JC. Studies on periarteritis nodosa. III. The differentiation between the vascular lesions of periarteritis nodosa and of hypersensitivity. Am J Pathol 1948;24:889–917.
45. Zeek PM. Periarteritis nodosa-a critical review. Am J Clin Pathol 1952;22: 777–90.
46. Zeek PM. Periarteritis nodosa and other forms of necrotizing angiitis. N Engl J Med 1953;248:764–72.
47. Arthus M, Breton M. Lesions cutanées produites par les injections de sérum de cheval chez le lapin anaphylactisé par et pour ce sérum. Compt Rend Soc de Biol 1903;55:1478–80.
48. Gairdner D. The Schönlein-Henoch syndrome (anaphylactoid purpura). QJM 1948;17:95–122.

49. Faille-Kuyber EH, Kater L, Kooiker CJ, et al. IgA-deposits in cutaneous blood-vessel walls and mesangium in Henoch-Schonlein syndrome. Lancet 1973;1: 892–3.
50. Conley ME, Cooper MD, Michael AF. Selective deposition of immunoglobulin A1 in immunoglobulin A nephropathy, anaphylactoid purpura nephritis, and systemic lupus erythematosus. J Clin Invest 1980;66:1432–6.
51. Mills JA, Michel BE, Bloch DA, et al. The American College of Rheumatology 1990 criteria for the classification of Henoch-Schönlein purpura. Arthritis Rheum 1990;33:1114–21.
52. Peru H, Soylemezoglu O, Bakkaloglu SA, et al. Henoch Schonlein purpura in childhood: clinical analysis of 254 cases over a 3-year period. Clin Rheumatol 2008;27:1087–92.
53. McDuffie FC, Sams WM, Maldonado JE, et al. Hypocomplementemia with cutaneous vasculitis and arthritis. Possible immune complex syndrome. Mayo Clin Proc 1973;48:340–8.
54. Zeiss CR, Burch FX, Marder RJ, et al. A hypocomplementemic vasculitic urticarial syndrome: Report of four new cases and definition of the disease. Am J Med 1980;68:867–75.
55. Wisnieski JJ, Naff GB. Serum IgG antibodies to C1q in hypocomplementemic urticarial vasculitis syndrome. Arthritis Rheum 1989;32:1119–27.
56. Buck A, Christensen J, McCarty M. Hypocomplementemic urticarial vasculitis syndrome: a case report and literature review. J Clin Aesthet Dermatol 2012; 5(1):36–46.
57. Behcet H, Matteson EL. On relapsing, aphthous ulcers of the mouth, eye and genitalia caused by a virus. 1937. Clin Exp Rheumatol 2010;28(Suppl 60):S2–5.
58. Wolf SM, Schotland DL, Phillips LL. Involvement of nervous system in Behçet's syndrome. Arch Neurol 1965;12:315–25.
59. Criteria for diagnosis of Behçet's disease. International Study Group for Behçet's Disease. Lancet 1990;335:1078–80.
60. Özen S. Pediatric onset Behcet disease. Curr Opin Rheumatol 2010;22:585–9.
61. Matsumoto T, Uekusa T, Fukuda Y. Vasculo-Behcet's disease: a pathologic study of eight cases. Hum Pathol 1991;22:45–51.
62. Mogan RF, Baumgarten CJ. Meniere's disease complicated by recurrent interstitial keratitis: excellent results following cervical ganglionectomy. West J Surg 1934;42:628.
63. Cogan DG. Syndrome of nonsyphilitic interstitial keratitis and vestibuloauditory symptoms. Arch Ophthal 1945;33:144–9.
64. Haynes BF, Kaiser-Kupfer MI, Mason P, et al. Cogan's syndrome: Studies in thirteen patients, long-term follow-up, and a review of the literature. Medicine 1980; 59:426–41.
65. Wintrobe MM, Buell MV. Hyperproteinemia associated with multiple myeloma. With report of a case in which an extraordinary hyperproteinemia was associated with thrombosis of the retinal veins and symptoms suggesting Raynauds disease. Bull Johns Hopkins Hosp 1933;52:156–65.
66. Brouet JC, Clauvel JP, Danon F, et al. Biologic and clinical significance of cryoglobulins: a report of 86 cases. Am J Med 1974;57:775–88.
67. Terrier B, Krastinova E, Marie I, et al. Management of noninfectious mixed cryoglobulinemia vasculitis: data from 242 cases included in the CryoVas survey. Blood 2012;119:5996–6004.
68. Cacoub P, Poynard T, Ghillani P, et al, for the MULTIVIRC Group. Extrahepatic manifestations of chronic hepatitis C. Arthritis Rheum 1999;42:2204–12.

69. Liou Y-T, Huang J-L, Ou L-S, et al. Comparison of cryoglobulinemia in children and adults. J Microbiol Immunol Infect 2013;46:59–64.
70. Terrier B, Cacoub P. Cryoglobulinemia vasculitis: an update. Curr Opin Rheumatol 2013;25:10–8.
71. Klemperer P. Diseases of the collagen system. Bull N Y Acad Med 1947;23: 581–8.
72. Klemperer P. The pathogenesis of lupus erythematosus and allied conditions. Ann Intern Med 1948;28:1–11.
73. Tan EM, Cohen AS, Fries JF, et al. The 1982 revised criteria for classification of systemic lupus erythematosus. Arthritis Rheum 1982;25:1271–7.
74. Johnson RT, Richardswon EP. The neurological manifestations of systemic lupus erythematosus. Medicine 1968;47:337–69.
75. Devinsky O, Petito CK, Alonso DR. Clinical and Neuropathological findings in systemic lupus erythematosus: the role of vasculitis, heart emboli, and thrombotic thrombocytopenic purpura. Ann Neurol 1988;23:380–4.
76. Feinglass EJ, Arnett FC, Dorsch CA, et al. Neuropsychiatric manifestations of systemic lupus erythematosus: diagnosis, clinical spectrum, and relationship to other features of the disease. Medicine 1976;55:323–39.
77. Mintz G, Fraga A. Arteritis in systemic lupus erythematosus. Arch Intern Med 1965;116:55–66.
78. Trevor RP, Sondheimer FK, Fessel WJ, et al. Angiographic demonstration of major cerebral vessel occlusion in systemic lupus erythematosus. Neuroradiology 1972;4:202–7.
79. Younger DS, Sacco R, Levine SR, et al. Major cerebral vessel occlusion in SLE due to circulating anticardiolipin antibodies. Stroke 1994;25:912–4.
80. Turesson C. Extra-articular rheumatoid arthritis. Curr Opin Rheumatol 2013;25: 360–6.
81. Turesson C, Jacobsson LT. Epidemiology of extra-articular manifestations in rheumatoid arthritis. Scand J Rheumatol 2004;33:65–72.
82. Scott DG, Bacon PA. Intravenous cyclophosphamide plus methylprednisolone in treatment of systemic rheumatoid vasculitis. Am J Med 1984;76:377–84.
83. Vollerstein RS, Conn DL, Ballard DJ, et al. Rheumatoid vasculitis: survival and risk factors. Medicine 1986;65:365–75.
84. Puéchal X, Said G, Hilliquin P, et al. Peripheral neuropathy with necrotizing vasculitis in rheumatoid arthritis. Arthritis Rheum 1995;38:1618–29.
85. Ramos M, Mandybur TI. Cerebral vasculitis in rheumatoid arthritis. Arch Neurol 1975;32:271–5.
86. Steiner JW, Gelbloom AJ. Intracranial manifestations in two cases of systemic rheumatoid disease. Arthritis Rheum 1959;2:537–45.
87. Kemper JW, Baggenstoss AH, Slocumb CH. The relationship of therapy with cortisone to the incidence of vascular lesions in rheumatoid arthritis. Ann Intern Med 1957;46:831–51.
88. Sokoloff L, Bunim JJ. Vascular lesions in rheumatoid arthritis. J Chronic Dis 1957;5:668–87.
89. Johnson RL, Smyth CJ, Holt GW, et al. Steroid therapy and vascular lesions in rheumatoid arthritis. Arthritis Rheum 1959;2:224–49.
90. Watson P, Fekete J, Deck J. Central nervous system vasculitis in rheumatoid arthritis. Can J Neurol Sci 1977;4:269–72.
91. Puéchal X, Gottenberg JE, Berthelot JM, et al. Rituximab therapy for systemic vasculitis associated with rheumatoid arthritis: Results from the Autoimmunity and Rituximab Registry. Arthritis Care Res 2012;64:331–9.

92. Bartolucci P, Ramanoelina J, Cohen P, et al. Efficacy of the anti-TNFαantibody infliximab against refractory systemic vasculitides: an open pilot stud on 10 patients. Rheumatology 2002;41:1126–32.

93. Puéchal X, Miceli-Richard C, Mejjad O, et al. Anti-tumor necrosis factor treatment in patients with refractory systemic vasculitis associated with rheumatoid arthritis. Ann Rheum Dis 2008;67:880–4.

94. Calabrese HL, Mallek JA. Primary angiitis of the central nervous system: report of 8 new cases, review of the literature, and proposal for diagnostic criteria. Medicine 1988;67:20–39.

95. Cupps TR, Moore PM, Fauci AS. Isolated angiitis of the central nervous system. Prospsective diagnostic and therapeutic experience. Am J Med 1983;74:97–105.

96. Younger DS, Hays AP, Brust JCM, et al. Granulomatous angiitis of the brain. An inflammatory reaction of diverse etiology. Arch Neurol 1988;45:514–8.

97. Younger DS, Calabrese LH, Hays AP. Granulomatous angiitis of the nervous system. Neurol Clin 1997;15:821–34.

98. Salvarani C, Brown RD Jr, Christianson TJH, et al. Adult primary central nervous system vasculitis: treatment and course. Arthritis Rheum 2015;67:1637–45.

99. De Boysson H, Arquizan C, Touze E, et al. Treatment and long-term outcomes of primary central nervous system vasculitis. Stroke 2018;49:1946–52.

100. Twilt M, Benseler SM. Central nervous system vasculitis in adults and children. Handb Clin Neurol 2016;133:283–300.

101. Benseler SM, deVeber G, Hawkins C, et al. Angiography-negative primary central nervous system vasculitis in children: a newly recognized inflammatory central nervous system disease. Arthritis Rheum 2005;52:2159–67.

102. Twilt M, Benseler SM. Childhood inflammatory brain diseases: pathogenesis, diagnosis and therapy. Rheumatology (Oxford) 2014;53:1359–68.

103. Walker DI, Bloor K, Williams G, et al. Inflammatory aneurysms of the abdominal aorta. Br J Surg 1972;59:609–14.

104. Rojo-Leyva F, Ratliff NB, Cosgrove DM, et al. Study of 52 patients with idiopathic aortitis from a cohort of 1,204 surgical cases. Arthritis Rheum 2000;43:901–7.

105. Hamamo H, Kawa S, Horiuchi A, et al. High serum IgG4 concentrations in patients with sclerosing pancreatitis. N Engl J Med 2001;344:732–8.

106. Hamano H, Kawa S, Ochi Y, et al. Hydronephrosis associated with retroperitoneal fibrosis and sclerosing pancreatitis. Lancet 2002;359:1403–4.

107. Sakata N, Tashiro T, Uesugi N, et al. IgG4-positive plasma cells in inflammatory abdominal aortic aneurysm: The possibility of an aortic manifestation of IgG4-related sclerosing disease. Am J Surg Pathol 2008;32:553–9.

108. Kasashima S, Zen Y, Kawashima A, et al. Inflammatory abdominal aortic aneurysm: close relationship to IgG4-releated periaortitis. Am J Surg Pathol 2008;32:197–204.

109. Ito H, Kalzaki Y, Noda Y, et al. IgG4-related inflammatory abdominal aortic aneurysm associated with autoimmune pancreatitis. Pathol Int 2008;58:421–6.

110. Khosroshahi A, Stone JR, Pratt DS, et al. Painless jaundice with serial multiorgan dysfunction. Lancet 2009;373:1494.

111. Stone JH, Khosroshahi A, Hilgenberg A, et al. IgG4-related systemic disease and lymphoplasmacytic aortitis. Arthritis Rheum 2009;60:3139–45.

112. Deshpande V, Zen Y, Chan JKC, et al. Consensus statement on the pathology of IgG4-related disease. Mod Pathol 2012;25:1181–92.

113. Kamisawa T, Okazaki K, Kawa S, et al. Japanese consensus guidelines for management of autoimmune pancreatitis: III. Treatment and prognosis of AIP. J Gastroenterol 2010;45:471–7.
114. Stone JH, Zeri Y, Deshpande V. IgG-4 related disease. N Engl J Med 2012;366:539–51.
115. Collins MP, Dyck PJ, Gronseth GS, et al. Peripheral Nerve Society Guideline on the classification, diagnosis, investigation, and immunsuppressive therapy of non-systemic vasculitis neuropathy: executive summary. J Peripher Nerv Syst 2010;15:176–84.
116. Hadden RDM, Collins MP, Zivkovic SA, et al, the Brighton Collaboration Vasculitic Peripheral Neuropathy Working Group. Vasculitic peripheral neuropathy: case definition for collection analysis, and presentation of immunization safety data. Vaccine 2017;35:1567–78.
117. Dyck PJ, Benstead TJ, Conn DL, et al. Nonsystemic vasculitic neuropathy. Brain 1987;110:843–53.
118. Torvik A, Berntzen AE. Necrotizing vasculitis without visceral involvement. Postmortem examination of three cases with affection of skeletal muscles and peripheral nerves. Acta Med Scand 1968;184:69–77.
119. Atkinson MA, Caclaren NK. The pathogenesis of insulin-dependent diabetes mellitus. N Engl J Med 1994;331:1428–36.
120. Grimaldi LME, Mertini G, Braghi S, et al. Heterogeneity of autoantibodies in stiff-man syndrome. Ann Neurol 1993;34:57–64.
121. Younger DS, Rosoklija G, Hays AP, et al. Diabetic peripheral neuropathy: a clinicopathologic and immunohistochemical analysis of sural nerve biopsies. Muscle Nerve 1996;19:722–7.
122. Younger DS. Diabetic neuropathy: a clinical and neuropathological study of 107 patients. Neurol Res Int 2010;2010:140379.
123. Dyck PJ, Norell JE, Dyck PJ. Non-diabetic lumbosacral radiculoplexus neuropathy: natural history, outcome and comparison with the diabetic variety. Brain 2001;124:1197–207.
124. Dyck PJB, Windebank AJ. Diabetic and nondiabetic lumbosacral radiculoplexus neuropathies: new insights into pathophysiology and treatment. Muscle Nerve 2002;25:477–91.
125. Younger DS. Diabetic lumbosacral radiculoplexus neuropathy: a postmortem studied patient and review of the literature. J Neurol 2011;258:1364–7.
126. Kissel JT, Slivka AP, Warmolts JR, et al. The clinical spectrum of necrotizing angiopathy of the peripheral nervous system. Ann Neurol 1985;18:251–7.
127. Said G, Lacroix-Ciaudo C, Fujimura H, et al. The peripheral neuropathy of necrotizing arteritis: a clinicopathologic study. Ann Neurol 1988;23:461–5.
128. Collins MP, Periquet MI, Mendell JR, et al. Nonsystemic vasculitis neuropathy. Insights from a clinical cohort. Neurology 2003;61:623–30.

Epidemiology of the Vasculitides

David S. Younger, MD, MPH, MS[a,b,*]

KEYWORDS

- Epidemiology primary • Secondary • Vasculitis • Autoimmune • Nervous system

KEY POINTS

- The epidemiology of vasculitis has witnessed extraordinary advances in the past decade.
- These advances have been influenced by the worldwide increased recognition and accurate classification and diagnosis of the vasculitides, and insights brought by genome-wide association studies and online genetic biological repositories that allow researchers to freely access a wide array of genetic and clinical resources.
- The result is improved understanding of the heritable factors of the systemic vasculitides.
- This article reviews the current knowledge of the epidemiology of vasculitides in different global regions.

INTRODUCTION

The publication of recent genome-wide association studies (GWAS) has brought awareness to the understanding of susceptibility factors designated genetic risk loci for many of the vasculitides, supporting the interplay of immunologic, environmental, and shared genetic susceptibility in the etiopathogenesis of vasculitic disorders, With an incidence and prevalence of primary systemic vasculitis that is steadily increasing and an impact that is being reported worldwide in developed countries, government and nongovernmental organizations, and other key stakeholders have not developed sufficient programs for the prevention and surveillance of these disorders. This article focuses on the epidemiology of the major large-vessel, medium-vessel, and small-vessel vasculitides shown in **Box 1**. A review of the epidemiology and classification of primary systemic vasculitides was published earlier.[1]

Disclosure Statement: The author has nothing to disclose.
[a] Department of Neurology, Division of Neuro-Epidemiology, New York University School of Medicine, New York, NY 10016, USA; [b] School of Public Health, City University of New York, New York, NY, USA
* 333 East 34th Street, Suite 1J, New York, NY 10016.
E-mail address: youngd01@nyu.edu
Website: http://www.davidsyounger.com

Neurol Clin 37 (2019) 201–217
https://doi.org/10.1016/j.ncl.2019.01.016
0733-8619/19/© 2019 Elsevier Inc. All rights reserved.

> **Box 1**
> **Classification of primary systemic vasculitides**
>
> *Large-Vessel Vasculitis*
>
> Giant cell arteritis (formerly temporal arteritis) (GCA)
>
> Takayasu arteritis (TAK)
>
> *Medium-Vessel Vasculitis*
>
> Kawasaki disease (KD)
>
> Polyarteritis nodosa (PAN)
>
> *Small-Vessel Vasculitis*
>
> Antineutrophil cytoplasmic antibody (ANCA)-associated vasculitis (AAV)
>
> Granulomatosis with polyangiitis (formerly Wegener granulomatosis) (GPA)
>
> Microscopic polyangiitis (formerly microscopic polyarteritis) (MPA)
>
> Eosinophilic granulomatosis with polyangiitis (formerly Churg-Strauss syndrome) (EGPA)

LARGE-SIZE VESSEL VASCULITIS
Giant Cell Arteritis

Background

Giant cell arteritis (GCA) is a chronic granulomatous vasculitis of large and medium-sized vessels that frequently affected the thoracic aorta and its branches, with a mean age of diagnosis of age 76 years and a male-to-female ratio of 1.5:1.[2] Both GCA and polymyalgia rheumatica (PMR), a related disorder, are probably polygenic diseases in which multiple environmental and genetic factors influence susceptibility and severity.[3] For both the purpose of epidemiologic studies and in clinical practice, GCA has been classified according to the 1990 American College of Rheumatology (ACR) criteria[4] and designed to discriminate between different types of vasculitides. The 5 discriminatory features include age older than 50 years at onset, new onset of localized headache, temporal artery tenderness or decreased temporal artery pulse, erythrocyte sedimentation rate greater than 50 mm/h, and biopsy of an artery showing necrotizing arteritis characterized by a predominance of mononuclear cells or a granulomatous process with multinucleated giant cells. Unrecognized and untreated or inadequately treated, there is a high likelihood of large-artery complications including increased morbidity and mortality,[5] especially as a result of aortic aneurysm and dissection and large-artery stenosis.

Epidemiology

The epidemiology of GCA was reviewed by Gonzalez-Gay and colleagues.[6] Since 2000, relatively large cohort studies exemplifying the epidemiologic aspects of GCA in different regions of the world have been reported from Australia,[7,8] Germany,[9] Israel,[10] Japan,[11] New Zealand,[12] Norway,[13,14] Spain,[15,16] Sweden,[17] the United Kingdom (UK),[18] and the United States (USA).[19] Smaller nonepidemiologic case series of patients with GCA have been reported from Brazil,[20] Saudi Arabia,[21] Mexico,[22] and Japan[11] where the incidence is very low, especially in Japan where a nationwide survey of GCA demonstrated a correspondingly low prevalence of 1.47 cases per 100,000 population. The global incidence and prevalence of GCA is summarized in **Table 1**.

Table 1
Global incidence and prevalence of GCA

Authors,[Ref.] Year	Country	Study Period	Incidence per 10^6	Prevalence per 10^6
Kobayashi et al,[11] 2003	Japan	1997	1.47	—
Herlyn et al,[9] 2004	Germany	2006	2.71	171
Dunstan et al.[7] 2014	Australia	1992–2011	3.20	—
Bas-Lando et al,[10] 2007	Israel	1980–2004	9.50	—
Gonzalez-Gay et al,[15] 2005; Gonzalez-Gay et al,[16] 2007	Spain	1981–2005	10.13	—
Mohammad et al,[17] 2014	Sweden	1997–2010	13.3	—
Salvarani et al,[19] 2004	USA	1950–1999	18.8	—
Smeeth et al,[18] 2006	UK	1990–2001	22.0	—
Haugeberg et al,[13] 2003; Haugeberg et al,[14] 2000	Norway Norway Norway	1992–1996 1992–1996 1992–1996	27.50 36.70 32.8	— — —

The highest known incidence of GCA was reported by Haugeberg and colleagues,[13,14] without major differences between northern and western Norway compared with southern Norway. By comparison, very low incidence rates of GCA were found in Saudi Arabian,[21] Mexican,[22] and Japanese populations.[11] Dustan and colleagues[7] found evidence of seasonal variation in the incidence of GCA in Australian Bureau of Statistics population data for South Australia, noting higher rates in the summer months ($P<.015$). Abdul-Rahman and coworkers[12] noted a cyclic annual incidence with peaks in 5 years between 1996 and 2005, and a statistically insignificant ($P<.9$) but suggestive seasonal variation nonetheless, with more cases diagnosed in the spring than in summer, fall, and winter. Bas-Lando and coworkers[10] noted more common onset of GCA in the late spring and early summer, with fluctuation in the annual incidence that included 3 distinctive peaks during the 25-year period of observation among 170 patients in Jerusalem between 1980 and 2014. Ninan and coworkers[8] noted that the relative survival for different follow-up periods in South Australian patients with GCA linked to birth, death, and marriage registry records showed mortality similar to that of the general population of age-matched and sex-matched controls. According to Herlyn and colleagues,[9] who studied inhabitants of the city of Luebeck and the rural region of Segeberg in northern Germany, GCA was the most prevalent systemic vasculitis in 2006, with 171 per million inhabitants, followed by granulomatosis with polyangiitis (GPA) with a prevalence rate of 98 per million inhabitants. The prevalence rate of GCA doubled in northern Germany for those aged 50 years or older from 240 to 440 per million inhabitants between 1994 and 2006, and from 87 to 171 per million population overall. There was a difference in both period prevalence and incidence rates between the urban and rural areas, with an incidence of GCA of 27.1 per million inhabitants per year in urban Luebeck compared with 14.7 per million inhabitants per year in rural Segeberg ($P = .2$), while respective prevalence rates were 237 and 116 per million population overall and 586 and 311 per million inhabitants of age 50 years or older.

Differences in incidence between regional populations of the world may be explained in part by immunogenetic and environmental factors that account for differences in susceptibility and may contribute to severity and outcome.[23] In 1980, Kemp and coworkers[24] performed human leukocyte antigen (HLA) tissue-type antigen determinations for the A, B, and C antigens in the sera of 88 mixed cases of clinical GCA and PMR with an overwhelming representation of women and only sporadic familial occurrence, demonstrating no significant deviation from a sample compared with 3164 blood donor controls. In 1983, Armstrong and colleagues[25] studied 55 patients with GCA and PMR, typed for HLA A, B, C, and DR loci, noting a significantly increased frequency of DR4, Cw3, and Cw6, with the increase in Cw3 possibly attributed to linkage disequilibrium to DR4. Among 128 DNA samples for 128 patients and 145 ethnically matched controls in a case-control association study to determine whether patients with GCA and PMR from a sample in Lugo, northwestern Spain, showed identical HLA class II associations, Dababneh and colleagues[26] found that the association of HLA-DRB 1*0401 and GCA reached statistical significance in the total GCA group of patients, but less so for DRG1*0101 and *0102. An association was also observed between the RA DRB1 shared epitope (SE) and GCA that was primarily accounted for by the presence of a single copy of the SE; moreover, an SE-bearing allele of DRB1 was observed in patients with jaw claudication and visual manifestations. The genetic susceptibility to GCA was supported by reports of the contribution of shared HLA class II gene polymorphisms in mannose-binding lectin variant alleles by Jacobsen and coworkers[27]; in DR4 by Jacobson,[27–29] Richardson,[30] and Barrier and colleagues[31]; in DR3 by Lowenstein and colleagues[32]; in DRB1 by Martinez-Taboda,[33] Weyand,[34,35] and Gonzalez-Gay and colleagues,[36] in Cw3 by Hansen and colleagues[37]; and in major histocompatibility complex (MHC) class I MICA and HLA-B gene polymorphisms by Gonzalez-Gay and coworkers.[38]

Takayasu Disease

Background

In contrast to GCA, Takayasu arteritis (TAK) occurs in individuals younger than age 40 years and presents with large vessel-sized vasculitis of the aorta and its branches. For the purpose of epidemiologic studies, the case definition has generally followed the ACR 1990 criteria for the classification of TAK.[39] The evolution and characterization of pediatric-specific vasculitis classification criteria and the associated clinical syndromes have been reviewed.[40,41] An understanding of the inflammatory lesions in TAK, like that of GCA, has been advanced by immunologic studies, revealing a clearer understanding of the pathophysiology, which may be affected by the genetic background of different global regions. The inflammatory cell infiltrate in aortic tissue specimens of affected patients is composed of neutrophils, macrophages, CD4$^+$ and CD8$^+$ T-cells, natural killer (NK) cells, and macrophages. Infiltrating $\alpha\delta$T cells and NK cells seems to facilitate endothelial cell apoptosis through production of perforin and killer cell lectin-like receptor subfamily K (NKG2D). The latter activating C-type lectin family receptor triggers NK cells and costimulates CD8$^+$ α/β T-cell receptor$^+$ T-cells, while CD4$^+$ T helper 1 (Th1) cells that secrete interferon-γ promote giant cell and granulomatous lesion formation.[42–45] Peripheral T-cells, notably Th1 and Th17, contribute to the pathophysiology of GCA and TAK[46,47] as do MHC I and II molecules and endothelial intracellular adhesion molecules, expressed in tissue lesions of the aorta with TAK.[42,48]

Epidemiology

Two GWAS conducted in TAK, respectively identifying 379 UK cases and 1985 controls[49] and 451 USA/Turkish cases and 1115 controls,[50] noted strong associations with IL12B located at the 5q33.3 chromosome locus (rs6871626), and susceptibility to the Max-like protein X (MAX) gene transcription factor-like 4 positioned at the

17q21.2 chromosome locus (rs665268),[49] whereas those in the UK alone[49] exhibited independent associations at the 6p21.32 chromosome locus in *HLA-DQB1/HLA-DRB1* (rs113452171; rs189754752). *HLA-DQB1* specifies the autoimmune response against insulin-producing islet cells that leads to insulin-dependent diabetes mellitus, while the function of *HLA-DRB1* is to present processed foreign antigens to T cells. The USA/Turkish group reported another susceptibility locus at the Fc fragment of immunoglobulin G (IgG) low-affinity IIa and IIIa receptors (*FCGR2A/3A*) at the 1q23.3 chromosome locus (rs10919543), leading to increased mRNA expression of *FCGR2A* and proteasome-assembling chaperone 1 (*PSMG1*). With receptors present on monocytes, macrophages, neutrophils, NK cells, and T and B lymphocytes, *FCGR2A/3A* play an essential role in the protection of the organism against foreign antigens by removing antigen-antibody complexes from the circulation, and participate in diverse functions such as phagocytosis of immune complexes and modulation of antibody production by B cells. Located at the 21q22.2 chromosome locus, *PSMG1* is involved in the maturation of the mammalian 20S proteasomes with a yet clear implication for TAK.

The global incidence and prevalence of TAK is summarized in **Table 2**. Watts and colleagues[51] using the primary care UK General Practice Research Database and the secondary care-based Norfolk Vasculitis Register from 2000 to 2005, applied the ACR 1990 criteria for incident cases[39], covering a population of 445,000. The authors identified 16 cases with a first diagnosis of TAK and an annual incidence of 0.8 per million, and calculated as the number of incident cases divided by the total person-years, which remained stable throughout the study period. The annual prevalence of TAK was 4.7 per million, with an increase during the course of the study period from 3.6 to 6.3 per million. Mohammad and Mandl[52] studied 3 health care districts of southern Sweden with a total population of 983,419 as of 2011 to identify incident cases of TAK among 5 hospitals in the study area and in all private rheumatology clinics between 1997 and 2011, noting 13 cases that fulfilled the ACR 1990 criteria for TAK.[39] Among them, 8 were of Swedish ancestry, 1 of Asian, 2 of Arab, 1 of African, and 1 of northern European descent. The annual incidence rate was estimated at 0.8 per million for the whole population. The point prevalence of TAK as of June 2012 was estimated at 13.2 per million for the whole population. The incidence findings were comparable with the reported incidence of 0.8, 0.5, and 0.4 per million, respectively, in previous studies from Sweden,[53] Germany,[54] and eastern Denmark,[55] although the prevalence of TAK was somewhat higher than the prevalence of 6.4 per million previously reported in Sweden.[53]

MEDIUM-SIZE VESSEL VASCULITIS
Polyarteritis Nodosa

The ACR 1990[56] and the Chapel Hill Consensus Conference (CHCC)[57] criteria for polyarteritis nodosa (PAN) have been used for the case definitions of most epidemiologic

Table 2
Global incidence and prevalence of TAK

Authors,[Ref.] Year	Country	Study Period	Incidence per 10^6	Prevalence per 10^6
Watts et al,[51] 2009	UK	2000–2005	0.8	4.7
Mohammad and Mandl,[52] 2013	Sweden	1997–2011	0.8	—
Waern et al,[53] 1983	Sweden	1969–1976	0.8	6.4
Reinhold-Keller et al,[54] 2005	Germany	1998–2000	0.5	—
Dreyer et al,[55] 2011	Demark	1990–2009	0.4	—

studies, as well as the criteria of other investigators[58,59] for adult cases, and the criteria of the Turkish Pediatric Vasculitis Study Group[60,61] for pediatric cases, stratified into cutaneous and classic PAN. This author was unable to find any GWAS for PAN.

The global incidence and prevalence of PAN is shown in **Table 3**. Mahr and colleagues[59] defined PAN as a predominantly medium-size-vessel disease that occurs alone or in association with hepatitis B virus (HBV) infection. These investigators angiographically documented aneurysms or histologic proof of vessel inflammation, without glomerulonephritis, lung hemorrhage, or Antineutrophil cytoplasmic antibody (ANCA) positivity, in a capture-recapture study in the calendar year 2000 in Seine-St Denis, a northeastern suburb of Paris with a population of 1,093,515 adults, 28% of whom were of non-European ancestry, from among general practitioners, departments of all of the public hospitals, 2 large private clinics, and the National Health Insurance System. The prevalence of PAN was estimated at 30.7 per million adults. However, previous studies based on the most restrictive and biopsy-dependent CHCC[57] criteria estimated PAN to be 9 per million adults, in comparison with 33 per million based on the less specific ACR criteria[56] that fail to discriminate between microscopic polyangiitis (MPA) and PAN. The total prevalence estimate for all disorders was 90.3 per million which, substratified for geographic origin, showed a 2-fold higher incidence rate for subjects of European than non-European ancestry, respectively, 104.7 compared with 52.5 per million. Not more than 30% of the PAN cases seemed to be HBV related, with most diagnosed during the 1980s, suggesting that the reported incidence of HBV-associated PAN of 77 per million noted in a small population of Alaskan Eskimos with high rates of HBV infection[62] was currently decreasing as a consequence of vaccination campaigns and the improved safety of blood products. Mohammad and colleagues[63] studied incident cases of PAN, GPA, MPA, and eosinophilic granulomatosis with polyangiitis (EGPA) in 2 health care districts of South Sweden (central and southwest Skåne) containing 14 municipalities with a population of 641,763 for the period 1997 to 2006 from hospital databases, identifying 144 cases of primary systemic vasculitis, of which 6 were PAN. The annual incidence rate was 21.8 per million for all patients and 0.9 per million for PAN. Watts and colleagues[64] studied incident cases of PAN, GPA, MPA, and EGPA in 2 regions of Europe, among general medical practices of the Norwich Health Authority (NHA) in Norfolk, UK covering 413,500 patients, and in the referral center of Lugo, Spain at the Hospital Xeral-Calde with a population of 250,000 people between 1988 and 1998. The study used the 2012 revised CHCC[57] and ACR criteria,[56] noting an overall incidence

Table 3
Global incidence and prevalence of PAN

Authors,[Ref.] Year	Country	Study Period	Incidence per 10^6	Prevalence per 10^6
Jennette et al,[57] 2013	USA	2012	—	30.7
Lightfoot et al,[56] 1990	USA	1990	—	9.0
Mohammad et al,[63] 2009	Sweden	1997–2006	0.9	—
Watts et al,[64] 2001	UK[a]	1988–1998	9.7	—
	Spain[b]	1988–1998	6.2	—
Omerod and Cook,[65] 2008	UK[a] + Spain[b]	1995–1999	2.3	—
	UK[a] + Spain[b]	2000–2004	1.1	—

[a] Norwich.
[b] Lugo.

of primary systemic vasculitis of 18.9 in Norwich compared with 18.3 per million in Spain, with a higher incidence of PAN in Norwich than in Spain, 9.7 versus 6.2 per million, respectively. Omerod and Cook[65] studied the prevalence and incidence of primary systemic vasculitides for the two 5-year periods of 1995 to 1999 and 2000 to 2004 in the Australian Capital Territory and the surrounding rural regions. Altogether, 41 cases of primary systemic vasculitides including PAN, GPA, MPA, and EGPA were identified between 1995 and 1999, and 67 between 2000 and 2004. This yielded a prevalence of 95 and 148 per million, with a similar annual incidence of 17 per million for Norwich, UK and Lugo, Spain; and a disease-specific incidence for PAN of 2.2 and 1.1 for the 2 successive periods.

Kawasaki Disease

Kawasaki disease (KD), or mucocutaneous lymph node syndrome, is an acute, self-limited systemic vasculitis of medium- and small-size vessels occurring predominantly in children aged 6 months to 5 years.[66] It is the second commonest childhood vasculitis and the leading cause of acquired childhood heart disease in developed countries.[67,68] The distribution is worldwide, with an incidence in Japanese populations 10-fold to 15-fold greater than in Caucasians.[69] Before revision of the criteria for KD, the classification was based on either Japanese[70] or the American Heart Association (AHA) classification.[71] The former criteria, applied in Japanese epidemiologic studies of KD, required the presence of 5 of the following 6 criteria: characteristic fever, bilateral conjunctivitis, changes in lips and oral cavity, polymorphous exanthema, changes of peripheral extremities, and cervical lymphadenopathy, whereas those of the latter, used in American and Caucasian studies, generally required fever plus 4 of the remaining 5 criteria. Two recent modifications to the criteria for KD made by the European League Against Rheumatism/Pediatric Rheumatology European Society consensus criteria conference,[61] which may alter the carriage of epidemiologic studies in the future, included the addition of perineal desquamation describing changes in the extremities; moreover, fewer than 4 of the remaining 5 criteria were deemed necessary in the presence of fever and coronary arterial involvement demonstrated by echocardiography. To emphasize pediatric vasculitis disease even before retrospective and prospective epidemiologic studies, a half-century of 1,335,045 postmortem examinations from the Annual of Pathologic Autopsy Cases in Japan from 1958 to 2008 identified 380 cases of vasculitis in children, more than one-half of which were KD and other disease entities including unclassified vasculitis, PAN, purpuric vasculitis, TAK, and others. Moreover, the postmortem findings for 24 of 125 childhood vasculitides performed before 1976 and diagnosed as non-KD were later consistent with KD.

The global incidence and prevalence of KD is shown in **Table 4**. Saundankar and colleagues[72] identified hospitalized patients in Western Australia with the diagnosis of KD, noting a steady increase in the mean annual incidence from 7.96 between 1990 and 1999 to 9.34 per 100,000 children younger than 5 years between 2000 and 2009, with the peak incidence of 15.7 per 100,000 in 2005. Lin and colleagues[73] identified hospitalized discharges with the diagnosis of KD in Ontario, noting a mean annual incidence of 26.2 per 100,000 for children younger than 5 years, 6.7 per 100,000 for 5- to 9-year old children, and 0.9 per 100,000 for those 10 to 14 years old, which steadily increased from 14.39 to 26.24 per 100,000 from 1995 to 2006. Ma and colleagues[74] studied all children sent to 1 of 50 hospitals in Shanghai, noting a mean annual incidence of 46.32 per 100,000 children younger than 5 years that steadily increased from 36.78 to 53.28 between 2003 and 2007. Li and coworkers[75] identified cases of KD in children younger than 5 years in 212 hospitals in Sichuan

Table 4
Global incidence and prevalence of KD

Authors,[Ref.] Year	Country	Study Period	Incidence per 10^6	Prevalence per 10^6
Saundankar et al,[72] 2014	Australia	1990–1999	7.96	—
	Australia	2000–2009	9.34	—
	Australia	2005	15.7	—
Lin et al,[73] 2010	Canada[a]	1995–2006	26.2[b]	—
	Canada[a]	1995–2006	6.8[c]	—
	Canada[a]	1995	14.39[d]	—
	Canada[a]	2006	26.24[d]	—
Ma et al,[74] 2010	China[e]	2003–2007	46.32[b]	—
	China[e]	2003	36.78[b]	—
	China[e]	2007	53.28[b]	—
Li et al,[75] 2008	China[f]	1997–2001	7.06[b]	—
	China[f]	1997	8.57[b]	—
	China[f]	2001	9.81[b]	—
Du et al,[76] 2007	China[g]	2000–2004	49.4[b]	—
	China[g]	2000	40.9[b]	—
	China[g]	2004	55.1[b]	—
Fischer et al,[77] 2007	Denmark	1981–2004	4.5–5.0	—
Holman et al,[78] 2010	Hawaii, USA	1996–2006	50.4	—
Ng et al,[79] 2011	Hong Kong	1994–1997	26.0	—
	Hong Kong	1994–1997	39.0	—
Singh et al,[80] 2011	North India	1994	0.51	—
	North India	2007	4.5	—
Nakamura et al,[81] 2012	Japan	2009	206.2	—
	Japan	2010	239.6	—
Park et al,[82] 2011	Korea	2006–2008	113.1	—
	Korea	2006	108.7	—
	Korea	2008	113.1	—
Schiller et al,[83] 1995	Sweden	1990–1992	2.9	—
	Sweden	1990–1992	6.2[b]	—
Lue et al,[84] 2013	Taiwan	2006	66.24[b]	—
Huang et al,[85] 2009	Taiwan	2003–2006	153.0	—
	Taiwan	2003–2006	69.0[b]	—
Harnden et al,[86] 2002	UK	1991	4.8	—
	UK	2000	9.2	—
Holman et al,[87] 2010	USA	2006	20.8	—

[a] Ontario.
[b] Age less than 5 years.
[c] Age 5 to 9 years.
[d] Age 10 to 14 years.
[e] Shanghai.
[f] Sichuan Provence.
[g] Beijing.

Province, noting a steady increase in the incidence from 8.57 to 9.81 per 100,000, with an average incidence throughout the latest 5 years of 7.06 per 100,000. Du and co-workers[76] conducted a hospital-based survey of KD in 45 Beijing hospitals, identifying 1107 KD patients with a mean annual incidence of 49.4 per 100,000 in children younger than 5 years, and a steady increase from 2000 to 2004 that ranged from

40.9 to 55.1 per 100,000. Fischer and colleagues[77] performed a population-based hospital study of KD children in Denmark from 1981 to 2004, identifying 360 cases of KD in children younger than 15 years and noting a mean annual incidence of 4.5 to 5 per 100,000 person-years, with a gradual increase over the study period. Holman and colleagues[78] conducted a retrospective analysis of children aged less than 18 years and focusing on those younger than 5 years hospitalized in Hawaiian hospitals from 1996 to 2006, noting a mean annual incidence of 50.4 per 100,000 children younger than 5 years, ranging from 45.5 to 56.5. Japanese children who had the highest mean annual incidence of 210.5 per 100,000 exceeded the mean Asian and Pacific pediatric annual incidence of 62.9 per 100,000 children, followed by native Hawaiian children with an incidence of 86.9, other Asian children with an incidence of 84.9, and Chinese children with an incidence of 83.2 per 100,000, exceeding that of whites with an KD incidence of 13.7 per 100,000 children. Ng and colleagues[79] conducted retrospective and prospective studies of KD in Hong Kong from 1994 to 1997 and then from 1997 to 2000, identifying 696 children younger than 15 years and noting a higher incidence of KD in the prospective period (39 versus 26 per 100,000 children). Singh and colleagues[80] analyzed the records of children younger than 15 years with KD in Chandigarh, North India, identifying 196 cases. There was an increasing incidence of disease from 0.51 to 4.5 cases during the period from 1994 to 2007. Nakamura and coworkers[81] conducted the 21st nationwide survey of 23,730 KD children treated between 2009 and 2010, noting an annual incidence rate of 206.2 and 239.6 per 100,000, establishing the highest rate ever for Japan in 2010. Park and coworkers[82] surveyed Korean hospitals for the period of 2006 to 2008, identifying 9039 KD children and noting an outbreak rate of 108.7 100,000 in 2006 that increased to 113.1 per 100,000 in 2008, with a mean annual incidence of 113.1 per 100,000 children. Schiller and colleagues[83] examined a national prospective study of KD children over a 2-year period from 1990 to 1992, recording an annual incidence rate of 2.9 per 100,000 children younger than 16 years, and a rate of 6.2 per 100,000 children younger than 5 years. Lue and colleagues[84] conducted nationwide hospital surveys of KD in Taiwan in 2006, noting an incidence of 66.24 per 100,000 children younger than 5 years, representing the highest of any preceding survey. Huang and colleagues[85] investigated the epidemiology of KD by using national insurance claims made between 2003 and 2006, noting an annual incidence of KD of 153 per 100,000 in children younger than 1 year with an overall incidence of 69 per 100,000 children younger than 5 years. Harnden and colleagues[86] analyzed hospital admission data for childhood KD in England for the period 1991 to 2000, identifying 2215 emergency admissions representing an incidence that increased from 4.8 to 9.2 per 100,000 in this time period. Holman and coworkers[87] performed a retrospective analysis of emergency childhood admission for KD in the USA using the Kids' Inpatient Database and a Nationwide Inpatient Sample for 2006, noting an incidence of 20.8 per 100,000 children.

Eight GWAS and linkage analysis studies of KD[88–92] have led to susceptibility genetic loci for KD. Onouchi and colleagues[88] performed a nonparametric GWAS of sib pairs on 75 full sib pairs, 3 sib trios, and 1 half-sib, applying Japanese criteria,[70] and identified a candidate gene locus at 12q24 (maximum logarithm-of-odds [LOD] score = 2.69), with possible linkage to 4q35, 5q35, 5q34, 6q27, 7p15, 8q24, 18q23, 19q13, Xp22, and Xq27. Moreover, 90 genes were believed to be expressed in organs related to immune function among the 128 genes that mapped within 1 LOD confidence interval of the linkage position on chromosome 12. Burgner and coworkers,[89] on behalf of the International Kawasaki Disease Genetics Consortium, investigated genetic determinants of KD susceptibility in a GWAS of 119 Caucasian KD patients and 135 matched controls using the AHA criteria.[71] The investigators[89] noted associations with 40 single-nucleotide polymorphisms (SNPs) and 6 haplotypes, most significantly at *NAALADL2* (rs17531088) and *ZRHX3* (rs7199343). The latter, also known as ATBF1, which encodes a large enhancer-binding transcription factor known to be polymorphic and interactive with several proteins including protein inhibitor of activated signal transducer and activator of transcription 3 (STAT3), is activated by interleukin (IL)-6 that is involved in innate immune reactivity. The function of the N-acetylated α-linked acidic dipeptidase-like 2 (NAALADI2) gene, which showed the greatest change in transcript levels between acute and convalescent KD, contributes to Cornelia de Lange syndrome, a multisystem malformation syndrome. Tsai and co-workers[90] conducted a GWAS in a Han Chinese population in 250 KD patients and 446 controls residing in Taiwan, using the AHA criteria.[71] The most strongly associated SNPs were detected in 3 novel loci close to the coatomer protein complex β-2 subunit (*COPB2*) gene (rs1873668, rs4243399, rs16849083), as well as in the intronic region of the endoplasmic reticulum aminopeptidase 1 (*ERAP1*) gene (rs14981). COPB2 coats non–clathrin-coated vesicles and is essential for Golgi budding and vesicular trafficking, whereas ERAP1 plays a role in trimming peptides to the optimal length for HLA)class I presentation, cleaving cell surface receptors for proinflammatory cytokines. Kim and coworkers, on behalf of the Korean Kawasaki Disease Genetics Consortium,[91] conducted a GWAS among 186 Korean KD patients and 600 controls, applying the disease definition according to the AHA,[71] and noted susceptibility loci for KD at the 1p31 region and 2p13.3 chromosomal loci. A putative KD susceptibility locus (rs5277409) mapped to chromosome 1p31, and the coronary artery lesion (CAL) locus (rs7604693) mapped to the Pellino 1 protein (*PELI1*) (rs7604693) gene in the 2p13.3 region encoding PEL1, an intermediate component in the signaling cascade initiated by toll-like receptors and the IL-1 receptor (*IL1R*) gene, which are associated with innate and adaptive immune responses. Khor and colleagues[92] performed a GWAS in 2173 KD patients of European and Asian descent, noting 2 significant loci in the Fc fragment of IgG, low-affinity 2A receptor (*FCGR2A*) (rs1801274), and for the rs2233152 SNP near the melanoma inhibitory activity (*MIA*), inositol 1,4,5-trisphosphate 3-kinase C (*ITPKC*) gene. Whereas the FCGR2A, present on monocytes, macrophages, neutrophils, NK cells, T-cells, and B-cells, participates in the phagocytosis of immune complexes and modulation of antibody production by B cells, ITPKC acts as a negative regulator of T-cell activation through the Ca^{2+}/NFAT signaling pathway; contributing to immune hyperactivity. Lee and coworkers[93] performed a GWAS in 622 KD patients and 1107 controls in a Han Chinese population residing in Taiwan, using the AHA criteria,[71] and noted 2 loci significantly associated with KD, including one at the B-lymphoid tyrosine kinase (*BLK*) gene and the other at *CD40*. Whereas the *BLK* gene seems to play an important role in the expression of B cell signaling, activation, and antibody secretion, *CD40* is instead a member of the tumor necrosis factor receptor superfamily, and its interaction with the CD40 ligand (CD40L) leads to cross-talk, integrating strong antigenic signals and microbial stimuli to induce IL-17-producing CD4[+] T-cells that contribute to inflammation and the development of autoimmune disease. Onouchi and coworkers[94,95] performed a GWAS in 428 Japanese KD patients and 3379 controls, noting significant associations in the *FAM167A-BLK* region at 8p22 to 23 (rs2254546) in the *HLA* region at 6p21.3 (rs2857151), and in the *CD40* region at 20q13 (rs48130030), also replicating the association of a functional SNP of *FCGR2A* (rs1801274). Although ubiquitously expressed, the function of *FAM167A* has not been well characterized. Yan and coworkers[95] analyzed variants of 6 SNPs in 358 Japanese KD patients and 815 controls, identifying 3, rs1801274, rs2857151, and rs22554546 respectively corresponding to *FCGR2A*, *HLA*, and *BLK* genes, noting a significant effect and stronger association on KD than single-locus, 2-loci, and 3-loci combinations; moreover, a significant association with CALs was noted in KD, with high-risk genotypes at both rs1801274 and rs2857151.

SMALL-SIZE VESSEL VASCULITIS
Antineutrophil Cytoplasmic Antibody-Associated Vasculitis

The classification of the ANCA-associated vasculitides (AAV) has been controversial[96] with existing systems developed by the ACR,[97,98] the CHCC,[57] and the European Medicines Agency algorithm[99] to provide a standardized method for their application in epidemiologic studies, each with separate deficiencies, especially when applied to unselected patients. These systems were developed as classification criteria and not as diagnostic criteria. As there were no validated diagnostic criteria for AAV, the Diagnostic and Classification Criteria for Vasculitis Study, developed by Watts and colleagues,[99] led to the consensus development and validation of diagnostic criteria by an algorithm to avoid inclusion of patients with other conditions. So defined, the investigators noted an annual incidence of 11.3 for GPA and 5.9 per million for MPA, with respective prevalence at the end of calendar year 2008 of 145.9 per million for GPA and 63.1 per million for MPA. Lyons and colleagues[100] conducted a GWAS in a cohort of 1233 UK subjects with AAV and 5884 controls, noting both MHC and non-MHC associations with AAV, with the strongest genetic association with the antigenic specificity of ANCA and not with the clinical syndrome. Those with anti-proteinase 3 (PR3) ANCA were associated with *HLA-DP* (rs3117242) at the 6p21.32 chromosome locus, as well as those encoding α1-antitrypsin (*SERPINA1* to *SERPINA11*) (rs7151526) at the 14q32 chromosome locus and proteinase 3 (*PRTN3*) (rs62132295) at the 19p13.3 chromosome locus, while anti-myeloperoxidase ANCA (MPO) was associated with *HLA-DQ* (rs5000634) at the 6p21.32 chromosome locus. These studies confirmed that the pathogenesis of AAV had a genetic component and that the genetic distinction between GPA and MPA was associated with ANCA specificity. Moreover, the response against the PR3 autoantigen was a central pathogenic feature of PR3-AAV, distinct from MPO-AAV.

The global incidence and prevalence of AAV is summarized in **Table 5**. Watts,[64,101] Ormerod,[65] Mohammad,[63] and Mahr and colleagues[59] evaluated the epidemiologic aspects of AAV globally in adults. In 2 regions of Europe, Norwich (UK) and Lugo (Spain), the incidence rate of GPA in Norwich was 10.6 per million compared with 4.9 per million in Lugo for 2008, with virtually equal age distribution of 34.1 per million between age 45 and 74 years, suggesting that environmental factors might be important in the their etiopathogenesis.[64] In a 10-year study of primary systemic vasculitis in the UK[101] in the NHA from 1988 to 1997, the annual incidence of GPA was 9.7, EGPA 2.7, and MPA 8.0 per million during the entire study period; however, a comparison of the periods 1988 to 1992 and 1993 to 1997 showed respective annual incidences toward an increase in all conditions (8.7 per million for GPA, 1.5 for EGPA, and 6.8 for MPA, compared with 10.3 for GPA, 3.7 for EGPA, and 8.9 for MPA). In a comparison of primary systemic vasculitis in the Australian Capital Territory and southeastern New South Wales between 1995 and 1999, and between 2000 and 2004, Ormerod and Cook[65] noted similar disease-specific incidences for each of the 2 periods, with 8.8 and 8.4 per million for GPA, 2.3 and 5.0 per million for MPA, and 2.3 and 2.2 per million for EGPA in the Australian Capital Territory in comparison with southeastern New South Wales, with a trend for higher values in MPA and GPA in rural areas. A similar relation was found in disease-specific prevalence for each of the 2 periods, with 64.3 and 95.0 per million for GPA, 17.5 and 39.1 per million for MPA, and 11.7 and 22.3 per million for EGPA in the Australian Capital Territory compared to southeastern

Table 5
Global incidence and prevalence of AAV

Authors,[Ref.] Year	Country	Study Period	Incidence per 10^6	Prevalence per 10^6
Watts et al,[101] 2000	UK	1988–1992	8.7[a]	—
	UK	1988–1992	6.8[b]	—
	UK	1988–1992	1.5[c]	—
	UK	1993–1997	10.3[a]	—
	UK	1993–1997	8.9[b]	—
	UK	1993–1997	3.7[c]	—
Ormerod and Cook,[65] 2008	Australia + UK	1995–1999	8.8[a]	64.3[a]
		2000–2004	8.4[a]	95.0[a]
		1995–1999	2.3[b]	17.5[b]
		2000–2004	5.0[b]	39.1[b]
		1995–1999	2.3[c]	11.7[c]
		2000–2004	2.2[c]	22.3[c]
Mahr et al,[59] 2004	France[d]	2000	—	23.7[a]
	France[d]	2000	—	25.1[b]
	France[d]	2000	—	10.7[c]
Mohammad et al,[63] 2009	Sweden	1997–2006	9.8[a]	—
	Sweden	1997–2006	10.1[b]	—
	Sweden	1997–2006	0.9[c]	—

[a] GPA.
[b] MPA.
[c] EGPA.
[d] Seine-St Denis County, Paris.

New South Wales. In incident cases of primary systemic vasculitis identified in the Seine-St Denis County of, Mahr and colleagues[59] estimated the prevalence of GPA as 23.7, MPA 25.1, and EGPA 10.7 per million adults in a population of 1,093,515, 28% of whom were of non-European ancestry, with an overall prevalence that was 2-fold higher for those of European (104.7 5 per million) compared with non-European ancestry (52.5 per million). Mohammad and colleagues[63] estimated incident cases of GPA, MPA, and EGPA in southern Sweden as 9.8, 10.1, and 0.9 per million, respectively, in a total population of 641,000 between 1997 and 2006, with a progressive increase in age-specific incidence rates over the study period.

REFERENCES

1. Scott DG, Watts RA. Epidemiology and clinical features of systemic vasculitis. Clin Exp Nephrol 2013;17:607–10.

2. Kermani TA, Warrington KJ, Crowson CS, et al. Large-vessel involvement in giant cell arteritis: a population based cohort study of the incidence-trends and prognosis. Ann Rheum Dis 2012;72:1989–94.

3. Salvarani C, Cantini F, Boiardi L, et al. Polymyalgia rheumatic and giant cell arteritis. N Engl J Med 2002;347:261–71.

4. Hunder GG, Bloch DA, Michel BA, et al. The American College of Rheumatology 1990 criteria for the classification of giant cell arteritis. Arthritis Rheum 1990;33: 1122–8.

5. Nuenninghoff DM, Hunder GG, Christianson TJH, et al. Incidence and predictors of large-artery complication (aortic aneurysm, aortic dissection, and/or

large artery stenosis) in patients with giant cell arteritis. Arthritis Rheum 2003;48: 3522–31.

6. Gonzalez-Gay MA, Vazquez-Rodriguez TR, Lopez-Diaz MJ, et al. Epidemiology of giant cell arteritis and polymyalgia rheumatica. Arthritis Rheum 2009;61: 1454–61.

7. Dunstan E, Lester SL, Rischmueller M, et al. Epidemiology of biopsy-proven giant cell arteritis in South Australia. Intern Med J 2014;44:32–9.

8. Ninan J, Nguyen AM, Cole A, et al. Mortality in patients with biopsy-proven giant cell arteritis: a south Australian population-based study. J Rheumatol 2011;38: 2215–7.

9. Herlyn K, Buckert F, Gross WL, et al. Doubled prevalence rates of ANCA-associated vasculitides and giant cell arteritis between 1994 and 2006 in northern Germany. Rheumatology (Oxford) 2014;53(5):882–9.

10. Bas-Lando M, Breuer GS, Berkun Y, et al. The incidence of giant cell arteritis in Jerusalem over a 25-year period: annual and seasonal fluctuations. Clin Exp Rheumatol 2007;25(Suppl 44):S15–7.

11. Kobayashi S, Yano T, Matsumoto Y, et al. Clinical and epidemiologic analysis of giant cell (temporal) arteritis from a nationwide survey in 1998 in Japan: the first government-supported nationwide survey. Arthritis Rheum 2003;49:594–8.

12. Abdul-Rahman AM, Molteno ACB, Bevin TH. The epidemiology of giant cell arteritis in Otago, New Zealand: a 9-year analysis. N Z Med J 2011;124:44–52.

13. Haugeberg G, Irgens KA, Thomsen RS. No major differences in incidence of temporal arteritis in northern and western Norway compared with reports from southern Norway. Scand J Rheumatol 2003;32:318–9.

14. Haugeberg G, Paulsen PQ, Bie RB. Temporal arteritis in Vest Agder County in southern Norway: incidence and clinical findings. J Rheumatol 2000;27:2624–7.

15. Gonzalez-Gay MA, Barros S, Lopez-Diaz MJ, et al. Giant cell arteritis: disease patterns of clinical presentation in a series of 240 patients. Medicine 2005;84: 269–76.

16. Gonzalez-Gay MA, Miranda-Filloy JA, Lopez-Diaz MJ, et al. Giant cell arteritis in northwestern Spain. A 25-year epidemiological study. Medicine 2007;86:61–8.

17. Mohammad AJ, Nilsson JA, Jacobsson LT, et al. Incidence and mortality rates of biopsy-proven giant cell arteritis in southern Sweden. Ann Rheum Dis 2014; 74(6):993–7.

18. Smeeth L, Cook C, Hall AJ. Incidence of diagnosed polymyalgia rheumatica and temporal arteritis in the United Kingdom, 1990-2001. Ann Rheum Dis 2006;65:1093–8.

19. Salvarani C, Crowson CS, O'Fallon M, et al. Reappraisal of the epidemiology of giant cell arteritis in Olmsted County, Minnesota, over a fifty-year period. Arthritis Rheum 2004;51:264–8.

20. De Souza AW, Okamoto KYK, Abrantes F, et al. Giant cell arteritis: a multicenter observational study in Brazil. Clinics (Sao Paulo) 2013;68:317–22.

21. Chaudhry IA, Shamsi FA, Elzaridi E, et al. Epidemiology of giant-cell arteritis in an Arab population: a 22-year study. Br J Ophthalmol 2007;91:715–8.

22. Alba MA, Mena-Madrazo JA, Reyes E, et al. Giant cell arteritis in Mexican patients. J Clin Rheumatol 2012;18:1–7.

23. Lane SE, Watts R, Scott DGI. Epidemiology of systemic vasculitis. Curr Rheumatol Rep 2005;7:270–5.

24. Kemp A, Marner K, Nissen SH, et al. HLA antigens in cases of giant cell arteritis. Acta Ophthalmol (Copenh) 1980;58:1000–4.

25. Armstrong RD, Behn A, Myles A, et al. Histocompatibility antigens in polymyalgia rheumatica and giant cell arteritis. J Rheumatol 1983;10:659–61.

26. Dababneh A, Gonzalez-Gay MA, Garcia-Porrua C, et al. Giant cell arteritis and polymyalgia rheumatica can be differentiated by distinct patterns of HLA class II association. J Rheumatol 1998;25:2140–5.

27. Jacobsen S, Baslund B, Madsen HO, et al. Mannose-binding lectin variant alleles and HLA-DR4 alleles are associated with giant cell arteritis. J Rheumatol 2002;29:2148–53.

28. Bignon JD, Ferec C, Barrier J, et al. HLA class II genes polymorphism in DR4 giant cell arteritis patients. Tissue Antigens 1988;32:254–8.

29. Bignon JD, Barrier J, Soulillou JP, et al. HLA DR4 and giant cell arteritis. Tissue Antigens 1984;24:60–2.

30. Richardson JE, Gladman DD, Fam A, et al. HLA-DR4 in giant cell arteritis: association with polymyalgia rheumatica syndrome. Arthritis Rheum 1987;30:1293–7.

31. Barrier J, Bignon JD, Soulillou JP, et al. Increased prevalence of HLA-DR4 in giant-cell arteritis. N Engl J Med 1981;305:104–5.

32. Lowenstein MB, Bridgeford PH, Vasey FB, et al. Increased frequency of HLA-DR3 and DR4 in polymyalgia rheumatica-giant cell arteritis. Arthritis Rheum 1983;26:925–7.

33. Martinez-Taboda VM, Bartolome MJ, Lopez-Hoyos M, et al. HLA-DRB1 allele distribution in polymyalgia rheumatica and giant cell arteritis: influence on clinical subgroups and prognosis. Semin Arthritis Rheum 2004;34:454–64.

34. Weyand CM, Hicok KC, Hunder GG, et al. The HLA-DRB1 locus as a genetic component in giant cell arteritis. Mapping of a disease-linked sequence motif to the antigen binding site of the HLA-DR molecule. J Clin Invest 1992;90:2355–61.

35. Weyand CM, Hunder NN, Hicok KC, et al. HLA-DRB1 alleles in polymyalgia rheumatica, giant cell arteritis, and rheumatoid arthritis. Arthritis Rheum 1994;37:514–20.

36. Gonzalez-Gay MA, Garcia-Porrua C, Llorca J, et al. Visual manifestations of giant cell arteritis. Trends and clinical spectrum in 161 patients. Medicine (Baltimore) 2000;79:283–92.

37. Hansen JA, Healey LA, Wilske KR. Association between giant cell (temporal) arteritis and HLA-Cw3. Hum Immunol 1985;13:193–8.

38. Gonzalez-Gay MA, Rueda B, Vilchez JR, et al. Contribution of MHC class I region to genetic susceptibility for giant cell arteritis. Rheumatology (Oxford) 2007;46:431–4.

39. Arend WP, Michel BA, Bloch DA, et al. The American College of Rheumatology 1990 criteria for the classification of Takayasu arteritis. Arthritis Rheum 1990;33:1129–34.

40. Ringold S, Wallace CA. Evolution of paediatric-specific vasculitis classification criteria. Ann Rheum Dis 2010;69:785–6.

41. Ruperto N, Ozen S, Pistorio A, et al. EULAR/PRINTO/PRES criteria for Henoch-Schönlein purpura, childhood polyarteritis nodosa, childhood Wegener granulomatosis and childhood Takayasu arteritis: Ankara 2008. Part 1: Overall methodology and clinical characterization. Ann Rheum Dis 2010;69:790–7.

42. Seko Y, Minota S, Kawasaki A, et al. Perforin-secreting killer cell infiltration and expression of a 65-kD heat-shock protein in aortic tissue of patients with Takayasu's arteritis. J Clin Invest 1994;93:750–8.

43. Wagner AD, Bjornsson J, Bartley GB, et al. Interferon-gamma-producing T cells in giant cell vasculitis represents a minority of tissue-infiltrating cells and are located distant from the site of pathology. Am J Pathol 1996;148:1923–33.

44. Sneller MC. Granuloma formation, implications for the pathogenesis of vasculitis. Cleve Clin J Med 2002;69(Suppl 2):SII40–3.

45. Weyand CM, Goronzy H. Medium- and large-vessel vasculitis. N Engl J Med 2002;349:160–9.

46. Deng J, Younge B, Olshen RA, et al. TH17 and Th1 T-cell responses in giant cell arteritis. Circulation 2010;121:906–15.

47. Terrier B, Geri G, Chaara W, et al. Interleukin-21 modulates Th1 and Th1 responses in giant cell arteritis. Arthritis Rheum 2012;64:2001–11.

48. Noguchi S, Numano F, Gravanis MB, et al. Increased levels of soluble forms of adhesion molecules in Takayasu arteritis. Int J Cardiol 1998;66(Suppl 1):S23–35.

49. Terao C, Yoshifuji H, Kimura A, et al. Two susceptibility loci to Takayasu arteritis reveal a synergistic role of the IL12B and HLA-B regions in a Japanese population. Am J Hum Genet 2013;93:289–97.

50. Saruhan-Direskeneli G, Hughes T, Aksu K, et al. Identification of multiple genetic susceptibility loci in Takayasu arteritis. Am J Hum Genet 2013;93:298–305.

51. Watts R, Al-Taiar A, Mooney J, et al. The epidemiology of Takayasu arteritis in the UK. Rheumatology 2009;48:1008–11.

52. Mohammad A, Mandl T. Takayasu's arteritis in southern Sweden. Presse Med 2013;42:719.

53. Waern AU, Andersson P, Hemmingsson A. Takayasu's arteritis: a hospital-region based study on occurrence, treatment and prognosis. Angiology 1983;34:311–20.

54. Reinhold-Keller E, Herlyn K, Wagner-Bastmeyer R, et al. Stable incidence of primary systemic vasculitides over five years: results from the German vasculitis register. Arthritis Rheum 2005;53:93–9.

55. Dreyer L, Faurschou M, Baslund B. A population-based study of Takayasu's arteritis in eastern Denmark. Clin Exp Rheumatol 2011;29(Suppl 64):S40–2.

56. Lightfoot RW Jr, Michel BA, Bloch DA, et al. The American College of Rheumatology 1990 criteria for the classification of polyarteritis nodosa. Arthritis Rheum 1990;33:1088–93.

57. Jennette JC, Falk RJ, Bacon PA, et al. International Chapel Hill consensus conference nomenclature of vasculitides. Arthritis Rheum 2013;65:1–11.

58. Guillevin L, Lhote F. Polyarteritis nodosa and microscopic polyangiitis. Clin Exp Immunol 1995;101(Suppl 1):22–3.

59. Mahr A, Guillevin L, Poissonnet M, et al. Prevalences of polyarteritis nodosa, microscopic polyangiitis, Wegener's granulomatosis, and Churg-Strauss syndrome in a French urban multiethnic population in 2000:A capture –recapture estimate. Arthritis Rheum 2004;51:92–9.

60. Ozen S, Bakkaloglu A, Dusunsel R, et al. Childhood vasculitides in Turkey: a nationwide survey. Clin Rheumatol 2007;26:196–200.

61. Ozen S, Ruperto N, Dillon MJ, et al. EULAR/PReS endorsed consensus criteria* for the classification of childhood vasculitides. Ann Rheum Dis 2006;65:936–41.

62. McMahon BJ, Heyward WL, Templin DW, et al. Hepatitis B-associated polyarteritis nodosa in Alaskan Eskimos: clinical and epidemiologic features and long-term follow-up. Hepatology 1989;9:97–101.

63. Mohammad AJ, Jacobsson LTH, Westman KWA, et al. Incidence and survival rates in Wegener's granulomatosis, microscopic polyangiitis, Churg-Strauss syndrome and polyarteritis nodosa. Rheumatology 2009;48:1560–5.

64. Watts RA, Gonzalez-Gay MA, Lane SE, et al. Geoepidemiology of systemic vasculitis: comparison of the incidence in two regions of Europe. Ann Rheum Dis 2001;60:170–2.

65. Ormerod AS, Cook MC. Epidemiology of primary systemic vasculitis in the Australian Capital Territory and south-eastern New South Wales. Intern Med J 2008;38:816–23.

66. Shulman ST, Rowley AH. Advances in Kawasaki disease. Eur J Pediatr 2004;63: 285–91.

67. Dillon MJ, Eleftheriou D, Brogan PA. Medium-size-vessel vasculitis. Pediatr Nephrol 2010;25:1641–52.

68. De Rosa G, Pardeo M, Rigante D. Current recommendations for the pharmacologic therapy in Kawasaki syndrome and management of its cardiovascular complications. Eur Rev Med Pharmacol Sci 2007;11:301–8.

69. Burns JC, Glode MP. Kawasaki syndrome. Lancet 2004;364:533–44.

70. Japan Kawasaki Disease Research Committee. Diagnostic guidelines for Kawasaki disease. 5th edition 2002. Tokyo. Available at: http://www.kawasaki-disease.org/diagnostic/index.html. Accessed November 1, 2018.

71. Newburger JW, Takahashi M, Gerber MA, et al. Diagnosis, treatment and long-term management of Kawasaki disease: a statement for health professionals from the Committee on Rheumatic Fever, Endocarditis, and Kawasaki Disease, Council on Cardiovascular Disease in the Young. Pediatrics 2004;114:1708–33.

72. Saundankar J, Yim D, Itotoh B, et al. The epidemiology and clinical features of Kawasaki disease in Australia. Pediatrics 2014;133:e1009–14.

73. Lin YT, Manlhiot C, Ching JC, et al. Repeated systematic surveillance of Kawasaki disease in Ontario from 1995 to 2006. Pediatr Int 2010;52:699–706.

74. Ma XJ, Huang M, Chen SB, et al. Epidemiologic features of Kawasaki disease in Shanghai from 2003 through 2007. Chin Med J 2010;123:2629–34.

75. Li XH, Li HJ, Xu M, et al. Epidemiological survey of Kawasaki disease in Sichuan Province of China. J Trop Pediatr 2008;54:133–6.

76. Du A-D, Zhao D, Du J, et al. Epidemiologic study on Kawasaki disease in Beijing from 2000 through 2004. Pediatr Infect Dis J 2007;26:449–51.

77. Fischer TK, Holman RC, Yorita KL, et al. Kawasaki syndrome in Denmark. Pediatr Infect Dis J 2007;26:411–5.

78. Holman RC, Christensen KY, Belay ED, et al. Racial/ethnic differences in the incidence of Kawasaki syndrome among children in Hawaii. Hawaii Med J 2010;69:194–7.

79. Ng YM, Sung RY, So LY, et al. Kawasaki disease in Hong Kong, 1994 to 2000. Hong Kong Med J 2005;11:331–5.

80. Singh S, Aulakh R, Bhalla AK, et al. Is Kawasaki disease incidence rising in Chandigarh, North India? Arch Dis Child 2011;96:137–40.

81. Nakamura Y, Yashiro M, Uehara R, et al. Epidemiologic features of Kawasaki disease in Japan: results of the 2009-2010 nationwide survey. J Epidemiol 2012;22:216–21.

82. Park YW, Han JW, Hong YM, et al. Epidemiologic features of Kawasaki disease in Korea, 2006-2008. Pediatr Int 2011;53:36–9.

83. Schiller B, Fasth A, Bjorkhem G, et al. Kawasaki disease in Sweden: incidence and clinical features. Acta Paediatr 1995;84:769–74.

84. Lue H-C, Chen L-R, Lin M-T, et al. Epidemiologic features of Kawasaki disease in Taiwan, 1976-2007: results of five nationwide questionnaire hospital surveys. Pediatr Neonatol 2013;55(2):92–6.

85. Huang WC, Huang LM, Chang IS, et al. Epidemiologic features of Kawasaki disease in Taiwan, 2003-2006. Pediatrics 2009;123:e401-5.
86. Harnden A, Alves B, Sheikh A. Rising incidence of Kawasaki disease in England: analysis of hospital admission data. BMJ 2002;324:1424-5.
87. Holman RC, Belay ED, Christensen KY, et al. Hospitalizations for Kawasaki syndrome among children in the United States, 1997-2007. Pediatr Infect Dis J 2010;29:483-8.
88. Onouchi Y, Tamari M, Takahashi A, et al. A genomewide linkage analysis of Kawasaki disease: evidence for linkage to chromosome 12. J Hum Genet 2007;52:179-90.
89. Burgner D, Davila S, Breunis WB, et al. A genome-wide association study identifies novel and functionally related susceptibility Loci for Kawasaki disease. PLoS Genet 2009;5:e1000319.
90. Tsai FJ, Lee YC, Chang JS, et al. Identification of novel susceptibility Loci for Kawasaki disease in a Han Chinese population by a genome-wide association study. PLoS One 2011;6:e16853.
91. Kim JJ, Hong YM, Sohn S, et al. A genome-wide association analysis reveals 1p31 and 2p13.3 as susceptibility loci for Kawasaki disease. Hum Genet 2011;129:487-95.
92. Khor CC, Davila S, Breunis WB, et al. Genome-wide association study identifies FCGR2A as a susceptibility locus for Kawasaki disease. Nat Genet 2011;43:1241-6.
93. Lee YC, Kuo HC, Chang JS, et al. Two new susceptibility loci for Kawasaki disease identified through genome-wide association analysis. Nat Genet 2012;44:522-5.
94. Onouchi Y, Ozaki K, Burns JC, et al. A genome-wide association study identifies three new risk loci for Kawasaki disease. Nat Genet 2012;44:517-21.
95. Yan Y, Ma Y, Liu Y, et al. Combined analysis of genome-wide-linked susceptibility loci to Kawasaki disease in Han Chinese. Hum Genet 2013;132:669-80.
96. Khan II, Watts RA. Classification of ANCA-associated vasculitis. Curr Rheumatol Rep 2013;15:383.
97. Leavitt RY, Fauci AS, Bloch DA, et al. The American College of Rheumatology 1990 criteria for the classification of Wegener's granulomatosis. Arthritis Rheum 1990;33:1101-7.
98. Masi AT, Hunder GG, Lie JT, et al. The American College of Rheumatology 1990 criteria for the classification of Churg-Strauss syndrome (allergic granulomatosis and angiitis). Arthritis Rheum 1990;33:1094-100.
99. Watts RA, Lane S, Hanslik T, et al. Development and validation of a consensus methodology for the classification of the ANCA-associated vasculitides and polyarteritis nodosa for epidemiological studies. Ann Rheum Dis 2007;66:222-7.
100. Lyons PA, Rayner TF, Watts RA, et al. Genetically distinct subsets within ANCA-associated vasculitis. N Engl J Med 2012;367:214-23.
101. Watts RA, Lane SE, Bentham G, et al. Epidemiology of systemic vasculitis. Arthritis Rheum 2000;43:414-9.

Genetic Basis of Vasculitides with Neurologic Involvement

Francisco David Carmona, PhD[a], Raquel López-Mejías, PhD[b],
Ana Márquez, PhD[c,d], Javier Martín, MD, PhD[d],
Miguel A. González-Gay, MD, PhD[b,e,f],*

KEYWORDS

- Vasculitis • Genetic risk factors • Polymorphisms
- Genome-wide association studies • Nervous system

KEY POINTS

- Vasculitides comprise a heterogeneous group of rare diseases with a complex etiology characterized by inflammatory lesions of blood vessels.
- Some forms of vasculitis are associated with severe neurologic complications that have an impact on the prognosis of the disease.
- An important progress in the elucidation of the genetic component of vasculitides has occurred during the last decade.
- Few genetic studies on specific clinical phenotypes of vasculitides have been published due to the difficulty in collecting well-powered case series.
- A better understanding of the genetic component leading to nervous system complications of patients with vasculitis would definitively help in their clinical management.

Disclosure Statement: The authors declare no conflicts of interest related to the subject matter discussed in this review.

[a] Departamento de Genética e Instituto de Biotecnología, Universidad de Granada, Granada, Spain; [b] Epidemiology, Genetics and Atherosclerosis Research Group on Systemic Inflammatory Diseases, Rheumatology Division, IDIVAL, Santander, Spain; [c] Systemic Autoimmune Diseases Unit, Hospital Clínico San Cecilio, Granada, Spain; [d] Instituto de Parasitología y Biomedicina 'López-Neyra', IPBLN-CSIC, PTS Granada, Granada, Spain; [e] School of Medicine, University of Cantabria, Santander, Spain; [f] Cardiovascular Pathophysiology and Genomics Research Unit, School of Physiology, Faculty of Health Sciences, University of the Witwatersrand, Johannesburg, South Africa

* Corresponding author. Epidemiology, Genetics and Atherosclerosis Research Group on Systemic Inflammatory Diseases, Rheumatology Division, IDIVAL, Avenida Cardenal Herrera Oria s/n, Santander 39011, Spain.
E-mail address: miguelaggay@hotmail.com

Neurol Clin 37 (2019) 219–234
https://doi.org/10.1016/j.ncl.2019.01.006
0733-8619/19/© 2019 Elsevier Inc. All rights reserved.

INTRODUCTION

The term "vasculitis" refers to a heterogeneous group of clinical entities in which blood vessels are damaged by inflammation-mediated processes. These conditions may be primary or secondary to other systemic diseases, and their pathologic manifestations depend on the caliber and location of the affected vessels.[1–3] Complications of the peripheral and central nervous system (CNS), such as ischemic or hemorrhagic lesions in different vascular territories of the brain, represent the most alarming injuries, because they may result fatal without an appropriate immunosuppressive therapy.

Vasculitides present a largely unknown multifactorial etiology in which the genetic causes seem to have a major role.[4] In particular, common variation of the human genome (especially single nucleotide polymorphisms [SNPs]) is responsible for the genetic effect on disease predisposition. Most vasculitides show a strong association with genetic factors located within the major histocompatibility complex (MHC) region (**Fig. 1**), supporting the autoinflammatory/autoimmune nature of these disorders.[4,5]

During the last decade, there has been a considerable leap in the understanding of the genetic landscape of many complex diseases, including vasculitides. This has been possible because of the unprecedented advance in the knowledge of the human genome architecture and the establishment of big consortia, which has allowed the analysis of robust study cohorts using very powerful technologies.

This review aims to provide an updated overview about the main genetic contributors to vasculitis susceptibility, with an especial focus on those involved in the most common neurologic complications of these conditions.

BEHÇET DISEASE

Behçet disease (BD) is a multisystem syndrome with a male preponderance characterized by inflammatory lesions of blood vessels of variable size throughout the body, leading to heterogeneous clinical manifestations. Oral and genital ulceration as well as ocular involvement (mainly uveitis) are the most frequent phenotypes.[6]

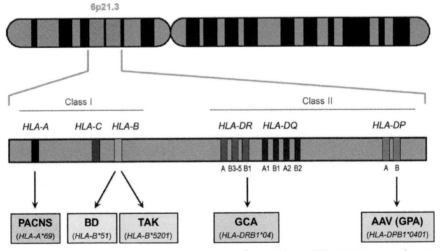

Fig. 1. Top HLA associations with different forms of vasculitis and their location on chromosome 6. AAV, antineutrophil cytoplasmic antibody-associated vasculitides; BD, Behçet disease; GCA, giant cell arteritis; GPA, granulomatosis with polyangiitis; PACNS, primary angiitis of the central nervous system; TAK, Takayasu arteritis.

Neurologic complications occur in around 10% to 30% of patients with BD, constituting the so-called neuro-Behçet syndrome (NB), which presents with fever, headache, aseptic meningeal irritation, and intracranial hypertension, amongst others.[7]

Associations with Behçet Disease Predisposition

Although we are still far from a complete understanding, the genetic component of BD is one of the best known amongst vasculitides. This has been possible thanks to the fulfillment of several large-scale genomic studies, including genome-wide association studies (GWAS) and Immunochip studies, in various ethnic groups.[8–16]

The primary genetic risk factor for BD corresponds to the human leukocyte antigen (HLA) class I haplotype *HLA-B*51* (especially *HLA-B51*01* and *HLA-B51*08*).[17] However, the causal allele of this association is still under debate, with different SNPs and amino acid models proposed to explain the observed effect.[12,18] Additional haplotypes with weaker but independent effects have been also proposed, such as *HLA-A*03*, *HLA-A*26*, *HLA-B*57*, and *HLA-Cw*1602*.[12,13,15]

Regarding the non-HLA genetic factors of BD, 10 loci have been already associated with disease predisposition at the genome-wide level of significance (most of them with key functions in the immune response), including interleukin (IL) 10 (*IL10*, encoding an antiinflammatory Th2 cytokine), the region of IL23 receptor/IL12 receptor beta 2 (*IL23R/IL12RB2*, involved in relevant pathways for Th1 and Th17 cell differentiation), guanosine-5'-triphosphatase IMAP family member 4 (*GIMAP4*, which may play a role in the regulation of lymphocyte apoptosis), CCR1 chemokine (C-C motif) receptor 1 (*CCR1*, encoding a member of the beta chemokine receptor family), signal transducer and activator of transcription 4 (*STAT4*, a key immunoregulatory gene for the adaptive response), a cluster of killer cell lectin-like receptor family member genes (*KLRK1-KLRC4*, encoding members of the NKG2 family that bind to a broad range of ligands leading to activation of natural killer cells), endoplasmic reticulum aminopeptidase 1 (*ERAP1*, encoding an aminopeptidase that processes peptides for HLA class I antigen binding), tumor necrosis factor alpha-inducible protein 3 (*TNFAIP3*, an important gene in the cytokine-mediated inflammatory response), IL12 alpha chain (*IL12A*, encoding a subunit of the IL-12 and IL-35 cytokines), and the jerky protein homolog-like (*JRKL*, with unknown function)/contactin 5 (*CNTN5*, encoding a member of the immunoglobulin superfamily) region.[8–11,13–15,19]

Highly affected biological pathways in BD identified through *in silico* analyses of GWAS data include inflammation processes (ie, focal adhesion as well as MAPK and TGF-β signaling), antigen processing, extracellular matrix-receptor interaction, and complement and coagulation cascades, highlighting the autoimmune and autoinflammatory nature of this condition.[20]

Associations with Neuro-Behçet Syndrome

Despite the high efforts dedicated to investigate the genetic basis of BD, few associations with clinical manifestations related to NB have been published to date.[21]

Human leukocyte antigen-B51

There is controversy about the possible role of *HLA-B51* in the development of neurologic symptoms in patients with BD. Some studies described that carriage of this HLA class I haplotype correlated with higher frequency of ocular involvement and lower frequency of neurologic involvement (and less disease severity in general).[22] However, a systematic review and a meta-analysis performed in 2012 of data from 72 published studies revealed no association of either *HLA-B51* or *HLA-B5* with NB, although a moderate association with ocular manifestations was suggested.[23] Two years later, Demirseren and colleagues[24] evaluated the correlations between clinical phenotypes of BD and *HLA-B51* subtypes in a Turkish population. The investigators observed that the *HLA-B51*03* haplotype may confer risk for NB development, although additional studies in bigger populations are required to confirm this finding.

Mannose binding lectin 2

The mannose binding lectin 2 (*MBL2*) gene encodes the soluble form of MBL that is present in the serum. This protein belongs to the C-type collectin family and it is involved in relevant processes of the innate response, such as binding of microbial surfaces through its lectin domains and activation of the classical complement pathway. *MBL2* gene polymorphisms have been associated with different immune-mediated diseases such as systemic lupus erythematosus and rheumatoid arthritis.[25] In 2009, Kim and collaborators analyzed different promoter and exonic *MBL2* alleles that were described to affect MBL2 functionality and serum concentrations in a Korean population. Although the frequencies of such polymorphisms did not differ between patients with BD and controls, they were significantly associated with development of NB and presence of ocular involvement. The variants producing wild-type protein and high protein levels were overrepresented in patients with BD showing those complications.[26] Contrarily, more recent studies in Chinese Han have reported that *MBL2* variation (in particular the nonsynonymous SNP rs1800450-p.Gly54Asp) may increase predisposition to overall BD instead of specific clinical phenotypes.[27] Therefore, further studies are required to clarify the exact role of *MBL2* polymorphisms in BD development and progression.

Paraoxonase 1

The serum enzyme encoded by paraoxonase 1 (*PON1*) is a component of the high-density lipoprotein that prevent accumulation of lipid peroxidation products.[28] Common genetic variation of *PON1* has been associated with reduced protein activity and predisposition to different forms of vasculitis.[29–31]

Dursun and colleagues[32] investigated the possible involvement of a *PON1* variant (*PON-1-L55M*) known to affect both mRNA levels and protein concentrations in BD development and clinical features. Although the statistical power of the study was considerably low, a significant difference in the allele frequencies of *PON-1-L55M* was observed between BD cases and controls. The effect size of the association was stronger when the subgroups of patients showing visual and neurologic involvement were compared against controls. The investigators speculated that the risk allele of *PON1* could affect those phenotypes by influencing the organophosphate toxicity in the nervous system.[32]

Mevalonate kinase

The *mevalonate kinase* (*MVK*) gene encodes a key peroxisomal enzyme in the signaling pathway involved in cholesterol biosynthesis. Genetic mutations of the gene causing MVK deficiency are responsible for the development of certain conditions such as mevalonic aciduria and hyperimmunoglobulin D syndrome.[33]

In a recent study, 3 *MKV* intronic mutations were described in a cohort of patients with BD from Turkey. One of them (rs104895331-c.769-3C>T) was found to be significantly more frequent in patients with NB than in patients with BD without neurologic involvement.[34] Although this finding needs confirmation in additional studies, this genetic association suggests that MKD could have some influence on the clinical presentations of BD, particularly those related to NB.

Ubiquitin-associated domain-containing protein 2

Although no association between BD and the ubiquitin-associated domain-containing protein 2 (*UBAC2*) gene at the genome-wide significance level has been published so far, there is consensus about considering this locus a confirmed BD risk factor,[35] the reason for which is the consistent *UBAC2* associations with BD susceptibility described in different ethnic groups since it was first suggested in a GWAS performed in 2009.[16,36–38] In addition, some of the associated SNPs were described to affect *UBAC2* expression.[36–38] This gene encodes an ubiquitination-related structural domain that plays a role in the ubiquitination process.[39]

Very recently, Yamazoe and collaborators confirmed *UBAC2* as a susceptibility region for BD predisposition in a well-powered Japanese population.[38] The most striking result of this study was the identification of an SNP, located in a nearby long noncoding RNA (rs9517723), specifically associated under the recessive model with visual and CNS lesions. The investigators also described that homozygosity of the risk allele correlated with enhanced *UBAC2* expression.[38] Therefore, *UBAC2* variation could be involved in both disease predisposition and clinical outcome.

LARGE VESSEL VASCULITIS

Large vessel vasculitides (LVV) are characterized by inflammatory lesions in large-sized vessels such as the aorta, the carotid, and their major branches. This group of vasculitides comprises giant cell arteritis (GCA) and Takayasu arteritis (TAK). Both conditions present a female preponderance, being GCA more frequent in people of European origin over the fifth decade of life and TAK in younger patients with a higher incidence in Asia and Latin America.[40,41]

Associations with Large Vessel Vasculitis Predisposition

The genetic component of LVV was thoroughly investigated during the last decades through many candidate gene studies.[42,43] However, because of the difficulty in establishing well-powered study cohorts, most of the suggested associations were not replicated in independent studies. More recently, the considerable increase in the sample sizes and the use of high-throughput genotyping platforms, including GWAS arrays and the Immunochip, led to the identification of robust genetic markers.[44–49] In this regard, *IL12B* (encoding the P40 subunit of IL-12 and IL-23) was identified as a common genetic factor for both types of LVV using Immunochip data.[49] Other disease-specific markers identified through the analysis of large-scale genomic data include protein tyrosine phosphatase, nonreceptor type 22 (*PTPN22*, one of the shared genetic master autoimmune genes with a critical role in T-cell and B-cell responses), plasminogen (*PLG*, encoding the precursor of plasmin and angiostatin), and prolyl 4-hydroxylase subunit alpha-2 (*P4HA2*, encoding the alpha subunit of the collagen prolyl 4-hydroxylase) for GCA, as well as *IL6* (involved in both proinflammatory and antiinflammatory responses with pleiotropic functions), the leukocyte immunoglobulin-like receptor B3 (*LILRB3*, involved in immunoregulatory processes of the innate and adaptive system) region, the Fc fragment of immunoglobulin G receptor IIa/IIIa (*FCGR2A/FCGR3A*, encoding cell-surface molecules of the immunoglobulin superfamily) loci, and a locus on chromosome 21 near proteasome assembly chaperone 1 (*PSMG1*, encoding a chaperone protein) for TAK.[44–48] The main differences between the genetic component of both forms of LVV rely on the HLA region, because GCA can be considered an archetypal HLA class II disease (with HLA-DRB1*04 as a major risk factor), whereas TAK is mainly associated with HLA class I molecules (mostly HLA-B*5201).[4,49]

Associations with Neurologic Complications of Giant Cell Arteritis

Unilateral or bilateral blindness (due to ischemic optic neuropathy) and stroke (due to cerebral infarction) are the most severe complications of GCA.[50] However, little is currently known about the genetic basis of such phenotypes, with just some insights from candidate gene studies performed in small populations.

Vascular endothelial growth factor

One of the proposed risk genes for neurologic involvement in GCA was vascular endothelial growth factor (*VEGF*). This gene was associated with severe ischemic manifestations (including transient or permanent visual loss, diplopia, cerebrovascular accidents, or jaw claudication, amongst others) of GCA in the Spanish population.[51] Consistent with this, increased circulating VEGF levels correlated with optic nerve ischemia in patients with GCA.[52] Associations between *VEGF* gene polymorphisms and susceptibility to developing GCA have been also described in several independent studies.[53,54] *VEGF* encodes an important proangiogenic signal protein involved in the adhesion of endothelial cells during vasculogenesis that induces pathogenic effector functions.[55,56] Therefore, the association between *VEGF* and GCA is in agreement with the formation of new *vasa vasorum* observed in the arterial walls from patients with this form of vasculitis, which has been suggested to act as a compensatory process for ischemia.[57,58]

Interferon gamma

GCA is a Th1 disease in which interferon gamma (IFNγ) producing Th1 cells represent crucial players of the pathogenic T-cell response within the arterial walls. Indeed, high expression levels of this proinflammatory cytokine have been measured in the vascular lesions of patients with GCA, even after treatment with corticosteroid therapy.[59–61] Consistently, hypomethylation of the *IFNG* gene has been detected in the cellular aggregates of GCA-affected arteries.[62] Because of all those evidences, there have been several attempts to identify genetic variants within the *IFNG* genomic region associated with GCA predisposition, with contradictory results across studies.[44,63,64] However, a relatively consistent association between a microsatellite dinucleotide repeat, located in the first intron of *IFNG*, and patients with GCA showing visual ischemic manifestations (including transient visual loss, amaurosis fugax, permanent visual loss, or diplopia) was described in a European population from Northwestern Spain. The associated allele was considerably overrepresented in the subgroup of patients with those visual phenotypes in comparison with the remaining ones (71.4% vs 44.4%, respectively).[64]

Associations with Neurologic Complications of Takayasu Arteritis

The occlusive lesions of TAK affecting the internal carotid artery and its main branches may cause neurologic dysfunction as the disease progresses, including ischemic optic neuropathy, transient ischemic attacks (leading to headache, syncope, and blurred vision), and stroke.[65] Indeed, studies of cerebral circulation in patients with TAK with noninvasive techniques evidenced a high proportion of vascular abnormalities in the intracranial cerebral vessels.[66] Nevertheless, as in GCA, the genetic component of such complications remains obscure.[42]

Human leukocyte antigen B/MHC class I polypeptide-related sequence A locus

Recently, Wen and colleagues[67] evaluated the effects on TAK susceptibility and severity of different tag polymorphisms located in the genomic region comprising *HLA-B* and MHC class I polypeptide-related sequence A (*MICA*) genes in the Chinese Han Beijing population. The allele frequencies of one SNP located upstream of

MICA (rs9366782) were significantly different between a subgroup of patients with TAK with ischemic brain disease and healthy controls. However, the investigators did not perform a case/case comparison between patients with TAK to discard TAK as a possible confounding factor. In any case, the fact that no association was observed with the overall disease suggested that it may represent a phenotype-specific association. The investigators speculated that rs9366782 could influence the function of the HLA system in antigen presentation within intracranial extensions of both the carotid and subclavian arteries.[67]

ANTINEUTROPHIL CYTOPLASMIC ANTIBODY-ASSOCIATED VASCULITIS

Antineutrophil cytoplasmic antibody (ANCA)-associated vasculitides (AAV) are primary systemic diseases of which major hallmark is a necrotizing inflammation of small blood vessels (arterioles, small arteries, capillaries and, venules) and presence of ANCAs against proteinase 3 (PR3) or myeloperoxidase (MPO). They include granulomatosis with polyangiitis (GPA, formerly Wegener granulomatosis), microscopic polyangiitis (MPA), and eosinophilic GPA (EGPA, formerly Churg–Strauss syndrome).[68]

Associations with Antineutrophil Cytoplasmic Antibody-Associated Vasculitis Predisposition

Although first candidate gene studies on AAV focused mainly on ANCA targets, many other genes involved in the immune response were evaluated and several associations were proposed.[69] However, the most relevant insights on the genetic basis of these forms of vasculitis were obtained from one large-scale genetic scan performed in Europeans (including patients with GPA and MPA) and 2 in North Americans (one including only patients with GPA and the other patients with GPA and MPA).[70–72] All 3 studies highlighted HLA-DPB1 as the major contributor of AAV genetic risk (particularly HLA-DPB1*0401 in GPA), although associations with other HLA class II genes (such as HLA-DPA1, HLA-DQA1 and HLA-DQB1) were also described. The higher association signals within the HLA region were detected when the analyses were carried out accordingly with the autoantibody status instead of the clinical subtype, suggesting a crucial role of the HLA system in the production of ANCAs (mostly anti-PR3).[70,72]

Outside the HLA region, genetic associations surpassing the genome-wide level of significance were described within serpin family A member 1 (SERPINA1, encoding a serine protease inhibitor that protects tissues against the enzymatic activity of inflammatory cells), PTPN22, proteinase 3 (PRTN3, encoding the autoantigen PR3), and semaphorin 6A (SEMA6A, encoding a transmembrane protein with unclear function).[70–72] Similar to that observed for the HLA system, SERPINA1 and PRTN3 showed stronger associations with the autoantibody status (anti-PR3 and anti-MPO) than with the clinical entities.[70,72]

Associations with Neurologic Complications of Antineutrophil Cytoplasmic Antibody-Associated Vasculitis

Despite the relatively high prevalence of neurologic complications in patients with AAV, the genetic component of these manifestations has been barely studied.[73,74] This is because most genetic studies on AAV have been focused on the different disease entities and on the autoantibody status, as previously stated.[69]

Protein tyrosine phosphatase, nonreceptor type 22

After a thorough search in the literature, only one study showing some firm evidence of genetic association with neurologic phenotypes in patients with AAV was found. The study was published in 2005 and followed a candidate gene strategy to evaluate the possible implication of the functional *PTPN22* variant rs2476601-R620W in GPA pre-disposition.[75] *PTPN22* encodes a tyrosine phosphatase with a pivotal role in different processes of the immune response, including both TCR and BCR signaling pathways. Consistently, the rs2476601-R620W variant represents one of most important contributor to disease risk in a wide range of autoimmune conditions, including AAV.[76] The study by Jagiello and colleagues[75] represented the first to report an association between this *PTPN22* allele and GPA (specifically in patients positive for ANCAs). The statistical significance considerably increased when the control group was compared against patients with visual and peripheral nervous system involvement. However, no replication of this finding is available and, therefore, it may be taken with caution.

POLYARTERITIS NODOSA

Polyarteritis nodosa (PAN) is a systemic vasculitis affecting mostly medium-sized arteries (generally related to the lungs' circulation but also to other internal organs such as the kidneys). Similar to AAVs, PAN involves necrotizing inflammation of blood vessels, although it is not associated with ANCA production.[77] Neurologic manifestations due to ischemia (which leads to thrombosis or bleeding) are relatively common in patients with PAN with an advance disease course. They include headache, memory dysfunction, sensory changes, aphasia, hemiplegia, visual manifestations, or mononeuritis multiplex, amongst others.[78]

Association with Deficiency of Adenosine Deaminase Type 2

Recent insights from whole-exome sequencing studies indicate that recessive mutations in all domains of the cat eye syndrome chromosome region candidate 1 (*CECR1*) gene are directly involved in the development of the clinical presentations of several systemic vasculitis, including PAN.[79–81] In this regard, the neurologic manifestations of central and peripheral nervous system represent the most severe phenotypes of these conditions. Those *CECR1* mutations cause a loss-of-function effect on the encoded protein, the adenosine deaminase type 2 (ADA2), disrupting protein dimerization, secretion, and enzymatic activity. Enzyme-replacement therapies and hematopoietic stem cell transplantation are being considered as promising targeted treatments for these vasculopathies associated with deficiency of ADA2.[82]

PRIMARY ANGIITIS OF THE CENTRAL NERVOUS SYSTEM

Primary angiitis of the CNS (PACNS), also known as primary CNS vasculitis, is a very rare vasculitis that involves low to medium caliber vessels of the brain, spinal cord, and the meninges, such as leptomeningeal, cortical, and subcortical arteries. The clinical manifestations range from headache to a variety of severe complications of CNS, such as behavioral dysfunction, transient ischemic attacks, or even coma.[83]

Association with Human Leukocyte Antigen Class I

Because of the low incidence of PACNS, little knowledge has been generated about its genetic component. In this regard, a recent candidate gene study performed in a small population of European origin evaluated the possible implication of the HLA system in the susceptibility to PACNS.[84] The frequencies of classical HLA haplotypes from the class I genes *HLA-A* and *HLA-B*, as well as the class II genes *HLA-DRB1* and *HLA-DQB1* were compared between biopsy-proven cases and controls. None of the analyzed alleles showed evidence of association except for the *HLA-A*69* variant, whose frequency was found significantly higher in the PACNS group in

Table 1
Most relevant non-HLA genetic risk factors for vasculitis predisposition

Vasculitis Form	Locus	Year	Analyzed Populations	N (Case/Control)	Strategy	SNP	Allele	P-Value	Odds Ratio	Reference
BD	IL10	2010	Turkish, Middle East, European, Asian	2430/2660	GWAS	rs1518111	A	3.54E-18	1.45	Remmers et al,[10] 2010
	IL23R/IL12RB2	2010	Japanese, Turkish, Korean	1945/2156	GWAS	rs1800871	T	1.00E-14	1.45	Mizuki et al,[9] 2010
		2010	Turkish, Middle East, European, Asian	2430/2660	GWAS	rs924080	A	6.69E-09	1.28	Remmers et al,[10] 2010
		2010	Japanese, Turkish, Korean	1945/2156	GWAS	rs1495965	G	1.90E-11	1.35	Mizuki et al,[9] 2010
		2016	European	278/1517	Immunochip	rs10889664	T	3.81E-12	2.00	Ortiz-Fernández et al,[13] 2016
	GIMAP4	2013	Korean	379/800	GWAS	rs1608157	C	6.01E-08[a]	2.53	Lee et al,[8] 2013
	ERAP1	2013	Turkish	790/1879	Imputed GWAS	rs17482078	T	4.73E-11[b]	4.56	Kirino et al,[11] 2013
	CCR1-CCR3	2013	Turkish, Japanese	2606/2580	Imputed GWAS	rs7616215	C	4.30E-13	0.72	Kirino et al,[11] 2013
	STAT4	2013	Turkish, Japanese	2583/2596	Imputed GWAS	rs7574070	A	1.29E-09	1.27	Kirino et al,[11] 2013
	KLRC4	2013	Turkish, Japanese	2545/2542	Imputed GWAS	rs2617170	T	1.34E-09	0.78	Kirino et al,[11] 2013
	TNFAIP3	2013	Han Chinese	722/1415	Candidate gene	rs9494885	C	8.35E-10	1.81	Li et al,[19] 2013
	IL12A	2015	European, Middle East, Turkish	2366/10,113	Meta-GWAS	rs17810456	G	1.12E-10	1.66	Kappen et al,[14] 2015
		2016	European	408/2117	Immunochip	rs1874886	A	1.62E-08	1.61	Ortiz-Fernández et al,[13] 2016
	JRKL/CNTN5	2016	European	408/2117	Immunochip	rs2848479	A	3.29E-10	1.66	Ortiz-Fernández et al,[13] 2016

(continued on next page)

Table 1
(continued)

Vasculitis Form	Locus	Year	Analyzed Populations	N (Case/Control)	Strategy	SNP	Allele	P-Value	Odds Ratio	Reference
GCA	PTPN22	2015	European	1651/15,306	Immunochip	rs2476601	A	1.73E-06	1.38	Carmona et al,[44] 2015
	PLG	2017	European	2134/9125	GWAS	rs4252134	C	1.23E-10	1.28	Carmona et al,[45] 2017
	P4HA2	2017	European	2134/9125	GWAS	rs128738	T	4.60E-09	1.32	Carmona et al,[45] 2017
TAK	IL12B	2013	Japanese	379/1985	GWAS	rs6871626	A	1.70E-13	1.75	Terao et al,[46] 2013
		2013	Turkish, European	451/2393	Immunochip	rs56167332	A	2.18E-08	1.54	Saruhan-Direskeneli et al,[47] 2013
	FCGR2A/FCGR3A	2013	Turkish, European	451/1115	Immunochip	rs10919543	G	5.89E-12	1.81	Saruhan-Direskeneli et al,[47] 2013
	IL6	2015	Turkish, European	693/1536	GWAS	rs2069837	G	6.70E-09	0.48	Renauer et al,[48] 2015
	RPS9/LILRB3	2015	Turkish, European	693/1536	GWAS	rs11666543	A	2.34E-08	0.61	Renauer et al,[48] 2015
	21q22	2015	Turkish, European	693/1536	GWAS	rs2836878	A	3.62E-10	0.56	Renauer et al,[48] 2015
AAV	SERPINA1	2012	European	2687/7550	GWAS	rs7151526	A	2.40E-09	0.59	Lyons et al,[70] 2012
		2017	European	1986/4723	GWAS	rs28929474	T	3.09E-12	2.18	Merkel et al,[72] 2017
	SEMA6A	2013	European	1020/2734	GWAS	rs26595	C	2.09E-08	0.74	Xie et al,[71] 2013
	PRTN3	2017	European	1986/4723	GWAS	rs62132293	G	8.60E-11	1.29	Merkel et al,[72] 2017
	PTPN22	2017	European	1986/4723	GWAS	rs6679677	A	1.88E-08	1.40	Merkel et al,[72] 2017

[a] Minor allele dominant model.
[b] Minor allele recessive model.

Table 2
Proposed genetic risk factors for neurologic manifestations in vasculitides

Vasculitis Form	Locus	Phenotype	Year	Analyzed Populations	N (Case/Control)	Strategy	SNP	Allele	P-Value	Odds Ratio	Reference
BD	MBL2	Neurologic involvement	2009	Korean	119/252	Candidate gene	54	A	1.00E-02	6.63	Kim et al,[26] 2009
	HLA-B	Parenchymal involvement	2012	Tunisian	178/125	Candidate gene	N/A	HLA-B51	9.00E-03	N/A	Hamzaoui et al,[22] 2012
		CNS involvement	2014	Turkish	51/44	Candidate gene	N/A	HLA-B51*03	1.50E-02	N/A	Demirseren et al,[24] 2014
	PON1	CNS involvement	2014	Turkish	50/50	Candidate gene	PON-1-L55M	M	2.00E-02	3.10	Dursun et al,[32] 2014
	MVK	Neurologic involvement	2014	Turkish	50/51	Candidate gene	rs104895331	T	1.20E-02	N/A	Arslan Tas et al,[34] 2014
	UBAC2	CNS involvement	2017	Japanese	611/737	Imputed GWAS	rs9517723	T	6.60E-03	2.78	Yamazoe et al,[38] 2017
GCA	IFNG	Visual manifestations	2004	Europeans	59/129	Candidate gene	microsatellite (intron 1)	3	1.00E-02	3.13	Gonzalez-Gay et al,[64] 2004
	VEGF	Visual manifestations	2005	Europeans	103/226	Candidate gene	rs2010963	C	2.10E-02	1.75	Rueda et al,[51] 2005
TAK	MICA	Ischemic brain disease	2018	Chinese	412/597	Candidate gene	rs9366782	T	3.00E-02	1.78	Wen et al,[67] 2018
AAV	PTPN22	Peripheral nervous system involvement in GPA	2005	Europeans	199/399	Candidate gene	rs2476601	A	8.00E-04	2.29	Jagiello et al,[75] 2005
PACNS	HLA-A	Whole disease	2017	Europeans	25/44	Candidate gene	N/A	HLA-A*69	2.00E-03	N/A	Kraemer et al,[84] 2017

comparison with the control one. Future large-scale genetic studies will inform about the exact effect size of this potential HLA association in the susceptibility to PACNS.

SUMMARY

The use of novel technologies for high-throughput genotyping and, most importantly, the establishment of large collaborative groups, have allowed a substantial increase in the understanding of the genetic network underlying vasculitis predisposition (**Table 1**). However, because most vasculitides are rare diseases with a complex etiology (in which genetic risk is conferred by hundreds of *loci* with a low effect independently), only a tiny fraction of their heritability has been unmasked despite the great efforts made. These limitations become even higher when the studies focus on the analysis of specific clinical manifestations, because the statistical power is considerably reduced. Because of it, very few associations with neurologic complications of vasculitides have been published to date and those reported have not been replicated in independent studies (**Table 2**). Therefore, combined efforts are still needed to successfully tackle the exciting challenge of deciphering the genetic influence of nervous system–related phenotypes in patients with vasculitis. Certainly, the results of such efforts will definitively help to improve the management of these severe clinical complications in the clinical practice, which will affect both the life expectancy and quality of many affected people.

ACKNOWLEDGMENTS

FDC was recipient of a grant from the "Ramón y Cajal" program of the Spanish Ministry of Economy and Competitiveness (RYC-2014-16458). RL-M and AM were recipients of a Miguel Servet type I program fellowship from the ISCIII, co-funded by the European Social Fund (ESF, "Investing in your future") (grants CP16/00033 and CP17/00008, respectively). JM and MAGG were founded by Instituto de Salud Carlos III (ISCIII), Spain, through the RETICS Programs RD16/0012/0004 and RD16/0012/0009 (RIER).

REFERENCES

1. Gonzalez-Gay MA, Garcia-Porrua C. Epidemiology of the vasculitides. Rheum Dis Clin North Am 2001;27:729–49.
2. Jennette JC, Falk RJ, Bacon PA, et al. 2012 revised International Chapel Hill consensus conference nomenclature of vasculitides. Arthritis Rheum 2013;65:1–11.
3. Sunderkotter CH, Zelger B, Chen KR, et al. Nomenclature of cutaneous vasculitis: dermatologic addendum to the 2012 revised international Chapel Hill consensus conference nomenclature of vasculitides. Arthritis Rheumatol 2018;70:171–84.
4. Carmona FD, Martin J, Gonzalez-Gay MA. Genetics of vasculitis. Curr Opin Rheumatol 2015;27:10–7.
5. Ramirez GA, Maugeri N, Sabbadini MG, et al. Intravascular immunity as a key to systemic vasculitis: a work in progress, gaining momentum. Clin Exp Immunol 2014;175:150–66.
6. Yazici H, Seyahi E, Hatemi G, et al. Behcet syndrome: a contemporary view. Nat Rev Rheumatol 2018;14:107–19.
7. Kidd DP. Neurological complications of Behcet's syndrome. J Neurol 2017;264: 2178–83.
8. Lee YJ, Horie Y, Wallace GR, et al. Genome-wide association study identifies GI-MAP as a novel susceptibility locus for Behcet's disease. Ann Rheum Dis 2013; 72:1510–6.

9. Mizuki N, Meguro A, Ota M, et al. Genome-wide association studies identify IL23R-IL12RB2 and IL10 as Behcet's disease susceptibility loci. Nat Genet 2010;42:703–6.
10. Remmers EF, Cosan F, Kirino Y, et al. Genome-wide association study identifies variants in the MHC class I, IL10, and IL23R-IL12RB2 regions associated with Behcet's disease. Nat Genet 2010;42:698–702.
11. Kirino Y, Bertsias G, Ishigatsubo Y, et al. Genome-wide association analysis identifies new susceptibility loci for Behcet's disease and epistasis between HLA-B*51 and ERAP1. Nat Genet 2013;45:202–7.
12. Hughes T, Coit P, Adler A, et al. Identification of multiple independent susceptibility loci in the HLA region in Behcet's disease. Nat Genet 2013;45:319–24.
13. Ortiz-Fernández L, Carmona FD, Montes-Cano MA, et al. Genetic analysis with the immunochip platform in Behcet Disease. Identification of residues associated in the HLA class I region and new susceptibility loci. PLoS One 2016;11: e0161305.
14. Kappen JH, Medina-Gomez C, van Hagen PM, et al. Genome-wide association study in an admixed case series reveals IL12A as a new candidate in Behcet disease. PLoS One 2015;10:e0119085.
15. Meguro A, Inoko H, Ota M, et al. Genetics of Behcet disease inside and outside the MHC. Ann Rheum Dis 2010;69:747–54.
16. Fei Y, Webb R, Cobb BL, et al. Identification of novel genetic susceptibility loci for Behcet's disease using a genome-wide association study. Arthritis Res Ther 2009;11:R66.
17. Wallace GR. HLA-B*51 the primary risk in Behcet disease. Proc Natl Acad Sci U S A 2014;111:8706–7.
18. Ombrello MJ, Kirino Y, de Bakker PI, et al. Behcet disease-associated MHC class I residues implicate antigen binding and regulation of cell-mediated cytotoxicity. Proc Natl Acad Sci U S A 2014;111:8867–72.
19. Li H, Liu Q, Hou S, et al. TNFAIP3 gene polymorphisms confer risk for Behcet's disease in a Chinese Han population. Hum Genet 2013;132:293–300.
20. Bakir-Gungor B, Remmers EF, Meguro A, et al. Identification of possible pathogenic pathways in Behcet's disease using genome-wide association study data from two different populations. Eur J Hum Genet 2015;23:678–87.
21. Salmaninejad A, Gowhari A, Hosseini S, et al. Genetics and immunodysfunction underlying Behcet's disease and immunomodulant treatment approaches. J Immunotoxicol 2017;14:137–51.
22. Hamzaoui A, Houman MH, Massouadia M, et al. Contribution of HLA-B51 in the susceptibility and specific clinical features of Behcet's disease in Tunisian patients. Eur J Intern Med 2012;23:347–9.
23. Maldini C, Lavalley MP, Cheminant M, et al. Relationships of HLA-B51 or B5 genotype with Behcet's disease clinical characteristics: systematic review and meta-analyses of observational studies. Rheumatology (Oxford) 2012;51: 887–900.
24. Demirseren DD, Ceylan GG, Akoglu G, et al. HLA-B51 subtypes in Turkish patients with Behcet's disease and their correlation with clinical manifestations. Genet Mol Res 2014;13:4788–96.
25. Turner MW, Hamvas RM. Mannose-binding lectin: structure, function, genetics and disease associations. Rev Immunogenet 2000;2:305–22.
26. Kim J, Im CH, Kang EH, et al. Mannose-binding lectin gene-2 polymorphisms and serum mannose-binding lectin levels in Behcet's disease. Clin Exp Rheumatol 2009;27:S13–7.

27. Yang Y, Tan H, Deng B, et al. Genetic polymorphisms of C-type lectin receptors in Behcet's disease in a Chinese Han population. Sci Rep 2017;7:5348.

28. Mackness MI, Arrol S, Durrington PN. Paraoxonase prevents accumulation of lipoperoxides in low-density lipoprotein. FEBS Lett 1991;286:152–4.

29. Espinola-Zavaleta N, Soto-Lopez ME, Carreon-Torres E, et al. Altered flow-mediated vasodilatation, low paraoxonase-1 activity, and abnormal high-density lipoprotein subclass distribution in Takayasu's arteritis. Circ J 2009;73:760–6.

30. Huesca-Gomez C, Soto ME, Castrejon-Tellez V, et al. PON1 gene polymorphisms and plasma PON1 activities in Takayasu's arteritis disease. Immunol Lett 2013; 152:77–82.

31. Yilmaz A, Emre S, Agachan B, et al. Effect of paraoxonase 1 gene polymorphisms on clinical course of Henoch-Schonlein purpura. J Nephrol 2009;22:726–32.

32. Dursun A, Cicek S, Keni FM, et al. The relation of PON1-L55M gene polymorphism and clinical manifestation of Behcet's disease. Acta Biochim Pol 2014; 61:271–4.

33. Mandey SH, Schneiders MS, Koster J, et al. Mutational spectrum and genotype-phenotype correlations in mevalonate kinase deficiency. Hum Mutat 2006;27: 796–802.

34. Arslan Tas D, Erken E, Yildiz F, et al. Mevalonate kinase gene mutations and their clinical correlations in Behcet's disease. Int J Rheum Dis 2014;17:435–43.

35. Gul A. Genetics of Behcet's disease: lessons learned from genomewide association studies. Curr Opin Rheumatol 2014;26:56–63.

36. Sawalha AH, Hughes T, Nadig A, et al. A putative functional variant within the UBAC2 gene is associated with increased risk of Behcet's disease. Arthritis Rheum 2011;63:3607–12.

37. Hou S, Shu Q, Jiang Z, et al. Replication study confirms the association between UBAC2 and Behcet's disease in two independent Chinese sets of patients and controls. Arthritis Res Ther 2012;14:R70.

38. Yamazoe K, Meguro A, Takeuchi M, et al. Comprehensive analysis of the association between UBAC2 polymorphisms and Behcet's disease in a Japanese population. Sci Rep 2017;7:742.

39. Zhang X, Smits AH, van Tilburg GB, et al. An interaction landscape of ubiquitin signaling. Mol Cell 2017;65:941–55.e8.

40. Gonzalez-Gay MA, Vazquez-Rodriguez TR, Lopez-Diaz MJ, et al. Epidemiology of giant cell arteritis and polymyalgia rheumatica. Arthritis Rheum 2009;61: 1454–61.

41. Mason JC. Takayasu arteritis–advances in diagnosis and management. Nat Rev Rheumatol 2010;6:406–15.

42. Renauer P, Sawalha AH. The genetics of Takayasu arteritis. Presse Med 2017;46: e179–87.

43. Carmona FD, Gonzalez-Gay MA, Martin J. Genetic component of giant cell arteritis. Rheumatology (Oxford) 2014;53:6–18.

44. Carmona FD, Mackie SL, Martin JE, et al. A large-scale genetic analysis reveals a strong contribution of the HLA class II region to giant cell arteritis susceptibility. Am J Hum Genet 2015;96:565–80.

45. Carmona FD, Vaglio A, Mackie SL, et al. A genome-wide association study identifies risk alleles in plasminogen and P4HA2 associated with giant cell arteritis. Am J Hum Genet 2017;100:64–74.

46. Terao C, Yoshifuji H, Kimura A, et al. Two susceptibility loci to Takayasu arteritis reveal a synergistic role of the IL12B and HLA-B regions in a Japanese population. Am J Hum Genet 2013;93:289–97.

47. Saruhan-Direskeneli G, Hughes T, Aksu K, et al. Identification of multiple genetic susceptibility loci in Takayasu arteritis. Am J Hum Genet 2013;93:298–305.

48. Renauer PA, Saruhan-Direskeneli G, Coit P, et al. Identification of susceptibility loci in IL6, RPS9/LILRB3, and an intergenic locus on chromosome 21q22 in takayasu arteritis in a genome-wide association study. Arthritis Rheumatol 2015; 67:1361–8.

49. Carmona FD, Coit P, Saruhan-Direskeneli G, et al. Analysis of the common genetic component of large-vessel vasculitides through a meta-Immunochip strategy. Sci Rep 2017;7:43953.

50. Gonzalez-Gay MA, Castaneda S, Llorca J. Giant cell arteritis: visual loss is our major concern. J Rheumatol 2016;43:1458–61.

51. Rueda B, Lopez-Nevot MA, Lopez-Diaz MJ, et al. A functional variant of vascular endothelial growth factor is associated with severe ischemic complications in giant cell arteritis. J Rheumatol 2005;32:1737–41.

52. Baldini M, Maugeri N, Ramirez GA, et al. Selective up-regulation of the soluble pattern-recognition receptor pentraxin 3 and of vascular endothelial growth factor in giant cell arteritis: relevance for recent optic nerve ischemia. Arthritis Rheum 2012;64:854–65.

53. Enjuanes A, Benavente Y, Hernandez-Rodriguez J, et al. Association of NOS2 and potential effect of VEGF, IL6, CCL2 and IL1RN polymorphisms and haplotypes on susceptibility to GCA–a simultaneous study of 130 potentially functional SNPs in 14 candidate genes. Rheumatology (Oxford) 2012;51:841–51.

54. Boiardi L, Casali B, Nicoli D, et al. Vascular endothelial growth factor gene polymorphisms in giant cell arteritis. J Rheumatol 2003;30:2160–4.

55. Neufeld G, Cohen T, Gengrinovitch S, et al. Vascular endothelial growth factor (VEGF) and its receptors. FASEB J 1999;13:9–22.

56. Wen Z, Shen Y, Berry G, et al. The microvascular niche instructs T cells in large vessel vasculitis via the VEGF-Jagged1-Notch pathway. Sci Transl Med 2017; 9(399) [pii:eaal3322].

57. Cid MC, Hernandez-Rodriguez J, Esteban MJ, et al. Tissue and serum angiogenic activity is associated with low prevalence of ischemic complications in patients with giant-cell arteritis. Circulation 2002;106:1664–71.

58. Kaiser M, Younge B, Bjornsson J, et al. Formation of new vasa vasorum in vasculitis. Production of angiogenic cytokines by multinucleated giant cells. Am J Pathol 1999;155:765–74.

59. Weyand CM, Hicok KC, Hunder GG, et al. Tissue cytokine patterns in patients with polymyalgia rheumatica and giant cell arteritis. Ann Intern Med 1994;121: 484–91.

60. Weyand CM, Tetzlaff N, Bjornsson J, et al. Disease patterns and tissue cytokine profiles in giant cell arteritis. Arthritis Rheum 1997;40:19–26.

61. Weyand CM, Younge BR, Goronzy JJ. IFN-gamma and IL-17: the two faces of T-cell pathology in giant cell arteritis. Curr Opin Rheumatol 2011;23:43–9.

62. Coit P, De Lott LB, Nan B, et al. DNA methylation analysis of the temporal artery microenvironment in giant cell arteritis. Ann Rheum Dis 2016;75:1196–202.

63. Amoli MM, Gonzalez-Gay MA, Zeggini E, et al. Epistatic interactions between HLA-DRB1 and interleukin 4, but not interferon-gamma, increase susceptibility to giant cell arteritis. J Rheumatol 2004;31:2413–7.

64. Gonzalez-Gay MA, Hajeer AH, Dababneh A, et al. Interferon-gamma gene microsatellite polymorphisms in patients with biopsy-proven giant cell arteritis and isolated polymyalgia rheumatica. Clin Exp Rheumatol 2004;22:S18–20.

65. Keser G, Aksu K, Direskeneli H. Takayasu arteritis: an update. Turk J Med Sci 2018;48:681–97.
66. Cantu C, Pineda C, Barinagarrementeria F, et al. Noninvasive cerebrovascular assessment of Takayasu arteritis. Stroke 2000;31:2197–202.
67. Wen X, Chen S, Li J, et al. Association between genetic variants in the human leukocyte antigen-B/MICA and Takayasu arteritis in Chinese Han population. Int J Rheum Dis 2018;21:271–7.
68. Chen M, Kallenberg CG. ANCA-associated vasculitides–advances in pathogenesis and treatment. Nat Rev Rheumatol 2010;6:653–64.
69. Ugarte-Gil MF, Espinoza LR. Genetics of ANCA-associated Vasculitides. Curr Rheumatol Rep 2014;16:428.
70. Lyons PA, Rayner TF, Trivedi S, et al. Genetically distinct subsets within ANCA-associated vasculitis. N Engl J Med 2012;367:214–23.
71. Xie G, Roshandel D, Sherva R, et al. Association of granulomatosis with polyangiitis (Wegener's) with HLA-DPB1*04 and SEMA6A gene variants: evidence from genome-wide analysis. Arthritis Rheum 2013;65:2457–68.
72. Merkel PA, Xie G, Monach PA, et al. Identification of functional and expression polymorphisms associated with risk for antineutrophil cytoplasmic autoantibody-associated vasculitis. Arthritis Rheumatol 2017;69:1054–66.
73. Imboden JB. Involvement of the peripheral nervous system in polyarteritis nodosa and antineutrophil cytoplasmic antibodies-associated vasculitis. Rheum Dis Clin North Am 2017;43:633–9.
74. Graf J. Central nervous system disease in antineutrophil cytoplasmic antibodies-associated vasculitis. Rheum Dis Clin North Am 2017;43:573–8.
75. Jagiello P, Aries P, Arning L, et al. The PTPN22 620W allele is a risk factor for Wegener's granulomatosis. Arthritis Rheum 2005;52:4039–43.
76. Carmona FD, Martin J. The potential of PTPN22 as a therapeutic target for rheumatoid arthritis. Expert Opin Ther Targets 2018;22:879–91.
77. Forbess L, Bannykh S. Polyarteritis nodosa. Rheum Dis Clin North Am 2015;41: 33–46, vii.
78. Younger DS. Vasculitis of the nervous system. Curr Opin Neurol 2004;17:317–36.
79. Zhou Q, Yang D, Ombrello AK, et al. Early-onset stroke and vasculopathy associated with mutations in ADA2. N Engl J Med 2014;370:911–20.
80. Navon Elkan P, Pierce SB, Segel R, et al. Mutant adenosine deaminase 2 in a polyarteritis nodosa vasculopathy. N Engl J Med 2014;370:921–31.
81. Caorsi R, Penco F, Grossi A, et al. ADA2 deficiency (DADA2) as an unrecognised cause of early onset polyarteritis nodosa and stroke: a multicentre national study. Ann Rheum Dis 2017;76:1648–56.
82. Meyts I, Aksentijevich I. Deficiency of adenosine deaminase 2 (DADA2): updates on the phenotype, genetics, pathogenesis, and treatment. J Clin Immunol 2018; 38:569–78.
83. Hajj-Ali RA, Calabrese LH. Diagnosis and classification of central nervous system vasculitis. J Autoimmun 2014;48-49:149–52.
84. Kraemer M, Becker J, Horn PA, et al. Association of primary central nervous system vasculitis with the presence of specific human leucocyte antigen gene variant. Clin Neurol Neurosurg 2017;160:137–41.

The Blood-Brain Barrier
Implications for Vasculitis

David S. Younger, MD, MPH, MS[a,b,*]

KEYWORDS

- Blood-brain barrier • Primary • Secondary • Vasculitis • Autoimmune
- Nervous system

KEY POINTS

- There has been extraordinary research in the blood-brain barrier over the past decade.
- The blood-brain barrier is fully functional in development and vital in cerebrovascular angiogenesis.
- The cellular components and other molecular constituents of the blood-brain barrier, contained in a neurovascular unit, protect the central nervous system from injury and systemic diseases.
- Blood-brain barrier disruption is now recognized as an important factor in a variety of primary neurologic diseases.
- This article reviews the history, neurodevelopment, ultrastructure, function, and clinico-pathologic correlation and relevance to central nervous system vasculitis.

INTRODUCTION

The past decade has witnessed an expansion of knowledge in the properties possessed by the blood-brain barrier (BBB) in health and disease summarized in several excellent recent reviews.[1–5] In essence, the neurovascular unit of the BBB is composed of capillary vascular and neural cells, extracellular matrix components, and a variety of immune cells that mediate local immunity contained in the neurovascular unit (NVU). The schematized and electron microscopic (EM) appearance of cerebral capillaries in the BBB, shown in **Figs. 1** and **2**, demonstrates layers of pericytes adherent to the abluminal or parenchymal surface of endothelial cells,

Disclosure Statement: The author has nothing to disclose.
[a] Department of Neurology, Division of Neuro-Epidemiology, New York University School of Medicine, New York, NY 10016, USA; [b] School of Public Health, City University of New York, New York, NY, USA
* 333 East 34th Street, Suite 1J, New York, NY 10016.
E-mail address: youngd01@nyu.edu
Website: http://www.davidsyounger.com

Neurol Clin 37 (2019) 235–248
https://doi.org/10.1016/j.ncl.2019.01.009
0733-8619/19/© 2019 Elsevier Inc. All rights reserved.

neurologic.theclinics.com

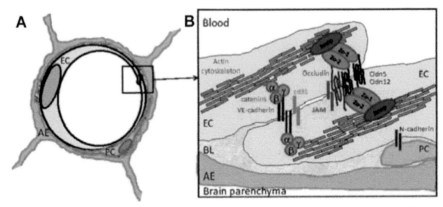

Fig. 1. (*A*) A capillary in the human BBB over an endothelial TJ. (*B*) The insert shows the molecular composition of tight and adherens junctions. See text for details. (*From* Daneman R. The blood-brain barrier in health and disease. Ann Neurol 2012;72:649; with permission.)

together surrounded by a layer of basal lamina composed of extracellular matrix protein molecules. The end-feet of neighboring astrocyte processes ensheathes the blood vessels. Monolayers of adjacent endothelial cells that form tight junction (TJ) strands, shown in **Fig. 1**, connect adjacent endothelial cells by adhesions of trans-membrane (occludin, claudin, and junctional associated molecules [JAM]) across the intercellular space, whereas cytoplasmic scaffolding and regulatory proteins, such as zona occludens type 1 and 2 (ZO-1, ZO-2), provide linkage to the actin cyto-skeleton and initiate several signaling mechanisms via protein-protein interactions. Endothelia BBB cells are also linked by adherens junctions composed of vascular

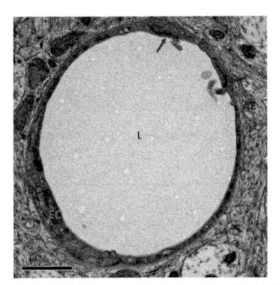

Fig. 2. EM of a capillary in the adult murine BBB. Endothelial cells are held together by TJs (*red arrow*). L, lumen. (*From* Daneman R. The blood-brain barrier in health and disease. Ann Neurol 2012;72:648–72; with permission.)

endothelial (VE)-cadherin, which mediates cell-cell adhesion interactions, linking adherens junctions to the actin cytoskeleton via catenins.[2,3] Perivascular macrophages that reside between astrocyte end-feet and the vessel wall, mast cells associated with specific regions of the central nervous system (CNS), resident microglia that act as antigen-presenting cells, circulating leukocytes that can penetrate the intact BBB via interactions with endothelial cell adhesion molecules (CAM) to mediate bidirectional cross-talk between immune cells and endothelium for normal surveillance, constitute the extended neurovascular unit.[2]

Breakdown or disruption of the BBB that accompanies a variety of inflammatory and autoimmune, neoplastic, infectious, and neurodegenerative CNS disorders, notably stroke, multiple sclerosis, brain trauma, human immune virus, infection, and Alzheimer disease. These disorders are associated with the abnormal entry of plasma components, immune molecules, and cellular elements that lead to further neural dysfunction and varying degrees of irreversible neural degeneration. Although there is little known about the role of BBB breakdown in primary and secondary CNS vasculitis, future progress could lead to improved understanding of primary and secondary forms of CNS vasculitis[6] with the prospect of even improving the outcome of 2 potentially devastating disorders, childhood and adult primary angiitis of the CNS.[7–9] According to Weiss and colleagues,[10] further understanding of the BBB could envision the use of new therapeutic strategies that bypass it, taking advantage of the selective expression of membrane-bound proteins expressed by brain endothelia cells or circulating leukocytes to target new drugs as well as improve the effectiveness of conventional systemic immunosuppression. This article reviews the history, neurodevelopment, ultrastructure, function, and clinicopathologic correlation and relevance to CNS vasculitis.

HISTORICAL BACKGROUND

In 1885, Ehrlich[11] provided the first suggestion of the presence of a barrier when a parenteral injection of vital dye into the bloodstream of mice penetrated practically every systemic organ except the brain, turning them dark purplish-blue, leaving the brain and spinal cord pale white-yellow. Ehrlich himself thought that this difference was due to a low binding affinity. The existence of a barrier at the level of the cerebral vessels was postulated by Bield and Kraus[12] and later by Goldman[13] and Lewandowsky[14] at the turn of the twentieth century, who jointly interpreted their experience in favor of a true BBB, later termed *Blut-Hirn-Schranke*. In 1967, Reese and Karnovsky[15] demonstrated a structural barrier to an intravenous injection of horseradish peroxidase (HRP) demonstrating exogenous peroxidase to the lumina of blood vessels and in some micropinocytotic vesicles within endothelial cells, but none beyond the vascular endothelium. The relatively scarce number of vesicles was a morphologic feature of a functioning BBB. Their findings localized at a fine structural level a barrier composed of the plasma membrane and the cell body of endothelial cells and TJ between adjacent cells of the cerebral cortex. In 1969, EM studies by Brightman and Reese[16] in the mouse conclusively demonstrated endothelial and epithelia TJ that occluded the interspaces between blood and parenchyma or cerebral ventricles, constituting the ultrastructural basis for the blood-brain and blood-cerebrospinal fluid barriers. Feder[17] noted active exclusion of the small electron-dense tracer microperoxidase by intact TJ after parenteral injection supplementing the findings of Reese and Karnovsky.[15] Nagy and colleagues[18] examined fracture faces of cerebral endothelium in normal and hyperosmolar mannitol-treated rat brains to elucidate the organization of TJ in various segments of the cerebral vascular bed and the structural basis of BBB opening in hyperosmotic conditions. Their findings provided no direct evidence for the structural basis of BBB opening in hyperosmolar mannitol-treated rat brains, noting extended TJ regions in capillaries and postcapillary venues. Shivers and co-workers[19] studied isolated rat brain capillaries using freeze-fracture images of interendothelial ZO revealing complex arrays of intramembrane ridges and grooves characteristic of TJ. The ZO of these capillary endothelial cells were considered very tight.

NEURODEVELOPMENT

In contrast to neuronal development, the vascular system undergoes blood vessel formation through the 2 distinct processes: vasculogenesis and angiogenesis. The former commences with endothelial differentiation from angioblasts to vascular plexuses, whereas the latter is associated with sprouting of new vessels from existing ones. Both vasculogenesis and angiogenesis are influenced by vascular endothelial growth factor (VEGF), a major attractive molecule for extending blood vessels, especially endothelial tip cells,[20] as well as by other molecules, blood flow, and contact with surrounding tissues. Found at the growing end of extending vessels, the shaft of extending endothelial tip cells is composed of an endothelial cell chain made of stalk cells similar to the axon growth cone and its associated axonal shaft. In vivo imaging using green fluorescent protein (GFP) depicts the advancing endothelial tip cell navigating the environment and sprouting from existing vasculature.[21]

Several experimental observations have suggested the importance of the neurodevelopment of the BBB.[5]

First, there are shared molecular and cellular mechanisms in both neurogenesis and angiogenesis.[22,23] Various axon guidance pathways from members of the 4 major families of axon guidance ligand-receptor pairs, including Slit/Robo, semaphoring/plexin/neuropilin, Netrin/Unc5/DCC, and Ephrin/Eph, that mediate complex cellular navigational programs within axons as both chemoattractants and repellents, also direct angiogenic tip cells toward their final destinations. Neuropilin-1 is necessary for endothelial tip cell guidance in the developing CNS.[24] Moreover, axonal terminal arborization parallels vessel sprouting. Similar to hypoxic tissue that secretes VEGF via hypoxia-inducible factor, a transcription factor that promotes cell survival through the downstream activation of numerous genes including VEGF,[25] axonal terminals devoid of synaptic input secrete nerve growth factor, the expression of which is downregulated when innervation occurs.

Second, there is coregulation of these 2 systems in developing embryonic and adult brains.[22,26,27] Stubbs and colleagues[26] found that blood vessels provided a supporting niche in regions of adult neurogenesis. The investigators[26] used Tbr2-GFP transgenic mice that served as a correlate for the expression of the intermediate progenitor cell (IPC) T-box transcription factor Tbr2, to examine the proximity of dividing cells in the subventricular zone (SVZ) and ventricular zone of the shaking rat Kawasaki and reeler mutant mouse in relation to blood vessels throughout neurogenesis. Their findings, which included the extension of neuritis toward and along labeled blood vessels, supported the notion of vascular-neuronal interactions in development. Javaherian and Kriegstein,[27] who likewise studied IPC in the SVZ of embryonic Swiss Webster mouse cortices, used confocal microscopy to image the vast network of capillaries in the SV and SVZ. The investigators[27] noted that Tbr2 cells divided near vascular branch points, suggesting endothelial tip cells contributed to the neurogenic niche for IPC, with ectopic overexpression of VEGF-A in a pattern that followed that of blood vessel development. These findings indicated that the developing cortical vasculature provided a microenvironment within the SVZ in which IPC accumulated and divided during neurogenesis.

Third, a structural and functional BBB complete with TJ appears as soon as cerebral vessels penetrate the CNS parenchyma.[28,29] Johansson and colleagues[28] explained that the widely held view that the BBB was immature during development stemmed from teleologic interpretations and experimental observations of high cerebrospinal fluid protein levels in fetal cerebrospinal fluid and the apparent passive passage of biomarkers during development. Instead, the blood–cerebrospinal fluid barrier, like the BBB, is functionally and morphologically mature from very early in development. The investigators maintain that inconsistent terminology used in the literature, such as leaky, immature, and developing, used to describe the barrier gives a connotation of TJ that is more permeable than their adult counterparts without evidence to support this concept. Mølgård and Saunders[30] noted well-formed complex TJ across cerebral endothelial cells in human embryos and fetuses by freeze fracture and thin-section EM by 8 weeks of age, commensurate with the differentiation of brain capillaries. Efflux transporters are likewise expressed in cerebral endothelial and choroid plexus epithelial cells early in the fetal and postnatal rats.[31] Ballabh and colleagues[32] studied the expression and quantification of endothelial TJ molecules, including claudin-5, occluding, and JAM, by immunohistochemistry and Western blot analysis in blood vessels of germinal matrix, cortex, and white matter of fetuses and premature infants gestational age 16 to 40 weeks. The investigators[32] noted no significant decrease in the expression of the endothelial TJ molecules claudin-5, occludin, and JAM-1 as a function of gestational age in germinal matrix compared with cortex and white matter, suggesting that they were unlikely to be responsible for germinal matrix fragility and vulnerability to hemorrhage in premature infants. These findings are consistent with the concept that TJ molecules develop and perhaps mature early during human gestation. Ballabh and colleagues[33] observed that a paucity of TJ or pericytes coupled with incomplete coverage of blood vessels by astrocyte end-feet, could instead account for the observed fragility of blood vessels in the germinal matrix of premature infants. Braun and colleagues[34] found that pericytes coverage and density were less in the germinal matrix vasculature than in the cortex or white matter in human fetuses, premature infants, and premature rabbit pups. Although VEGF suppression significantly enhanced pericyte coverage in germinal matrix, it remained less than in other brain regions.

NEUROBIOLOGY AND CELLULAR INTERACTIONS
Endothelial Cell Interactions

The existence of the endothelial cell was first surmised by William Harvey, first observed by Marcello Malpighi in blood capillaries using compound microscopy in the nineteenth century, and later by EM in the mid-twentieth century, revealing the presence of plasmalemmal vesicles or caveolae. The ability to culture EC later permitted even more detailed investigation of their activation and function in vivo. Derived from mesoderm via the differentiation of hemangioblasts and angioblasts, there are a few protein/messenger RNA marker candidates, including platelet/endothelial cell adhesion molecule (PECAM)-1 in monocytes and VE-cadherin in fetal stem cells. Endothelial cells of the BBB not only provide a physical barrier between the systemic circulation and the brain but also assure the selective inward passage of ions, nutrients, and neuropeptides via specialized transport mechanisms. Sodium, potassium, chloride, hydrogen, bicarbonate, and calcium ions are transported across the BBB via transporters located mainly along the luminal surface of endothelial cells, including the sodium and potassium adenosine triphosphate (ATP) -dependent transport pump, the sodium-potassium-chloride cotransporter, sodium-proton, chloride-bicarbonate, and sodium calcium exchanges that assure optimal levels of brain electrolyte levels and intracellular pH. The transport of essential nutrients is assured by members of the solute-linked carriers (SLC) superfamily, located variably along the luminal and abluminal membrane, including glucose transporter-1, monocarboxylic acid-1, excitatory, organic acid, cation, amine, and choline transporters, respectively, to transport lactate and ketone bodies as alternative energy neuronal sources, and sodium-independent or -dependent removal of glutamate, aspartate, glutamine, histidine, and asparagine from the interstitial compartment of the brain. Other specific carrier-mediated transporters mediate the passage of transferrin, low-density lipoproteins, leptin, immunoglobulin G, insulin, and growth factors via receptor-mediated transcytosis via binding of the protein to specific receptors on the endothelial cell surface followed by endocytosis of the ligand-receptor complex with passage across the cytoplasm and exocytosis at the opposite side of the cell[35] and via the formation of caveolae or vesicle formation for the transport of macromolecules.[36] Transmigration of cellular elements across endothelial cells of the BBB during inflammation, including leukocytes, neoplastic cells, and pathogenic viruses, bacteria and yeasts, investigated in experimental animal models using HRP, highlighted the role of caveolae as minitransporters of the CNS.[36] Unique systems of modified caveolae that fuse together forming transendothelial cell channels and later vesiculocanalicular or vesiculotubular structures or vesiculovacuolar organelles appear to be an important gateway to the CNS in damaged endothelial cell populations.[36] Transportation of potentially toxic endogenous or xenobiotic lipid-soluble nonpolar molecules from the brain to the blood is accomplished by transporters located along the luminal membrane, such as the ATP binding cassette transporter P-glycoprotein 1 (multidrug resistance protein 1 or ATP-binding cassette subfamily B member 1), respectively, important in the distribution of CNS tumor drug treatment[37] and the active efflux of the anti–human immunodeficiency virus type 1 (HIV1) nucleoside drug abacavir at the BBB,[38–40] and breast-cancer resistance protein and multidrug resistance related protein (MRP) 1, 2, 4, and 5 efflux transporter pumps that serve as defense mechanisms and determinate bioavailability and concentration of many CNS drugs important in the treatment of CNS cancers,[41] such as the novel tyrosine kinase inhibitor dasatinib,[42] and the efflux transportation of the protease inhibitor lopinavir that contributes to its poor oral bioavailability in the treatment of HIV1.[43] The neuroinflammation and progression of damage associated with focal cerebral ischemia appear to be modulated by upregulation of other MRP protein molecules that activate Toll-like receptor signaling contributing to neuroinflammation and progression of ischemic cerebral damage.[44]

Transendothelial migration of circulating leukocytes involves a multistep process. Leukocyte adhesion molecules expressed on the surface of EC initiate binding of leukocytes as a beginning step in the in their entry in brain tissue, which later includes rolling adhesion to EC, firm adhesion, and transmigration. Although less well understood, the molecular mechanism is thought to involve endothelial CAM, including CD99, PECAM-1/CD31, vascular CAM-1 (VCAM-1) (important in firm adhesion); junctional adhesion molecule-1; and expression of leukocyte adhesion molecules E- and P-selectin (rolling adhesion); cytokine responsiveness so noted in situ and in cell culture,[45,46] and expression of the integrins alpha-4 and beta-2. Inflamed capillary endothelia support transmigration of different subsets of leukocytes. There are 2 routes for leukocytes to pass through endothelial cells: the so-called paracellular route, or through the endothelial cell itself or transcellular route. The BBB with its abundance of TJ complexes relies primarily on the transcellular route as it does for solute and fluid transport. *Neutrophil recruitment is partially dependent on ICAM-1, and express L-selectin and lymphocyte function-associated antigen-1 but not chemokine C motif receptor 7 may explain why granulocytes roll but do not arrest for transmigration in high endothelial venules.

Pericyte Interactions

Brain endothelial cells are exposed to a myriad of pericyte interactions[47] in the regulation of brain angiogenesis, endothelial cell TJ formation, as well as the differentiation, microvascular vasodynamic capacity, structural stability, and neuroimmunologic network operations of the intact BBB.[48] Rouget[49] first ascribed capillary contractility to pericytes, but Zimmerman[50] named the cell and described its morphologic aspects. The presence of smooth muscle cells in association with pericytes and the absence of a smooth muscle layer from capillaries and postcapillary venues influenced early views ascribing contractile properties to narrow capillaries, hence regulating microvascular flow even though several subsequent experimental studies failed to substantiate it.[51,52] Smooth muscle actin was conclusively demonstrated in pericytes by immunocytochemistry using smooth muscle α-actin isoform-specific antibodies and immunogold labeling in conjunction with EM, noting that smooth muscle α-actin expression in capillaries was limited exclusively to pericytes and not present in endothelial cells.[53] Because the histochemical localization of smooth muscle α-actin is demonstrated in precapillaries and not in midcapillaries, it has been suggested that smooth muscle α-actin–containing capillaries are involved in contractility and the control of capillary blood flow in the BBB.[54]

Unlike other perivascular cells, they lie within the microvessel basal lamina and contribute to its formation, and typical CNS pericytes are flattened or elongated, stellate-shaped solitary cells with multiple cytoplasmic processes encircling the capillary endothelium and contacting a large abluminal vessel area. Brain pericytes are characterized by granular deposits present in lysosomes that strongly react with acid phosphatase, a finding that led to consideration of a phagocytic role.[55] They rapidly phagocytose an intravenous injection of HRP, which can be used as a pericyte histochemical stain. The number of granular lysosomes in brain pericytes increases with disruption of the BBB. Several other markers have been used in the identification of pericytes, including smooth muscle α-actin, desmin, polydendrocytes (NG2 cells), platelet-derived growth factor receptor-β, aminopeptidase A and N, regulator of G-protein signaling 5, and the promoter trap transgene *XlacZ4*.[56]

An active role of pericytes in the BBB was inferred from the localization of γ-glutamyl transpeptidase (GGTP) in brain capillary endothelial cells and pericytes, both in vivo and in vitro.[57] This heterodimeric glycoprotein distributed on the external surface of the cell catalyzes the transfer of γ-glutamyl from glutathione to accept peptides and functionally appears to be concerned with transport of large neutral amino acids across the BBB. Detectable amounts of GGTP are found in other regions of the brain with an intact BBB but not in those that lack one, such as the median eminence. Abnormal platelet-derived growth factor (PDGF)-B and PDGF-β signaling play a critical role in the recruitment of pericytes to newly formed vessels, and when deficient, as in knockout of *pdgfb* and *pdbfrb*, lead to perinatal death due to vascular dysfunction with associate vascular leakage and hemorrhage.

Pericyte-endothelia cell signaling factors have been identified. Sphingosine-1-phosphate signaling triggers cytoskeletal, adhesive, and junctional changes, affecting cell migration, proliferation, and survival.[58] Angiopoietin-Tie2 signaling in the vascular wall is involved in reciprocal communication between endothelial cell and pericytes, such as may be seen in *ang1*-or *tie2*-null mice deficient in Ang1, which leads to defective angiogenesis and poorly organized BM and reduced coverage and detachment of pericytes. Conversely, overexpression of Ang1 leads to expanded and stabilized leakage-resistant microvasculature.[59,60]

The importance of CNS pericytes has been underscored by their proposed role in neuroimmunologic networks associated with BBB function. First, CNS pericytes may be actively involved in the regulation of leukocyte transmigration, antigen presentation, and T-cell activation. They constitutively express low levels of VCAM-1 and ICAM-1, which have costimulatory activity in main histocompatibility cell class II dependent antigen presentation, and leukocytes cluster on pericytes in culture,[48] suggesting a role in inflammation. Smooth muscle pericytes present antigen in vivo and differentially activate Th1 and Th2 CD4$^-$ T cells. Moreover, CNS pericytes produce several immunoregulatory cytokines, including interleukin (IL) 1β and granulocyte-macrophage colony stimulatory factor.[61] Transforming growth factor (TGF)-β produced in an active form in pericytes/endothelial cocultures may function as an endogenous immunoregulator at the BBB.[62] It is therefore of interest that TFG-β1 inhibits cytokine-induced CNS endothelial cell activation in isolated rat CNS microvessels.[63] To further emphasize the importance of pericyte interactions in association with endothelial cells, there are no known genetic human diseases due to pericytes deficiency.

Astrocyte Interactions

The intimate relationship of astrocytes and blood vessels was appreciated by Ramon y Cajal[64] and Golgi[65] in the late nineteenth century. Since then, ultrastructural studies have shown that astrocytic end-feet in the perivascular astroglial sheath leads to a complete covering of brain microvessels.[66] Signaling at the gliovascular interface is facilitated by astrocyte-specific proteins and channels in astrocyte end-feet, including acquaporin-4, connexin 43, purinergic receptors, and potassium channels.[67] Moreover, ultrastructural studies have demonstrated that processes of vasoactive neurons for the regulation of cerebrovascular tone, in particular, those expressing noradrenaline, synapse onto astrocytes rather than directly onto blood vessels.[68] Altogether, these findings support the observation that astrocytes, one of the more numerous cells in the CNS, are important determinants of the intact BBB and crucial as well for ionic homeostasis, neurotransmitter uptake, synapse formation, and neurodevelopment. Zhang and Barres[69] have reviewed the differences in astrocyte morphology, developmental origin, gene expression profile, physiologic properties, function, and response to injury and disease. Two essential roles of astrocytes, in neurovascular coupling and the regulation of lymphocyte trafficking across the BBB, have been extensively studied.

All signaling molecules targeted to the cerebral vasculature must first act on or pass through astrocytes in order to reach smooth muscle cells in the vessel wall. It is now recognized that neurotransmitter-mediated signaling has a key role in regulating cerebral blood flow, and that much of this control is mediated by astrocytes[70]; moreover, cerebral blood flow may be controlled by capillaries as well as by arterioles. The glial and neuronal control of cerebral blood flow has been studied in brain slices.[71] Koehler and colleagues[72] demonstrated that electrical field stimulations in brain slices led to an increase in intracellular calcium in astrocyte cell bodies, which, when transmitted to perivascular end-feet, was followed by a decrease in vascular smooth muscle calcium oscillations and arteriolar dilation. The increase in astrocyte calcium after neuronal activation was in part mediated by activation of metabotropic glutamate receptors. Calcium signaling in vitro was influenced by adenosine acting on A2B receptors and by epoxyeicosatrienoic acids (EET) shown to be synthesized in astrocytes. Moreover, prostaglandins, EET, arachidonic acid, and potassium ions are candidate mediators of communication between astrocyte end-feet and vascular smooth muscle. Astrocytes appear to be capable of transmitting signals to pial arterioles on the brain surface to ensure adequate blood flow to feeding arterioles; therefore, these cells play an important role in the coupling of dynamic changes in cerebral blood flow in association with neuronal activity.

Koehler and colleagues[72] have provided insight into the morphologic aspects of neurovascular coupling at the capillary level of the BBB. At least one astrocyte end-foot process contacts a blood vessel, and those abutting capillaries and larger vessels express connexin-43 and puringeric P2Y receptors, which together permit Ca^{2+} increases to be transmitted 60 μm or more along the abluminal side of the vessel wall. Astrocytic cells are therefore in a unique position for sensing neuronal activity, integrating that information, and communicating with blood vessels in brain parenchyma. Although neurons do not directly innervate intraparenchymal vascular smooth muscle, subpopulations of GABAergic interneurons come into close contact with astrocyte foot processes and elicit vasodilation. Such neurons might modulate vascular function through stimulation of nitric oxide synthase activity, release of vasoactive peptides, or an astrocyte signaling mechanism.

Hudson and coworkers[73] studied trafficking of peripheral blood mononuclear cells (PBMC) across feline brain endothelial cells (FBEC) in cell culture system after the addition of combinations of different configurations of astrocytes and microglia in a model of feline immunodeficiency virus. The addition of astrocytes to FBEC significantly increased the adherence of PBMC, which was suppressed by the addition of microglia, whereas the latter alone had no effect on PBMC adherence. Whereas all PBMC showed some level of trafficking across FBEC, monocytes and B cells were significantly increased if astrocytes were present. The exposure of astrocytes notably increased the percentage of trafficking CD8 T cells from 24% to 64%, whereas microglia led to a significant reversal in the preferential trafficking of CD8 cells in the presence of astrocytes. Astrocytes are capable of secreting various cytokines and chemokines in the upregulation of adhesion molecules and T-cell ligands in intact endothelial cells, such as ICAM, VCAM, E-selectin, and PECAM. Human cocultured human endothelial cells and astrocytes increase the expression of ICAM-1 due to inflammatory activation by hypoxia in vitro.[74] Other studies have demonstrated that astrocytes are a source of IL-6, tumor necrosis factor-α, and monocyte chemoattractant protein-1, which contribute to the CNS inflammatory response.[75] Trafficking of PBMC along the endothelial cell of the BBB is a complex mechanism that involves major subsets of immune cells and relies heavily on astrocyte, microglia, and endothelial cell interactions; moreover, astrocytes appear to be an active factor in the recruitment of immune cells, whereas microglia appear to curtail this activity.

IMPLICATIONS FOR CEREBRAL VASCULITIS

There is an extensive literature of BBB biology in health and in widely differing neurologic disorders, including stroke,[76] epilepsy,[77] multiple sclerosis,[78] Alzheimer disease,[79] motor neuron disease,[80] Parkinson disease,[81] trauma,[82] glioblastoma,[83] HIV encephalitis,[84] and neuropsychiatric systemic lupus erythematosus (NPSLE).[85] Between 40% and 70% of patients with SLE have involvement of the CNS,[86] yet unlike systemic and primary CNS vasculitides, the role of the BBB in CNS lupus has been the subject of intense study using animal models and human clinical data.

The BBB is crucial because it maintains the brain internal milieu constant, allowing optimal neuronal function. Loss of BBB integrity leads to influx of inflammatory cells, and molecules, such as autoantibodies, causing brain injury. Earlier studies using the well-established MRL/lpr mouse model that reflects the events that occur in human CNS lupus revealed loss of BBB integrity with worsening disease[87,88] due to chronic activation of the complement cascade with the generation of the anaphylatoxins, C3a and C5a, and aggravated C5a/C5aR signaling. In cell culture, C5a causes neuronal cells to become apoptotic and binds to 2 receptors, the G-coupled, C5aR1, and the alternate receptor, C5aR2.[89] C5a/C5aR1 signaling mediates several biological processes, including chemotaxis and degranulation of mast cells, basophils, neutrophils, and eosinophils. It increases vascular permeability, increases generation of reactive oxygen species, and enhances production of cytokines from monocytes and macrophages. Whether C5a/C5aR signaling is protective or neurotoxic depends on the setting, with increases in circulating C5a leading to poor outcomes in CNS lupus.[89]

Hopkins and colleagues[90] measured levels of complement anaphylatoxin split products, C3a and C5a, in the circulation of patients with SLE who were followed serially. Means complement levels were significantly higher during periods of lupus flare compared with those during a stable period, with the highest levels seen in patients with CNS involvement. Pathologic specimens from 2 cases who died during an acute lupus flare revealed neutrophils occluding the cerebral and systemic intestinal vessels.

C5a also contributes to cellular apoptosis in lupus,[91] wherein treatment with the C5aRant, inhibiting C5a/C5aR signaling, results in significant and substantial decreases in brain pathologic condition in MRL/lpr mice, leaving upstream potentially protective complement activation events intact. There was evidence for a relationship between complement activation, inflammation, and neuronal viability in lupus brain tissue. C5aR1 is present predominantly on blood myeloid cells, but is also constitutively expressed on several brain cell types, including endothelial cells, which contribute to BBB integrity. Such studies show the possible neuroprotective role for C5aR antagonists in MRL/lpr mice and indicate potential future avenues of research for systemic and primary CNS vasculitides.

SUMMARY

There has been extraordinary research in the BBB over the past decade. Once considered a static anatomic barrier to the traffic of molecules in and out of the CNS, the BBB of children and adults is now recognized to be fully functional and vital to both cerebrovascular angiogenesis and normal homeostatic maintenance. The cellular components and other molecular constituents of the BBB, contained in the NVU, protect the CNS from injury and disease by limiting the passage of toxins, pathogens, and inflammatory effectors of the immune system. The implications of BBB disruption in cerebral vasculitis have yet to be appreciated; however, comparisons to CNS lupus may lead to a better understanding of the neural mechanisms involved in disease pathogenesis and BBB integrity, and efficacious neuroprotective treatment strategies.

REFERENCES

1. Daneman R. The blood-brain barrier in health and disease. Ann Neurol 2012;72:648–72.
2. Benarroch EE. Blood-brain barrier. Neurology 2012;78:1268–76.
3. Hawkins BR, Davis TP. The blood-brain barrier/Neurovascular unit in health and disease. Pharmacol Rev 2005;57:173–85.
4. Weiss N, Miller F, Cazaubon S, et al. The blood-brain barrier in brain homeostasis and neurological diseases. Biochim Biophys Acta 2009;1788:842–57.

5. Neuwelt EA, Bauer B, Fahlke C, et al. Engaging neuroscience to advance translational research in brain barrier biology. Nat Rev Neurosci 2011;12:169–82.
6. Younger DS. Adult and childhood vasculitis of the nervous system. In: Younger DS, editor. Chapter 14. Motor disorders. 3rd edition. New York: Rothstein Publishing; 2013. p. 235–80.
7. Twilt M, Benseler SM. The spectrum of CNS vasculitis in pediatrics and adults. Nat Rev Rheumatol 2011;8:97–107.
8. Hajj-Ali RA, Singhal AB, Benseler S, et al. Primary angiitis of the CNS. Lancet Neurol 2011;10:561–72.
9. Salvarani C, Brown RD Jr, Calamia KT, et al. Primary central nervous system vasculitis: analysis of 101 patients. Ann Neurol 2007;62:442–51.
10. Weiss N, Miller F, Cazaubon S, et al. Implications of the blood-brain barrier in neurological diseases: part II. Rev Neurol (Paris) 2009;165:1010–22 [in French].
11. Ehrlich P. The requirement of the organism for oxygen. An analytical study with the aid of dyes. In: Himmelweit F, Marquardt M, Dale H, editors. The collected papers of Paul Ehrlich. London: Pergamon Press; 1957. p. 433–96 [English translation].
12. Bield A, Kraus B. Über eine bisher unbekannte toxische Wirkung der Gallensauren auf das Zentralnervensystem. Zhl Inn Med 1898;19:1185–200.
13. Goldmann EE. Vitalfarbung am Zentral-nervensystem. Abh Preuss Akad Wissensch. Physkol Mathem Klasse 1913;1:1–60.
14. Lewandowsky M. Zür lehre der cerebrospinal flüssigkeit. Z Klin Med 1900;40:480–94.
15. Reese TS, Karnovsky MJ. Fine structural localization of a blood-brain barrier to exogenous peroxidase. J Cell Biol 1967;34:207–17.
16. Brightman MW, Reese TS. Junctions between intimately apposed cell membranes in the vertebrate brain. J Cell Biol 1969;40:648–77.
17. Feder N. Microperoxidase: an ultrastructural tracer of low molecular weight. J Cell Biol 1971;51:339–43.
18. Nagy Z, Peters H, Huttner I. Fracture faces of cell junctions in cerebral endothelium during normal and hyperosmotic conditions. Lab Invest 1984;50:313–22.
19. Shivers RR, Betz AL, Goldstein GW. Isolated rat brain capillaries possess intact, structurally complex, interendothelial tight junctions: freeze-fracture verification of tight junction integrity. Brain Res 1984;324:313–22.
20. Gerhardt H, Golding M, Fruttiger M, et al. VEGF guides angiogenic sprouting utilizing endothelial tip cell filopodia. J Cell Biol 2003;161:1163–77.
21. Lawson ND, Weinstein BM. In vivo imaging of embryonic vascular development using transgenic zebrafish. Dev Biol 2002;248:307–18.
22. Tam SJ, Watts RJ. Connecting vascular and nervous system development: angiogenesis and the blood-brain barrier. Annu Rev Neurosci 2010;33:379–408.
23. Carmeliet P, Tessier-Lavigne M. Common mechanisms of nerve and blood vessel wiring. Nature 2005;436:193–200.
24. Gerhardt H, Ruhrberg C, Abramsson A, et al. Neuropilin-1 is required for endothelial tip cell guidance in the developing central nervous system. Dev Dyn 2004;231:503–9.
25. Pugh CW, Ratcliffe PJ. Regulation of angiogenesis by hypoxia: role of the HIF system. Nat Med 2003;9:677–84.
26. Stubbs D, DeProto J, Nie K, et al. Neurovascular congruence during cerebral cortical development. Cereb Cortex 2009;19:i32–41.
27. Javaherian A, Kriegstein A. A stem cell niche for intermediate progenitor cells of the embryonic cortex. Cereb Cortex 2009;19:i70–7.

28. Johansson PA, Dziegielewska KM, Liddelow SA, et al. The blood-CSF barrier explained: when development is not immaturity. Bioassays 2008;30:237–48.
29. Ek CJ, Dziegielewska KM, Stolp H, et al. Functional effectiveness of the blood-brain barrier to small water soluble molecules in developing and adult opossum (*Monodelphis domestica*). J Comp Neurol 2006;496:13–26.
30. Møllgård K, Saunders NR. The development of human blood-brain and blood-CSF barriers. Neuropathol Appl Neurobiol 1986;12:337–58.
31. Ek CJ, Wong A, Liddelow SA, et al. Efflux mechanisms at the developing brain barriers: ABC-transporters in the fetal and postnatal rat. Toxicol Lett 2010;197:51–9.
32. Ballabh P, Hu F, Kumarasiri M, et al. Development of tight junction molecules in blood vessels of germinal matrix, cerebral cortex, and white matter. Pediatr Res 2005;58:791–8.
33. Ballabh P, Braun A, Nedergaard M. The blood-brain barrier: an overview. Structure, regulation, and clinical implications. Neurobiol Dis 2004;16:1–13.
34. Braun A, Xu H, Hu F, et al. Paucity of pericytes in germinal matrix vasculature of premature infants. J Neurosci 2007;27:12012–24.
35. Kreuter J. Drug delivery to the central nervous system by polymeric nanoparticles: What do we know? Adv Drug Deliv Rev 2014;71:2–14.
36. Lossinsky AS, Shivers RR. Structural pathways for macromolecular and cellular transport across the blood-brain barrier during inflammatory conditions. Histol Histopathol 2004;19:535–64.
37. Dai H, Marbach P, Lemaire M, et al. Distribution of ST1-571 to the brain is limited by P-glycoprotein-mediated efflux. J Pharmacol Exp Ther 2003;304:1085–92.
38. Shaik N, Giri N, Pan G, et al. P-glycoprotein-mediated active efflux of the anti-HIV1 nucleoside abacavir limits cellular accumulation and brain distribution. Drug Metab Dispos 2007;35:2076–85.
39. Zhang C, Kwan P, Zuo Z, et al. The transport of antiepileptic drugs by P-glycoprotein. Adv Drug Deliv Rev 2012;64:930–42.
40. Aronica E, Sisodiya SM, Gorter JA. Cerebral expression of drug transporters in epilepsy. Adv Drug Deliv Rev 2012;64:919–29.
41. Kerb R, Hoffmeyer S, Brinkmann U. ABC drug transporters: hereditary polymorphisms and pharmacological impact in MDR1, MRP1 and MRP2. Pharmacogenomics 2001;2:51–64.
42. Chen Y, Agarwal S, Shaik NM, et al. P-glycoprotein and breast cancer resistance protein influence brain distribution of dasatinib. J Pharmacol Exp Ther 2009;330:956–63.
43. Agarwal S, Pai D, Mitra AK. Both P-gp and MRP2 mediate transport of lopinavir, a protease inhibitor. Int J Pharm 2007;339:139–47.
44. Ziegler G, Prinz V, Albrecht MW, et al. Mrp-8 and -14 mediate CNS injury in focal cerebral ischemia. Biochim Biophys Acta 2009;1792:1198–204.
45. Petzelbauer P, Bender JR, Wilson J, et al. Heterogeneity of dermal microvascular endothelial cell antigen expression and cytokine responsiveness in situ and in cell culture. J Immunol 1993;151:5062–72.
46. Milstone DS, O'Donnell PE, Stavrakis G, et al. E-selectin expression and stimulation by inflammatory mediators are developmentally regulated during embryogenesis. Lab Invest 2000;80:943–54.
47. Armulik A, Abramssson A, Betsholtz C. Endothelial/pericytes interactions. Circ Res 2005;97:512–23.
48. Balabanov R, Dore-Duffy P. Mini-review. Role of the CNS microvascular pericytes in the blood-brain barrier. J Neurosci Res 1998;53:637–44.

49. Rouget C. Mémoire sur le dévelopement, la structure et les propriéties physiolo- giques des capillaires sanguins et lymphatiques. Arch Physiol Normale Pathol 1873;5:603–61.

50. Zimmerman K. Die feinere Bau der Blutcapillaren. A Anat Entwickl 1923;68: 29–109.

51. Diaz-Flores LR, Gutierrez H, Varela N, et al. Microvascular pericytes: a review of their morphological and functional characteristics. Histol Histopathol 1991;6: 269–86.

52. Tilton RG. Capillary pericytes: perspectives and future trends. J Electon Microsc Tech 1991;19:327–44.

53. Bandopadhyay R, Orte C, Lawrenson JG, et al. Contractile proteins in pericytes at the blood-brain and blood-retinal barriers. J Neurocytol 2001;30:35–44.

54. Boado RJ, Pardridge WM. Differential expression of α-actin mRNA and immuno- reactive protein in brain microvascular pericytes and smooth muscle cells. J Neurosci Res 1994;39:430–5.

55. Farrell CR, Steward PA, Farrell CL, et al. Pericytes in human cerebral microvascu- lature. Anat Rec 1987;218:466–9.

56. Gerhardt H, Betsholtz C. Endothelial-pericyte interactions in angiogenesis. Cell Tissue Res 2003;314:15–23.

57. Frey AB, Meckelein H, Weiler-Guttler B, et al. Pericytes of the brain microvascu- lature express γ-glutamyl transpeptidase. Eur J Biochem 1991;202:421–9.

58. Allende ML, Proia RL. Sphingosine-1-phosphate receptors and the development of the vascular system. Biochim Biophys Acta 2002;1582:222–7.

59. Suri C, McClain J, Thurston G, et al. Increased vascularization in mice overex- pressing angiopoietin-1. Science 1998;282:468–71.

60. Thurston G, Suri C, Smith K, et al. Leakage-resistant blood vessels in mice tran- genically overexpressing angiopoietin-1. Science 1999;286:2511–4.

61. Fabry Z, Fitzsimmons K, Herlein J, et al. Production of cytokines interleukin 1 and 6 by murine brain microvessel endothelium and smooth muscle pericytes. J Neuroimmunol 1993;47:23–34.

62. Dore-Duffy P, Balabanov R, Rafols J, et al. The recovery phase of acute experi- mental autoimmune encephalomyelitis in rats corresponds to development of endothelial cell unresponsiveness to interferon gamma activation. J Neurosci Res 1996;44:223–34.

63. Dore-Duffy P, Balabanov R, Washington R, et al. Transforming growth factor-β1 inhibits cytokine-induced CNS endothelial cell activation. Mol Chem Neuropathol 1994;22:161–75.

64. Ramon y Cajal S. Algunas conjeturas sobre el mecanismo anatomico de la idea- cion, asociacion y atencion. Rev Med Cir Pract 1895;36:497–508.

65. Golgi C. Sulla fina anatomia degli organi central del sistema nervosa. Milan (Italy): Hoepli; 1986.

66. Mathiisen TM, Lehre KP, Danbolt NC, et al. The perivascular astroglial sheath pro- vides a complete covering of the brain microvessels: an electron microscopic 3D reconstruction. Glia 2010;58:1094–103.

67. Price DL, Ludwig JW, Mi H, et al. Distribution of rSlo Ca2+-activated K+ channels in rat astrocyte perivascular endfeet. Brain Res 2002;956:183–93.

68. Hamel E. Perivascular nerves and the regulation of cerebrovascular tone. J Appl Physiol (1985) 2006;100:1059–64.

69. Zhang Y, Barres BA. Astrocyte heterogeneity: an underappreciated topic in neurobiology. Curr Opin Neurobiol 2010;20:588–94.

70. Petzold GC, Murthy VN. Role of astrocytes in neurovascular coupling. Neuron 2011;71:782–97.
71. Attwell D, Buchan AM, Charpak S, et al. Glial and neuronal control of brain blood flow. Nature 2010;468:232–43.
72. Koehler RC, Gebremedhin D, Harder DR. Role of astrocytes in cerebrovascular regulation. J Appl Physiol (1985) 2006;100:307–17.
73. Hudson LC, Bragg DC, Tompkins MB, et al. Astrocytes and microglia differentially regulate trafficking of lymphocyte subsets across brain endothelial cells. Brain Res 2005;1058:148–60.
74. Zhang W, Smith C, Howlett D, et al. Inflammatory activation of human brain endothelial cells by hypoxic astrocytes in vitro is mediated by IL-1beta. J Cereb Blood Flow Metab 2000;20:967–78.
75. Dong Y, Benveniste EN. Immune function of astrocytes. Glia 2001;36:180–90.
76. Jiao H, Wang Z, Liu Y, et al. Specific role of tight junction proteins claudin-5, occluding, and ZO-1 of the blood brain barrier in a focal cerebrovascular ischemic insult. J Mol Neurosci 2011;44:130–9.
77. Oby E, Janigro D. the blood-brain barrier and epilepsy. Epilepsia 2006;47:1761–74.
78. Alvarez JI, Cayrol R, Prat A. Disruption of central nervous system barriers in multiple sclerosis. Biochim Biophys Acta 2011;1812:252–64.
79. Bowman GL, Kaye JA, Moore M, et al. Blood-brain barrier impairment in Alzheimer disease: stability and functional significance. Neurology 2007;68:1809–14.
80. Garbuzova-Davis S, Haller E, Saporta S, et al. Ultrastructure of blood-brain barrier and blood-spinal barrier in SOD1 mice modeling ALS. Brain Res 2007;1157:126–37.
81. Faucheux BA, Bonnet AM, Agid Y, et al. Blood vessels change in the mesencephalon of patients with Parkinson's disease. Lancet 1999;353:981–2.
82. Tompkins O, Shelef I, Kaizerman I, et al. Blood-brain barrier disruption in post-traumatic epilepsy. J Neurol Neurosurg Psychiatry 2008;79:774–7.
83. Ishihara H, Kubota H, Lindberg RL, et al. Endothelial cell barrier impairment induced by glioblastoma and transforming growth factor beta2 involves matrix metalloproteinases and tight junction proteins. J Neuropathol Exp Neurol 2008;67:435–48.
84. Roberts TK, Buckner CM, Berman JW. Leukocyte transmigration across the blood-brain barrier: perspectives on neuroAIDS. Front Biosci 2010;15:478–536.
85. Huizinga TW, Diamond B. Lupus and the central nervous system. Lupus 2008;17:376–9.
86. Mahajan SD, Tutino VM, Redae Y, et al. C5a induces caspase-dependent apoptosis in brain vascular endothelial cells in experimental lupus. Immunology 2016;148:407–19.
87. Jacob A, Hack B, Chen P, et al. C5a/CD88 signaling alters blood–brain barrier integrity in lupus through nuclear factor-κB. J Neurochem 2011;119:1041–51.
88. Jacob A, Hack B, Chiang E, et al. C5a alters blood–brain barrier integrity in experimental lupus. FASEB J 2010;24:1682–8.
89. Mahajan SD, Tutino VM, Redae Y, et al. C5a induces caspase-dependent apoptosis in brain vascular endothelial cells in experimental lupus. Immunology 2016;148:407–19.
90. Hopkins P, Belmont HM, Buyon, et al. Increased levels of plasma anaphylatoxins in systemic lupus erythematosus predict flares of the disease and may elicit vascular injury in lupus cerebritis. Arthritis Rheum 1988;31:632–41.
91. Jacob A, Hack B, Bai T, et al. Inhibition of C5a receptor alleviates experimental CNS lupus. J Neuroimmunol 2010;221:46–52.

Imaging the Vasculitides

David S. Younger, MD, MPH, MS[a,b],*

KEYWORDS

- Neuroimaging • Computerized tomography • Magnetic resonance imaging
- Single-photon emission tomography • Positron emission tomography
- Cerebral angiography

KEY POINTS

- Neuroimaging plays a vital role in the diagnosis of primary and secondary vasculitic disorders.
- There are a multiplicity of neuroimaging options available to accurately describe the underlying clinical deficits of involved cases.
- Noninvasive neuroimaging modalities provide less risk and when interdigitated, form the basis for a more conclusive understanding of the disease process.
- There are instances in which invasive cerebral angiography may be needed to image the intricate and at times, small involved vessels.
- Neuroradiologists should be included in the multidisciplinary team of physicians caring for patients with vasculitides and in research to provide more sensitive and safe modalities for the accurate diagnosis thereof.

INTRODUCTION

Vasculitis is a term used to describe a diverse spectrum of diseases characterized by inflammation of the blood vessels that may progress to ischemic injury of the central nervous system (CNS) resulting in a myriad of focal and generalized neurologic symptoms. The injury is usually secondary to mural changes resulting in vessel stenosis or occlusion. Endothelial inflammation promotes intraluminal coagulation and thrombosis.[1] Perivascular inflammatory changes and edema contribute to the pathologic picture. Arterial and venous components may be involved separately or together and dural sinuses may be affected. Generalized inflammatory processes may produce a secondary encephalitis or myelitis. The radiological aspects of CNS vasculitis have evolved in the past decade.[2] No one single imaging modality is sufficient or

Disclosure Statement: The author has nothing to disclose.
[a] Department of Neurology, Division of Neuro-Epidemiology, New York University School of Medicine, New York, NY 10016, USA; [b] School of Public Health, City University of New York, New York, NY, USA
* 333 East 34th Street, Suite 1J, New York, NY 10016.
E-mail address: youngd01@nyu.edu
Website: http://www.davidsyounger.com

Neurol Clin 37 (2019) 249–265
https://doi.org/10.1016/j.ncl.2019.01.010
0733-8619/19/© 2019 Elsevier Inc. All rights reserved.

neurologic.theclinics.com

preeminent; a combination of studies is typically required for a confident diagnosis of CNS vasculitis.

OVERVIEW AND CLASSIFICATION

With an estimated worldwide incidence of 20 per million for eosinophilic granulomatosis with polyangiitis (EGPA), also known as Churg-Strauss syndrome, 10 per million for granulomatosis with polyangiitis (GPA) or Wegener granulomatosis, 2.6 per million for Takayasu arteritis (TAK), and 0.9 per million for polyarteritis nodosa (PAN),[3,4] and only a fraction of patients presenting with CNS involvement, it is important for clinicians to be familiar with the clinical and neuroradiologic presentations of the vasculitides. This is especially important in young and middle-aged adults in whom the prevalence of atherosclerotic disease is low.[5–9]

The historical aspects of the classification of the vasculitides are reviewed elsewhere in this issue. To illustrate the clinical importance placed on the radiologic manifestations of the PAN group of primary systemic vasculitides, the narrative should begin with Citron and colleagues[10] who described multiorgan arteritis of the CNS in a highly publicized report of 14 Los Angeles multidrug abusers with a common denominator of intravenous methamphetamine abuse by all but 2 patients, and exclusively by 1. Acute vessel lesions included fibrinoid necrosis of the media and intima with infiltration of polymorphonuclear cells, eosinophils, lymphocytes, and histiocytes, followed by vascular elastic and vascular smooth muscle destruction resulting in lesions considered typical for PAN. Substantiation of necrotizing arteritis was present in only 4 of the 14 patients. Citron and Peters[11] responded to the criticism from Baden[12] that he had not observed a causal relation between drug abuse and necrotizing arteritis at the Office of Chief Medical Examiner of New York City for the past one-half century among thousands of autopsied drug abusers, with the countering opinion that evidence of aneurysms noted in 13 of the 14 patients was ample proof of arteritis.

The contribution of angiography to the designation of CNS vasculitis commenced with the identification of angiographic beading and a sausagelike appearance of cerebral vessels at sites of presumed arteritis first in 1964 by Hinck and coworkers[13] in giant cell arteritis (GCA). In 1983, Cupps and colleagues[14] established the utility of cerebral angiography in the diagnosis of histologically proven isolated angiitis or primary angiitis of the CNS (PACNS). As giant cells and epithelioid cells usually found at postmortem examination in such patients were an inconsistent finding in a meningeal and brain biopsy and therefore considered unnecessary for antemortem diagnosis, Moore and Cupps[15] considered angiography necessary for the diagnosis of PACNS. This prevailing opinion was shared by Calabrese and Mallek,[16] who proposed criteria for the diagnosis of PACNS, and Hajj-Ali and Calabrese[17] who later separated PACNS from the reversible cerebral vasoconstrictive syndrome (RCVS), characterized instead by transient nonvasculitic narrowing of intracranial vessels.

By 1990, Hunder and colleagues[18] on behalf of the American College of Rheumatology (ACR) noted that the goal in classification was to identify sets of sensitive criteria that recognized a high proportion of patients with a particular form of vasculitis, while specifically excluding a high proportion of those with other diseases. Although highly specific and sensitive classification criteria might prove useful in the depiction of patients for epidemiologic studies and therapeutic trials, such criteria might not necessarily include the full spectrum of manifestations of a particular vasculitic disease, which was instead the role of formal diagnostic criteria. Lie[19] noted that although a definitive diagnosis of vasculitis almost invariably required histologic documentation, the interpretation of a diagnostic tissue sample was subject to variables as diverse as the pathologist's experience, tissue selection, sample size, chronologic age of the disease, and any prior treatment at the time of the biopsy. The angiographic appearance of aneurysms or occlusions of visceral arteries not due to arteriosclerosis, fibromuscular dysplasia, or other noninflammatory causes, were useful in the classification of PAN[20] with a sensitivity of 73.5% and specificity of 89.2%. The angiographic features of narrowing, aneurysm, or occlusion of the aorta or its primary branches, were useful criteria for the classification of TAK[21] with sensitivities and specificities of 85.5% and 81.2%, 20.3% and 95.9%, and 51.6% and 86.1%, respectively. In the same 1990 volume of the journal, *Arthritis and Rheumatism*, the ACR Subcommittee on Classification of Vasculitis noted no diagnostic features of angiography useful in the classification criteria of EGPA, GPA, hypersensitivity vasculitis, immunoglobulin A vasculitis (IgAV) and GCA.[22–26]

Jennette and colleagues[27] held 2 Chapel Hill Consensus Conferences (CHCCs) beginning in 1994 with a 2012 revision,[28] establishing the nomenclature or nosology of systemic vasculitides. However, different from the ACR Subcommittee on Classification of Vasculitis,[18] Jennette and colleagues[27,28] incorporated prevailing knowledge about etiology, pathogenesis, pathology, demographics, and clinical manifestations, and used a model of the predominant caliber of involved vessel that delineated the 3 major categories of systemic vasculitis including large-size vessel vasculitis (LVV), medium-size vessel vasculitis (MVV), and small-sized vessel vasculitis (SVV) types, adding further distinctions as to the structural and functional characteristics of particular vascular beds, as well as the known biochemical and functional properties that rendered them susceptible to vasculitic injury. With approximately 26 recognized vasculitides in the 2012 revised CHCC, many of which demonstrate overlap in affected involved arteries, coupled with advances in the neuroradiologic techniques for discerning CNS involvement, there has been heightened interest in imaging the cerebral vasculature.

Küker[29] differentiated the entities of extracranial LVV and intracranial MVV and SVV, noting that vasculitic involvement of the internal carotid (ICA), common carotid (CCA), M1 and A1 segments of the middle (MCA) and anterior cerebral arteries (ACA), intracranial vertebral and basilar arteries, and P1 segment of the posterior cerebral artery (PCA), generally regarded as intracranial LVV, would instead be considered systemic MVV by 2012 Revised CHCC nomenclature.[28] Moreover, vasculitic involvement along arterial vessels distal to the MCA bifurcation, as well as communicating vessels such as the anterior and posterior communicating arteries, were still considered MVV systemically although intracranial. They may not be demonstrable along with intracranial LVV by MRI, magnetic resonance angiography (MRA), or computed tomographic angiography (CTA), and may require conventional angiography (CA) for luminal irregularity to be visualized.

The smallest muscular arteries and arterioles in the brain parenchyma, as well as the capillaries and proximal venules, all considered intracranial SVV by their lumen size, corresponded to a caliber of 200 to 500 μm or less,[30,31] and were considered beneath the resolution of invasive and noninvasive neuroimaging, requiring tissue biopsy to diagnose vasculitic involvement. The radiologic findings of nonvasculitic inflammatory vasculopathies, such as systemic lupus erythematosus (SLE), and other noninflammatory vasculopathies, such as RCVS (**Fig. 1**), cerebral atherosclerosis, and spontaneous dissection may mimic PACNS (**Fig. 2**).

NEURORADIOLOGIC APPROACH TO CENTRAL NERVOUS SYSTEM VASCULITIS

Küker[29] described 3 steps in the diagnostic evaluation of CNS vasculitis beginning with the demonstration of brain lesions by T_2-weighted and diffusion-weighted and

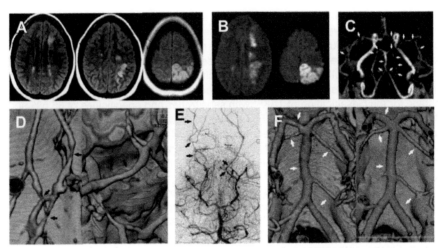

Fig. 1. RCVS. (*A*) MRI FLAIR imaging on presentation demonstrates multifocal abnormal hyperintense signal within the bilateral hemispheric white matter, more prominent in the parietal and occipital lobes where it extends to the cortex. (*B*) T_2-diffusion imaging demonstrates restricted diffusion consistent with acute ischemia. The white matter distribution within the left hemisphere straddles the anterior, middle, and posterior cerebral vascular territories, a "watershed" distribution. (*C*) MRA at admission demonstrates short-segment multifocal narrowing within the distal bilateral vertebral arteries, the basilar artery, and bilateral middle and posterior cerebral vasculature (*white arrows*). (*D*) CTA demonstrates moderate narrowing within the right PCA P2 segment and a more severe narrowing distally within the P3 parieto-occipital segment (*left, black arrows*). Mild narrowing is present within the ACA A1 segment (*right, black arrow*). (*E*) CA confirms multifocal narrowing within the bilateral posterior cerebral arteries (*black arrows*). (*F*) Follow-up CTA (at presentation on the left, 5 months' follow-up on the right) reveals complete resolution of the original findings (*white arrows*). (*Courtesy of* Adam Davis, MD New York, NY.)

perfusion-weighted MRI, followed by the delineation of underlying vascular pathology by 1.5-T MRA to study the entire course of the carotid and vertebral arteries, as well as the circle of Willis. Time-of-flight (TOF) MRA sequences permit detection of more subtle stenoses and improve spatial resolution, as well as mural thickness in basal brain arteries with MRA source images; moreover, MRI may discern mural enhancement. Conventional angiography with digital subtraction (DSA) is used to evaluate medium-sized and small brain vessels and the status of cerebral hemodynamics and assessment of brain perfusion.

Gomes[32] divided available neuroimaging studies into 3 groups, including the brain parenchyma, vessel lumen, and vessel wall. Parenchymal findings, although least specific, were necessary to detect the presence of disease as well as to follow progression and remission status. Vessel lumen and wall abnormalities, although highly suggestive for systemic vasculitis when present, were considered nonspecific and insensitive in the diagnosis of intracranial SVV.

Parenchymal Imaging

The MRI findings of CNS vasculitis have been previously described,[33–36] the commonest of which are T_2/fluid-attenuated inversion recovery (FLAIR) hyperintense lesions secondary to ischemia distributed throughout subcortical and deep white matter, the deep gray nuclei, and the cortices. The MCA territory is the commonest involved

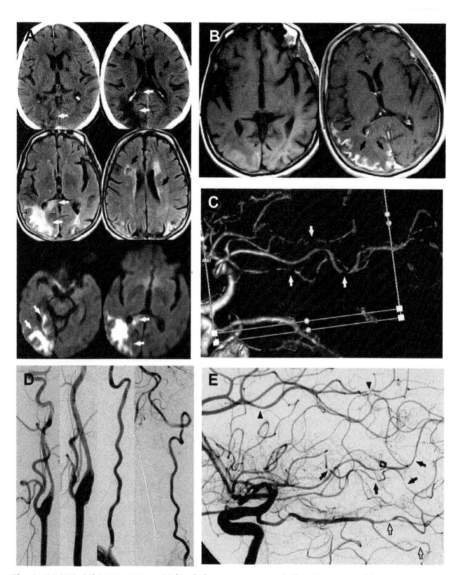

Fig. 2. PACNS. (*A*) Noncontrast CT (*top*) demonstrates multifocal regions of low attenuation. Those in the right frontal subcortical white matter and left basal ganglia (*black arrows*) are sharply defined, without mass effect and likely reflect old infarctions. Both the cortex and underlying white matter of the right occipital lobe are involved, as is the right splenium of the corpus callosum (*white arrows*). In these locations, the margins are more ill-defined and there is subtle mass effect characterized by sulcal and ventricular effacement, suggesting acute ischemia in the right PCA territory. MRI FLAIR imaging (*middle*) demonstrates central low and peripheral high signal intensity within the frontal and periventricular white matter lesions (*black arrows*) consistent with chronic encephalomalacia from old infarctions. The FLAIR hyperintense signal within the right occipital lobe is more confluent and extends to the posterior temporal lobe and splenium, involving both cortex and white matter (*white arrows*) and better delineates the extent of the acute infarct. DWI (*bottom*) demonstrates restricted diffusion consistent with acute ischemia. (*B*) T_1-weighted imaging before and after gadolinium demonstrates extensive leptomeningeal enhancement along

in CNS vasculitis.[37,38] Diffusion-weighted imaging (DWI) helps to distinguish acute, subacute, and chronic ischemia and is thus mandatory. Lesions are frequently bilateral and of differing ages. Involvement of multiple vascular territories or lesions within a frankly nonvascular territorial distribution may be clues to the diagnosis of CNS vasculitis, although they also can be seen in association with thrombophilic and cardiogenic multiple embolic process that produce ischemia. Ischemic lesions are present in up to one-half of patients with PACNS.[35] Nonspecific white matter changes, which may be the only finding in symptomatic patients,[39,40] are unlikely findings of atherosclerotic hypertensive disease in young patients, yet sometimes difficult to distinguish from CNS demyelinating disease.

Intraparenchymal and subarachnoid hemorrhages may be presenting or associated radiographic features of CNS vasculitis,[41] although they occur less commonly than ischemic lesions so noted in up to 40% of patients with PACNS as compared with hemorrhage that occurred in only 4% to 12% of patients.[42–44] There is uncertainty regarding the significance of microscopic hemorrhage in patients with CNS vasculitis. T_2-weighted gradient-echo MRI, which depicts chronic blood or hemosiderin products as regions with marked signal intensity loss (susceptibility effect), was useful in demonstrating multiple silent petechial hemorrhages scattered throughout both cerebral hemispheres located in cortical-subcortical regions in a patient with stereotypic tingling spells in the right hand followed by acute mutism due to histological-proven PACNS. Brain computed tomography (CT) showed a small hematoma in the left parietal lobe and 1.5-T T_1-weighted, turbo spin-echo T_2-weighted, and FLAIR brain MRI demonstrated acute hemorrhage in the left parietal lobe as well as subacute hemorrhage in the right frontal lobe.[42] However, T_2-weighted gradient-echo images showed multiple small hemorrhages scattered throughout the cerebral hemispheres located in the cortical-subcortical regions sparing the basal ganglia, thalamus, and brain stem. Conversely, neither large nor small silent cortical hemorrhages were found among 25 patients with intracranial vasculitis using T_2*-weighed MRI.[45]

Leptomeningeal enhancement by MRI was noted in up to 9% of patients with PACNS,[34,44] often in association with cognitive disturbances, normal MRA and conventional or catheter angiography (CA), granulomatous angiitis histopathology and small-vessel involvement.[44]

Delayed perfusion and reduced cerebral blood volume may be seen on brain CT and MRI in patients with cerebral vasculitis.[34,45,46] Magnetic resonance spectroscopy reveals elevated glutamate and glutamine levels and reduced N-acetyl aspartate (NAA) content in cerebral vasculitis,[46,47] and absence of a choline peak.[46–48]

High-Resolution MRI

High-resolution MRI (hrMRI), using gadolinium-enhanced fat-saturation T_1 spin-echo techniques, provides useful information of possible inflammatory changes in those with suspected systemic LVV. More recently, the use of vessel wall imaging has increased due to the multiple applications in vivo, such as the differentiation between

---

the cortical surface of the posterior temporal and occipital lobes. (*C*) CTA demonstrates multifocal vascular narrowing within several branches of the MCA (*white arrows*) with intervening regions of normal-appearing vasculature. At the bottom of the image, vascular narrowing within the PCA (not marked) is present. (*D, E*) CA reveals completely normal extracranial vasculature. The ACA (*black arrowheads*), MCA (*black arrows*), and PCA (*black outlined arrows*) demonstrate mild to severe short-segment stenoses. (*Courtesy of* Adam Davis, MD and Tibor Bescke, MD.)

atherosclerosis and vasculitis, the visualization of intracranial dissection, and to determine which aneurysm has ruptured in patients with acute subarachnoid hemorrhage and multiple aneurysms. The arterial wall enhancement in patients with vasculitis is probably related to contrast leakage from the lumen into the arterial wall, given the increased permeability of the endothelium; it is also possible that the presence of dilated neovessels in the wall is responsible for the increased contrast enhancement. It is important to keep in mind that there may be a discordance between the MRI findings and the clinical vasculitis activity.[49]

In 26 patients with TAK and 16 healthy subjects so studied,[50] contrast-enhanced T_1-weighted spin-echo MRI using small fields of view and thin slices showed enhancement of thickened aortic wall compared with myocardium, suggesting active TAK. The degree of disease activity was concordant with laboratory measures of disease activity in 88.5% of patients, including erythrocyte sedimentation rates (ESRs) and C-reactive protein (CRP). The measured signal intensity of the aortic wall relative to that of myocardium during the early phase of contrast-enhanced MRI, which was significantly correlated with serologic markers of inflammation, provided a useful assessment of disease activity in TAK. Notably, T_2-weighted signal intensity changes were less sensitive than enhanced images. In 64 consecutive patients with suspected GCA, Bley and colleagues[51] assessed mural thickness, lumen diameter, and mural contrast-enhancement scores by T_1-weighted spin-echo images with sub-millimeter in-plane spatial resolution. Their findings demonstrated that evaluation of the mural inflammatory MRI signs for diagnosing vasculitis resulted in a sensitivity of 80.6% and a specificity of 97.0%, in comparison to histologic results alone, which demonstrated a sensitivity of 77.8% and specificity of 100%. Some positive MRI results were associated with biopsy-negative histopathology for GCA, presumably due to sampling errors with skip lesions predominating in the tissue biopsy. Among patients with GCA who received treatment with corticosteroids less than 10 days, sensitivity of hrMRI ranged from 81% to 85%, whereas others receiving corticosteroids for more than 10 days demonstrated a sensitivity of 33%. Notwithstanding, hrMRI still should provide sensitive and specific information when neuroimaging is performed within days following the initiation of immunosuppressive treatment. In addition, in GCA, Geiger and colleagues[52] demonstrated how mural contrast enhancement of the ophthalmic arteries could be demonstrated using a 3-T MRI examination and they showed that it is a common finding in patients with GCA with suspicious ophthalmic arteries involvement.

hrMRI findings of intracranial vasculitis include concentric and asymmetric vessel wall thickening, an eccentric or narrowed vessel lumen, and vessel wall enhancement. Enhancement may be limited to the vessel wall or extend to adjacent leptomeninges. For intracranial large vessel disease, direct vascular wall inflammatory wall changes provide greater specificity than indirect luminal imaging findings. The degree and persistence of vessel wall enhancement helped to differentiate PACNS from RCVS because mural enhancement is less prominent in RCVS and resolves in nearly all restudied patients at 3 months while those with PACNS demonstrate an increased vessel wall enhancement that persists for greater than a year.

An additional role of wall imaging MRI is to help selecting the appropriate target for biopsy in cases of suspected vasculitis.

Indirect Vessel Imaging Techniques

Indirect imaging techniques that characterize changes in the vessel lumen leading to ischemia, infarction, and hemorrhage in cerebral vasculitis can be obtained by MRA, CTA, and CA; however, these do not provide direct evidence of the associated underlying mural and perivascular inflammation. Catheter angiography provides up to 0.2 mm of spatial resolution and 0.5 to 0.25 seconds of temporal resolution in a typical study, exceeding MRA and CTA.[30] The spatial resolution of multidetector CTA, which is dependent on detector row thickness, is approximately 0.4 to 0.75 mm. CA provides detailed information regarding hemodynamics that is generally absent from both CTA and MRA. Dynamic 320-section CTA provides limited hemodynamic information with a temporal resolution of 1 second and a spatial resolution of 0.5 mm.[53] Indices for MRA spatial resolution are even less precise than these other techniques.

Magnetic resonance angiography

This noninvasive nonionizing indirect vessel wall imaging study does not require intravenous contrast administration for the assessment of intracranial stenoses and vascular occlusions in suspected CNS vasculitis. MRA may overestimate vascular stenosis secondary to diminished signal intensity from vessel tortuosity and slow flow. The more subtle finding of intracranial vessel irregularity is more difficult to assess due to lower spatial resolution. Among 9 arteries from 14 young patients with clinical and radiological suspicion of cerebral vasculitis, the sensitivity for detecting a stenosis by 3-dimensional TOF MRA or DSA varied from 62% to 79% for MRA, and 76% to 94% for DSA. The specificity for detecting a stenosis varied from 83% to 87% for MRA and from 83% to 97% for DSA. Using the criterion of greater than 2 stenoses in 2 or more separate vascular distributions as a true positive criterion for cerebral vasculitis, the false-positive rate for MRA and DSA were comparable.[54] When more than 2 stenoses are noted on MRA, DSA is unlikely to add further diagnostic precision in a given patient with suspected cerebral vasculitis, but yet might be useful when MRA is normal or discloses fewer than 3 stenoses.[54]

Computed tomography angiography

Indirect vessel wall imaging using CTA has been used in TAK, GCA, PAN, and CNS vasculitis. The efficacy of CTA in TAK, a chronic idiopathic LVV that primarily affects large vessels such as the aorta and its major branches, as well as the pulmonary and coronary arteries, is well established.[55] Nonspecific inflammation of involved vessels leads to concentric wall thickening, fibrosis, and thrombus formation. These produce the characteristic neuroradiologic findings of focal stenosis, occlusion, dilatation, and luminal irregularity with a characteristic distribution and severity of involvement. The relative sensitivity and specificity of CTA for TAK was respectively 93% to 95% and 98% to 100%.[56] The salient CTA features of TAK include mural thickening, luminal changes, collateral vessels, and other findings usually with respect to the pulmonary and coronary arteries. In the early stages of TAK, mural inflammatory changes may precede luminal contour changes, an important advantage of CTA as compared with DSA.

CTA is useful in patients with GCA in whom LVV occurs in 25% of patients,[57] especially in those with confirmed biopsy pathology to screen for the presence of stenosis, dissection, and aneurysms, and to assess the extent of arterial involvement or monitor vascular lesions for signs of progression.[58] Intramural leaky microvessels, which give rise to delayed enhancement of the arterial wall, are consistent with, but not specific for inflammatory vasculopathy. Moreover, generally irreversible wall thickening and increased intrawall blood pooling despite immunosuppressant treatment should not be used to assess the inflammatory burden or disease activity.[56] Aneurysm formation along gastrointestinal and renal arteries and other systemic medium-sized vessels so noted on CTA, particularly in the absence of aortic involvement, are useful neuroradiologic signs of PAN and the differential diagnosis of TAK.[59,60]

An entity considered by some to be part of the GCA spectrum, and often diagnosed with a CTA of the neck, is carotidynia, a clinical entity first described by Fay in 1927, that manifests as unilateral tenderness and pain in the neck at the level of the carotid bifurcation. These 2 clinical signs of carotidynia are not specific, and other causes of neck pain can have the same clinical presentation. It is thought to be caused by perivascular inflammation as suggested by the increase of the ESR or CRP and ipsilateral lymph node enlargement and pharyngeal or laryngeal inflammation. The findings on CT include perivascular infiltration, defined as soft amorphous tissue replacing the fat surrounding the carotid artery. A relationship with GCA has not been demonstrated, however in a series of 47 patients, 8 patients had an autoimmune disease, such as rheumatoid arthritis, SLE, ankylosing spondylarthritis, Graves disease, Sjögren syndrome and Hashimoto thyroiditis.[61] The newly proposed name for the condition is transient perivascular inflammation of the carotid artery (TIPIC) syndrome.

CTA also provides useful assessment of stenotic, dilated, and focally occluded vessels of the circle of Willis and the second-order and third-order branches of the ACA, MCA, and PCA involved by CNS vasculitis. However, the resolution of luminal irregularity is less well appreciated on CTA compared with CA, because the former modality, which is less dynamic, requires the inference of collateral flow and angio-architecture from opacified vessels. The radiation dose penalty, which is slightly greater than a routine head CT, makes CTA suitable as an initial screening modality for CNS vasculitis in adults, but less desirable in children and young adults. CT readily identifies abnormal mural thickening as defined by thickness greater than 1 mm in 93% of patients with clinical evidence of TAK along the ascending aorta, arch of aorta, and descending thoracic aorta.[55] Up to 73% of patients with TAK demonstrate changes within the cervicocerebral vessels, most commonly the arch and descending thoracic aorta, brachiocephalic artery, and common carotid artery where wall thickening varied from 1 mm to 10 mm. Once considered the gold standard for detecting abnormal vasculature, CA may be falsely negative in the early stages of TAK.[47,55] This is an important consideration, as the disease is most effectively treated with immunosuppressive therapy during the earliest phase of the illness; a time when CA may be nondiagnostic. CTA is an excellent option in these circumstances, as it provides not only information regarding luminal abnormalities, including stenosis, occlusion, aneurysmal dilatation, and contour irregularities similar to CA, but direct diagnostic findings, including wall thickening, calcification, and abnormal enhancement.[47,55] Although nonspecific to the cerebrovascular circulation, Yamada and colleagues[56] demonstrated a sensitivity and specificity of 95% and 100%, respectively, for CTA in the diagnosis of TAK, with claims of positive correlation of vessel wall changes to the histopathologic findings.[47] Heterogeneous mural enhancement and an inner concentric low-attenuation ring that enhanced at delayed imaging likewise demonstrated a positive correlation with the acute phase of histopathologic findings of vascularization and intimal swelling in the tunica media.

Catheter angiography

Although CA has been the gold standard for diagnosis of cerebral vasculitis, it occupies a less important role compared with MRA and CTA in the initial evaluation of suspected patients. The classic angiographic features of CNS vasculitis are multifocal luminal narrowing, vascular contour irregularity, and vascular dilatations with the appearance of a string of beads often along multiple vessels and in differing vascular territories, although ectasia and normal luminal diameter also may occur. The affected vessel may demonstrate a smooth or irregular luminal contour and vascular stenosis, which is classically a discrete short segment or elongated. The size of the vessels affected, and the distribution of lesions within each of the vessels varies with the vasculitic etiology and may be a clue to the proximate cause. Extracranial large vessel narrowing and undulation of long segments with variable luminal angiographic involvement occurs in GCA, whereas variable intracranial skull–based and medium cortical vessel involvement occurs in anti-neutrophil cytoplasm antibody–associated vasculitides, SLE, and PACNS. There is no predilection for vessel branch points in PACNS in contrast to atherosclerosis and hypertensive disease.[62] Whereas luminal narrowing along vascular regions of laminar flow disruption and high shear stress, such as the ICA bulb, petro-cavernous junction, and cavernous segments, suggests atherosclerosis, multifocal stenosis and luminal irregularity within the same vessel segment with intervening normal vessel contours, and isolated stenosis within separate vascular territories and otherwise normal vessel contours favors vasculitis. Multiple emboli generally present with more obstructive than stenotic lesions, and tend not to occur as discretely along multiple vascular territories or in tandem along the same vessel in contrast to CNS vasculitis. Angiographic features that favor MVV involvement due to systemic vasculitis and autoimmune disease in contrast to PACNS include abrupt vascular truncation, occlusion, and microaneurysm formation.[63] The collateral circulation should be investigated and quantified by CT and MR perfusion imaging in patients with severe luminal narrowing and vascular occlusion of medium and large vessels, as should abnormal cerebral hemodynamics typified by slow anterograde flow, diminished distal luminal size, and prolonged circulation time. Vascular dissection, which rarely occurs in intracranial vasculitis, is much more common in the extracranial vasculature in GCA.

The sensitivity of CA for PACNS is 40% to 100%,[34,35,38,40,62–66] and the specificity no higher than 37% for CA in the diagnosis of PACNS[67]; however, they may vary depending on the particular clinical, radiographic, and histopathologic definitions used. SVV involvement is typically beneath resolution of CA. Children especially with so-called angiography negative, biopsy positive, small-vessel childhood PACNS,[68] who present with negative angiography and a positive MRI, are generally considered to be candidates for cerebral and leptomeningeal biopsy to confirm the presence of vasculitis.

There is a poor correlation between neuroradiologic findings on MRI and CA in PACNS.[38,63] Whereas two-thirds of lesions detected by MRI showed a CA lesional correlate, 44% of lesions detected by CA were conversely identified on MRI. Of 41 territories involved by MRI in a series of patients with PACNS, CA correlated with 15%, whereas among 50 vascular territories involved by CA, a correlate was found in only 34% of MRI studies.

The risk of transient neurologic injury is 10%, and permanent morbidity occurs in approximately 1% of patients undergoing CA for the evaluation of CNS vasculitis.[69] Intravenous corticosteroids administered before CA may ameliorate the risk of injury and reduce complications.

NUCLEAR MEDICINE IMAGE MODALITIES
PET

Nuclear medicine evaluation of neurovasculitis remains promising but problematic. Conceptually the ability to monitor metabolic activity within the vessel wall should be a good indicator of inflammatory activity. PET with ^{18}Fluorodeoxyglucose (FDG-

PET) has been the best studied radionuclide for this indication, particularly in systemic LVV. One meta-analysis[70] demonstrated a wide variability of diagnostic sensitivity for TAK ranging from 28% to 100%, whereas the range of specificity was 50% to 100%. Fused PET and CT images provide superior anatomic localization and improved sensitivity and specificity of 91% and 89% for TAK. A greater diagnostic sensitivity of 80% and specificity of 89% in those studied by FDG-PET were noted for GCA.[71] Nonetheless, the specificity of FDG-PET is degraded by the presence of atherosclerosis, as active inflammatory plaques may produce false-positive findings.[72] The utility of FDG-PET for monitoring disease activity in these patients may be problematic. Some patients with TAK deemed inactive by clinical criteria may in fact demonstrate biopsy-proven active inflammation.[73] Studies indicate that FDG-PET may be a sensitive and helpful diagnostic study for identifying these patients with subclinical active disease, with 83% of patients with biopsy-proven GCA demonstrating positive FDG-PET studies.[74] The sensitivity and specificity of FDG-PET in the identification of active vasculitic disease compared with clinical signs and laboratory criteria lead to respective rates of 100% and 89%.[75] The fusion of MRI for morphology and volumetric assessment, and FDG-PET for metabolic analysis of the brain, has been used to investigate the autoimmune encephalitides, and may have a role in the investigation of CNS vasculitides.[76]

Single-Photon Emission Computed Tomography

Single-photon emission computed tomography (SPECT) uses multiplanar nuclear medicine imaging for the investigation of regional CNS perfusion abnormalities. It provides direct information about the pathophysiology and cerebral metabolism in cerebral vasculitides at the level of capillary endothelium in the blood-brain barrier (BBB) microcirculation beyond the resolution of MRA, CTA, and CA.[77,78]

There are claims of the utility of brain SPECT imaging in the clinical diagnosis and management of cerebral vasculitis associated with SLE,[79,80] Kawasaki disease,[81] IgAV,[82] neurologic Behçet disease,[83] GPA,[84] and brain irradiation.[85,86] Apart from the direct impact of vascular narrowing and occlusion resulting from necrotizing arteritis and vascular infiltration, other explanations for an abnormal brain SPECT include circulating immune complexes on the BBB,[87] and neurotoxic effects of antibodies and brain antigenic targets,[81] glial cell interactions,[86] and pathogenic hypersensitivity responses to brain antigens released during vascular-mediated tissue necrosis.[86]

The results of brain SPECT imaging were described in one patient with histologically verified cerebral vasculitis.[88] This 71-year-old man with later-proven granulomatous angiitis of the brain underwent Tc-99m hexamethylpropyleneamine oxime brain SPECT 3 weeks after onset of CNS disease. There was irregular radiotracer uptake throughout both cerebral hemispheres with scattered multiple areas of hypoperfusion, further demonstrated in surface volumetric images. Postmortem examination showed fibrinoid necrosis, inflammatory cells, mainly lymphocytes, histiocytes, and a few multinucleated giant cells involving medium-to-small meningeal and parenchymal vessels with intramural vascular deposits of amyloid, without systemic vasculitis.

Color Doppler Ultrasonography

Color Doppler ultrasonography and color duplex imaging provide direct imaging and evaluation of superficial arteries and their vessel walls. It has been most extensively studied in systemic LVV, such as GCA and TAK. It provides a high-resolution imaging of the walls of deep-seated vessels as compared with MRI, detecting wall thickness and edema, the latter of which produces a hypoechoic signal on color Doppler ultrasonography as a halo sign. In a meta-analysis of 998 patients with 17 studies, the sensitivity of the halo sign for biopsy-proven GCA was only 75%, but specificity was 83%. Concentric homogeneous mural thickening, stenosis, and occlusion of the aorta and brachiocephalic branches are typical ultrasonography features of GCA and TAK,[72,89,90] which may be differentiated from atherosclerotic disease by the absence of plaque formation, concentric long segment involvement, and location. Ultrasonography revealed subtle mural changes characterized by a homogeneous, circumferential mid-echoic wall thickening within the subclavian and carotid arteries in the early stages of TAK preceding abnormalities detected by CA,[91] with overall greater wall thickness of the CCA and ICA in the vasculitic vessels compared with controls. The CCA intima-to-medial thickness ratio was increased in patients with TAK compared with normal controls,[92] yielding respective sensitivity and specificity rates of 82% and 70%.

The wall diameters of common, frontal, and parietal division of the superficial temporal artery were significantly greater in patients with GCA than in symptomatic patients without the disease, as well as asymptomatic age-matched controls.[93] A hypoechoic halo surrounding a patent vessel lumen was found in 73% of patients with biopsy-proven vasculitis, but not in symptomatic patients without GCA and asymptomatic controls. The histopathologic finding of mural cellular infiltration did not correlate with a hypoechoic halo albeit attributed to edema. The halo disappeared at a mean of 16 days after effective treatment. Similar findings are present in the occipital arteries,[94] although the sensitivity is less when compared with the superficial temporal arteries. The halo examination is useful for symptomatic patients presenting with nuchal pain, occipital headache, or occipital scalp tenderness, especially when occipital artery involvement may be the only imaging manifestation of the disease.

SUMMARY

The neuroimaging evaluation of vasculitis may seem complex and nonspecific, particularly for PACNS and the primary systemic autoimmune vasculitides. When all imaging modalities, including those that provide parenchymal, luminal, and mural evaluation, are brought to bear on a given patient with suspected vasculitis, the entire constellation of findings typically brings clarity to the situation. When imaging is combined with the clinical and laboratory results, this diagnostic triad becomes more predictable even in the most difficult of clinical cases.

ACKNOWLEDGMENTS

The author acknowledges the assistance of Eytan Raz, MD, PhD, Department of Radiology, Division of Neuro-Radiology, New York University School of Medicine, New York, NY, who provided valuable edits, advice, and figures (as noted) to this article. Adam Davis, MD, formerly of the, Department of Radiology, Division of Neuro-Radiology, New York University School of Medicine, New York, NY, provided imaging studies (as noted).

REFERENCES

1. Giannini C, Salvarani C, Hunder G, et al. Primary central nervous system vasculitis: pathology and mechanisms. Acta Neuropathol 2012;123:759–72.
2. Wynne PJ, Younger DS, Khandji A, et al. Radiographic features of central nervous system vasculitis. Neurol Clin 1997;15:779–804.

3. Marsh EB, Zeiler SR, Levy M, et al. Diagnosing CNS vasculitis: the case against empiric treatment. Neurologist 2012;18:233–8.
4. Weyand CM, Goronzy JJ. Giant-cell arteritis and polymyalgia rheumatica. Ann Intern Med 2003;139:505–15.
5. Adams HP, Kapelle J, Biller J, et al. Ischemic stroke in young adults. Iowa registry of stroke in young adults. Arch Neurol 1995;52:491–5.
6. Gemmete JJ, Davagnanam I, Toma AK, et al. Arterial ischemic stroke in children. Neuroimaging Clin N Am 2013;23:781–98.
7. Younger DS. Adult and childhood vasculitis of the nervous system. Chapter 14. In: Younger DS, editor. Motor disorders. 3rd edition. New York: David S. Younger MD PC; 2013. p. 235–80.
8. Younger DS, Kass RM. Vasculitis and the nervous system. Neurol Clin 1997;15: 737–58.
9. Cupps TR, Fauci AS. The vasculitides. Major Probl Intern Med 1981;21:1–5.
10. Citron BP, Halpern M, McCarron M, et al. Necrotizing angiitis associated with drug abuse. N Engl J Med 1970;283:1003–11.
11. Citron B, Peters R. Angiitis in drug abusers [letter]. N Engl J Med 1971;284: 111–3.
12. Baden M. Angiitis in drug abusers [letter]. N Engl J Med 1971;284:111.
13. Hinck V, Carter C, Rippey C. Giant cell (cranial) arteritis. A case with angiographic abnormalities. Am J Roentgenol Radium Ther Nucl Med 1964;92:769–75.
14. Cupps TR, Moore PM, Fauci AS. Isolated angiitis of the central nervous system. Prospective diagnostic and therapeutic experience. Am J Med 1983;74:97–105.
15. Moore PM, Cupps TR. Neurological complications of vasculitis. Ann Neurol 1983; 14:155–67.
16. Calabrese HL, Mallek JA. Primary angiitis of the central nervous system: report of 8 new cases, review of the literature, and proposal for diagnostic criteria. Medicine 1988;67:20–39.
17. Hajj-Ali RA, Calabrese LH. Central nervous system vasculitis. Curr Opin Rheumatol 2009;21:10–8.
18. Hunder GG, Arend WP, Bloch DA, et al. The American College of Rheumatology 1990 criteria for the classification of vasculitis. Introduction. Arthritis Rheum 1990; 33:1065–7.
19. Lie JT. Illustrated histopathologic classification criteria for selected vasculitis syndrome. Arthritis Rheum 1990;33:1074–87.
20. Lightfoot RW Jr, Michel BA, Bloch DA, et al. The American College of Rheumatology 1990 criteria for the classification of polyarteritis nodosa. Arthritis Rheum 1990;33:1088–93.
21. Arend WP, Michel BA, Bloch DA, et al. The American College of Rheumatology 1990 criteria for the classification of Takayasu arteritis. Arthritis Rheum 1990;33: 1129–34.
22. Masi AT, Hunder GG, Lie JT, et al. The American College of Rheumatology 1990 criteria for the classification of Churg-Strauss syndrome (allergic granulomatosis and angiitis. Arthritis Rheum 1990;33:1094–100.
23. Leavitt RY, Fauci AS, Bloch DA, et al. The American College of Rheumatology 1990 criteria for the classification of Wegener's granulomatosis. Arthritis Rheum 1990;33:1101–7.
24. Calabrese LH, Michel BEA, Bloch DA, et al. The American College of Rheumatology 1990 criteria for the classification of hypersensitivity vasculitis. Arthritis Rheum 1990;33:1108–13.

25. Mills JA, Michel BA, Bloch DA, et al. The American College of Rheumatology 1990 criteria for the classification of Henoch-Schönlein purpura. Arthritis Rheum 1990;33:1114–21.
26. Hunder GG, Bloch DA, Michel BA, et al. The American College of Rheumatology 1990 criteria for the classification of giant cell arteritis. Arthritis Rheum 1990;33: 1122–8.
27. Jennette JC, Falk RJ, Andrassy K, et al. Nomenclature of systemic vasculitides. Proposal of an international consensus conference. Arthritis Rheum 1994;37: 187–92.
28. Jennette JC, Falk RJ, Bacon PA, et al. 2012 revised International Chapel Hill consensus conference nomenclature of vasculitides. Arthritis Rheum 2013;65: 1–11.
29. Küker W. Cerebral vasculitis: imaging signs revisited. Neuroradiology 2007;49: 471–9.
30. Kaufman TJ, Kallmes DF. Diagnostic cerebral angiography: archaic and complication-prone or here to stay for another 80 years? AJR Am J Roentgenol 2008;190:1435–7.
31. Hajj-Ali RA, Calabrese LH. PACNS. Autoimmun Rev 2013;12:463–6.
32. Gomes LJ. The role of imaging in the diagnosis of central nervous system vasculitis. Curr Allergy Asthma Rep 2010;10:163–70.
33. Lie JT. Vasculitis associated with infectious agents. Curr Opin Rheumatol 1996;8: 26–9.
34. Zuccoli G, Pipitone N, Haldipur A, et al. Imaging findings in primary central nervous system vasculitis. Clin Exp Rheumatol 2007;29(Suppl 64):S104–9.
35. Salvarani C, Brown RD Jr, Calamia KT, et al. Primary central nervous system vasculitis: analysis of 101 patients. Ann Neurol 2007;62:442–51.
36. Kuker W. Imaging of cerebral vasculitis. Int J Stroke 2007;2:184–90.
37. Wasserman BA, Stone JH, Hellman, et al. Reliability of normal findings on MR imaging for excluding the diagnosis of vasculitis of the central nervous system. AJR Am J Roentgenol 2001;177:455–9.
38. Pomper M, Miller T, Stone J, et al. CNS vasculitis in autoimmune disease: MR imaging findings and correlation with angiography. AJNR Am J Neuroradiol 1999; 20:75–85.
39. Rossi CM, Comite G. The clinical spectrum of the neurological involvement in vasculitides. J Neurol Sci 2009;285:13–21.
40. Neel A, Pangnoux C. Primary angiitis of the central nervous system. Clin Exp Rheumatol 2009;27:S95–107.
41. Spitzer C, Mull M, Rohde V, et al. Non-traumatic cortical subarachnoid haemorrhage: diagnostic work-up and etiological background. Neuroradiology 2005; 47:525–31.
42. Ay H, Sahin G, Saatci I, et al. PACNS and silent cortical hemorrhages. AJNR Am J Neuroradiol 2002;23:1561–3.
43. Miller DV, Salvarani C, Hunder GG, et al. Biopsy findings in PACNS. Am J Surg Pathol 2009;33:35–43.
44. Salvarani C, Brown RD Jr, Gene G. Adult primary central nervous system vasculitis. Lancet 2012;380:767–77.
45. Küker W, Gaertner S, Nägele T, et al. Vessel wall contrast enhancement: a diagnostic sign of cerebral vasculitis. Cerebrovasc Dis 2008;26:23–9.
46. Muccio CF, DiBlasi A, Espositio G, et al. Perfusion and spectroscopy magnetic resonance imaging in a case of lymphocytic vasculitis mimicking brain tumor. Pol J Radiol 2013;78:66–9.

47. Park MS, Marlin AE, Gaskill SJ. Angiography-negative primary angiitis of the central nervous system in childhood. J Neurosurg Pediatr 2014;13:62–7.
48. Sundgren PC, Jennings J, Attwood JT, et al. MRI and 2D-CSI MR spectroscopy of the brain in the evaluation of patients with acute onset of neuropsychiatric systemic lupus erythematosus. Neuroradiology 2005;47:576–85.
49. Mandell DM, Mossa-Basha M, Qiao Y. Vessel wall imaging Study Group of the American Society of Neuroradiology. Intracranial vessel wall MRI: principles and expert consensus recommendations of the American Society of Neuroradiology. AJNR Am J Neuroradiol 2017;38(2):218–29.
50. Choe YH, Han BK, Koh EM, et al. Takayasu's arteritis: assessment of disease activity with contrast-enhanced MR imaging. AJR Am J Roentgenol 2000;175:505–51.
51. Bley TA, Uhl M, Carew J, et al. Diagnostic value of high-resolution MR imaging in giant cell arteritis. AJNR Am J Neuroradiol 2007;28:1722–7.
52. Geiger J, Ness T, Uhl M, et al. Involvement of the ophthalmic artery in giant cell arteritis visualized by 3T MRI. Rheumatology (Oxford) 2009;48(5):537–41.
53. Brouwer PA, Bosman T, van Walderveen MA, et al. Dynamic 320-section CT angiography in cranial arteriovenous shunting lesions. AJNR Am J Neuroradiol 2010;31:767–70.
54. Demaerel P, De Ruyter N, Maes F, et al. Magnetic resonance angiography in suspected cerebral vasculitis. Eur Radiol 2004;14:1005–12.
55. Khandelwal N, Kalra N, Garg MK, et al. Multidetector CT angiography in Takayasu's arteritis. Eur J Radiol 2011;77:369–74.
56. Yamada I, Nakagawa T, Himeno Y, et al. Takayasu's arteritis: evaluation of the thoracic aorta with CT angiography. Radiology 1998;209:103–9.
57. Kermani TA, Warrington KJ, Crowson CS, et al. Large-vessel involvement in giant cell arteritis: a population-based cohort study of the incidence-trends and prognosis. Ann Rheum Dis 2013;72:1989–94.
58. Weyand CM, Goronzy JJ. Giant-cell arteritis and polymyalgia rheumatica. N Engl J Med 2014;4:371, 50-57.
59. Zhu FP, Luo S, Wang ZJ, et al. Takayasu arteritis: imaging spectrum at multidetector CT angiography. Br J Radiol 2012;85:e1282–92.
60. Mnif N, Chaker M, Oueslati S, et al. Abdominal polyarteritis nodosa: angiographic features. J Radiol 2004;85:635–8.
61. Lecler A, Obadia M, Savatovsky J, et al. TIPIC syndrome: beyond the myth of carotidynia, a new distinct unclassified entity. AJNR Am J Neuroradiol 2017;38:1391–8.
62. Birnbaum J, Hellman DB. Primary angiitis of the central nervous system. Arch Neurol 2009;66:704–9.
63. Cloft HJ, Phillips CD, Dix JE, et al. Correlation of angiography and MR imaging in cerebral vasculitis. Acta Radiol 1999;40:83–7.
64. Alrawi A, Trobe JD, Blaivas M, et al. Brain biopsy in primary angiitis of the central nervous system. Neurology 1999;53:858–60.
65. Harris KG, Tran DD, Sickels WJ, et al. Diagnosing intracranial vasculitis: the roles of MR and angiography. AJNR Am J Neuroradiol 1994;15:317–30.
66. Duna GF, Calabrese LH. Limitations of invasive modalities in the diagnosis of primary angiitis of the central nervous system. J Rheumatol 1995;22:662–7.
67. Chu CT, Gray L, Goldstein LB, et al. Diagnosis of intracranial vasculitis: a multidisciplinary approach. J Neuropathol Exp Neurol 1998;57:30–8.

68. Benseler SM, deVeber G, Hawkins C, et al. Angiography-negative primary central nervous system vasculitis in children: a newly recognized inflammatory central nervous system disease. Arthritis Rheum 2005;52:2159–67.

69. Hellmann DB, Roubenoff R, Healy RA, et al. Central nervous system angiography: safety and predictors of a positive result in 125 consecutive patients evaluated for possible vasculitis. J Rheumatol 1992;19:568–72.

70. Cheng Y, Lu N, Wang Z, et al. 18F-FDG-PET in assessing disease activity in Takayasu's arteritis: a meta-analysis. Clin Exp Rheumatol 2013;31:S22–7.

71. Besson FL, Arienti JJ, Bienvenu B, et al. Diagnostic performance of 18Fuorodeoxyglucose positron emission tomography in giant cell arteritis: a systematic review and meta-analysis. Eur J Nucl Med Mol Imaging 2011;38:1764–72.

72. Amezcua-Guerra LM, Pineda C. Imaging studies in the diagnosis and management of vasculitis. Curr Rheumatol Rep 2007;9:320–7.

73. Direskeneli H, Aydın SZ, Merkel PA. Assessment of disease activity and progression in Takayasu's arteritis. Clin Exp Rheumatol 2011;29:S86–91.

74. Blockmans D, de Ceuninck L, Vander-Schueren S, et al. Repetitive 18F-fluorodeoxyglucose positron emission tomography in giant cell arteritis: a prospective study of 35 patients. Arthritis Rheum 2006;55:131–7.

75. Karapolat I, Kalfa M, Keser G, et al. Comparison of 18F-FDG PET/CT findings with current clinical disease status in patients with Takayasu's arteritis. Clin Exp Rheumatol 2013;31:S15–21.

76. Bacchi S, Franke K, Wewegama D, et al. Magnetic resonance and positron emission tomography in anti-NMDA receptor encephalitis: a systemic review. J Clin Neurosci 2018;52:54–9.

77. Yuh WTC, Ueda T, Maley JE, et al. Diagnosis of microvasculopathy in CNS vasculitis: value of perfusion and diffusion imaging. J Magn Reson Imaging 1999;10:310–3.

78. Masdeu JC, Brass LM, Holman BL, et al. Brain single-photon emission computed tomography. Neurology 1994;44:1970–7.

79. Meusser S, Rubbert A, Manger B, et al. 99m-Tc-HMPAO-SPECT in diagnosis of early cerebral vasculitis. Rheumatol Int 1996;16:37–42.

80. Zhang X, Zhu A, Zhang F, et al. Diagnostic value of single-photon-emission computed tomography in severe central nervous system involvement of systemic lupus erythematosus: a case-control study. Arthritis Rheum 2005;53:845–9.

81. Sato T, Ushiroda Y, Oyama T, et al. Kawasaki disease-associated MERS: pathological insights from SPECT findings. Brain Dev 2012;34(34):605–8.

82. Suh J-S, Hahn W-H, Cho R-S, et al. A rare case of cerebral vasculitis in Henoch-Schönlein purpura with emphasis on the diagnostic value of magnetic resonance angiography (MRA) and single-photon emission computed tomography (SPECT) given normal magnetic resonance imaging (MRI). Int J Dermatol 2010;49:803–5.

83. Sener RN. Neuro-Behcet's disease: diffusion MR imaging and proton MR spectroscopy. AJNR Am J Neuroradiol 2003;24:1612–4.

84. Marienhagen J, Geissler A, Lang B. High resolution single photon emission computed tomography of the brain in Wegener's granulomatosis. J Rheumatol 1996;23:1828–30.

85. Groothuis DR, Mikhael MA. Focal cerebral vasculitis associated with circulating immune complexes and brain irradiation. Ann Neurol 1986;19:590–2.

86. Rottenberg DA, Chernik NL, Deck MEF, et al. Cerebral necrosis following radiotherapy of extracranial neoplasms. Ann Neurol 1977;1:339–57.

87. Faust TW, Chang EH, Kowal C, et al. Neurotoxic lupus antibodies alter brain function through two distinct mechanisms. Proc Natl Acad Sci U S A 2010;107: 18569–74.
88. Shih W-J, Wilson D, Stipp V, et al. Heterogeneous uptake on brain SPECT. Semin Nucl Med 1999;29:85–8.
89. Gotway M, Araoz PA, Macedo TA, et al. Imaging findings in Takayasu's arteritis. AJR Am J Roentgenol 2004;184:1945–50.
90. Kissin EY, Merkel PA. Diagnostic imaging in Takayasu's arteritis. Curr Opin Rheumatol 2004;16:31–7.
91. Schmidt WA, Nerenheim A, Seipelt E, et al. Diagnosis of early Takayasu's arteritis with sonography. Rheumatology (Oxford) 2002;41:496–502.
92. Seth S, Goyal NK, Jagia P, et al. Carotid intima–medial thickness as a marker of disease activity in Takayasu's arteritis. Int J Cardiol 2006;108:385–90.
93. Schmidt WA, Kraft HE, Vorpahl K, et al. Color duplex ultrasonography in the diagnosis of temporal arteritis. N Engl J Med 1997;337:1336–42.
94. Pfadenhauer K, Weber H. Giant cell arteritis of the occipital arteries: a prospective color coded duplex sonography study in 78 patients. J Neurol 2003;250: 844–9.

Granulomatous Angiitis
Twenty Years Later

David S. Younger, MD, MPH, MS[a,b,*]

KEYWORDS

- Central nervous system • Stroke • Vasculitis • Granulomatous angiitis

KEY POINTS

- The vasculitides are diseases characterized by inflammation of blood vessels and inflammatory leukocytes in vessel walls.
- Granulomatous angiitis refers to distinctive clinicopathologic disorders with the essential features of granulomatous inflammation of cerebral and spinal arteries.
- No typically abnormal laboratory study excludes or makes the diagnosis except a positive brain and meningeal biopsy specimen.
- Therapy is aimed at preventing infarction or hemorrhage from inflamed or scarred vessels.

HISTORICAL CASES

Harbitz[1] first described primary central nervous system (CNS) vasculitis (PCNSV) due to granulomatous angiitis in 1922 in 2 patients, one with worsening headaches, mental change, and ataxia culminating in stupor, spastic paraparesis, coma, and death in 2 years. A second patient presented with hallucinations and confusion progressing to gait difficulty, stupor, coma, and death in 9 months. At postmortem examination, both had granulomatous vasculitis of the meninges comprising lymphocytes, multinucleated giant cells, and epithelioid cells with vessel necrosis and extension into the brain along involved veins and arteries of varying caliber.

Over the ensuing quarter century, additional patients with granulomatous angiitis of the brain (GAB) or the equivalent team, granulomatous angiitis, reported under the rubric of allergic angiitis and granulomatosis,[2] giant cell arteritis (GCA),[3] and sarcoidosis[4] were described. Cravioto and Fegin[5] delineated the clinicopathologic syndrome of noninfectious granulomatous angiitis; for 2 more decades, rare affected patients were identified in life, but there was no effective treatment. The identification of

Disclosure Statement: The author has nothing to disclose.
[a] Department of Neurology, Division of Neuro-Epidemiology, New York University School of Medicine, New York, NY 10016, USA; [b] School of Public Health, City University of New York, New York, NY, USA
* 333 East 34th Street, Suite 1J, New York, NY 10016.
E-mail address: youngd01@nyu.edu
Website: http://www.davidsyounger.com

angiographic beading and a sausagelike appearance of cerebral vessels at sites of presumed arteritis was noted by Hinck and coworkers[6] in GCA, and later by Cupps and Fauci[7] in so-called isolated angiitis of the CNS (IACNS). The judged efficacy of a combination immunosuppressive regimen of oral cyclophosphamide and alternate day prednisone in 3 patients with IACNS defined angiographically, and in another with biopsy-proven granulomatous angiitis of the filum terminale, led to prospective diagnostic and therapeutic recommendations.[8] At that time, investigators regarded IACNS[7] and other cases typified by granulomatous angiitis as interchangeable terms with the former term emphasizing the restricted nature of the vasculitis, and the latter term emphasizing the granulomatous histology. The thinking was that giant cells and epithelioid cells, usually found at autopsy in cases of granulomatous angiitis, were an inconsistent finding in leptomeningeal and brain or spinal cord biopsy tissues and therefore considered unnecessary for antemortem diagnosis.

In 1988, Calabrese and Mallek[9] proposed criteria for the diagnosis of primary angiitis of the central nervous system vasculitis (PACNS) among 6 adults and 2 children aged 10 and 12 years. Seven patients, including both children, recovered either spontaneously (1 child) or with intensive immunosuppressant therapy (6 patients), empirically (4 patients) or based on a positive leptomeningeal and brain biopsy for vasculitis, although one died of autopsy-confirmed spinal cord vasculitis. Among 3 cases studied at postmortem (cases 4, 5, and 7), 2 had positive leptomeningeal biopsies, among them one with a normal cortex; a third had vasculitis of the spinal cord. The histopathology of case 5 was consistent with granulomatous small-vessel vasculitis affecting meningeal veins (**Fig. 1**) with proliferation of epithelioid cells along vascular walls, sparing the cortex. Cerebral angiography in that patient was negative, showing tortuosity and irregularity of the lumen of intracranial vessels without segmental or alternating stenosis and ectasia typical of arteritis.

Contemporaneously, Younger and colleagues[10] described the limits of GAB in 4 postmortem and 74 literature cases, all of which met the selection criteria of pathologic evidence of cerebral blood vessel inflammation by giant cells or epithelioid cells. Granulomatous giant cell or epithelioid cell infiltration was detected in the walls of larger named vessels in the first patient who had concomitant varicella herpes zoster virus ophthalmicus (HZO); in large and small leptomeningeal vessels together in the second patient with no other condition; in small leptomeningeal vessels in the third patient with Hodgkin lymphoma (**Fig. 2**); and leptomeningeal and cortical veins in the fourth patient with neurosarcoidosis, all with varying degrees of vessel wall destruction and necrosis. None had evidence of systemic vasculitis at autopsy. Brain infarcts were widespread, involving both brainstem and cerebral hemispheres. Spinal cord lesions were seen in other patients with clinical myelopathy. No typically abnormal laboratory study excluded, or made the diagnosis of GAB in a living patient except a "positive" CNS biopsy specimen.

Although some authorities[8] cite diagnostic changes on cerebral arteriography, this seems to be a dubious contention because vessel narrowing, beading, multiple dilatations, aneurysms, avascular mass lesions, and normal studies were all seen in granulomatous angiitis and in angiitis of other origins.[11] Polyarteritis nodosa, amphetamine abuse, and rheumatoid arthritis cause arteriographic changes that resemble granulomatous angiitis, but the lesions in these diseases characteristically do not include giant cells or epithelioid cells. Because the changes were associated with diverse and dissimilar diseases and pathologic alterations, no particular arteriographic finding could be considered diagnostic of granulomatous angiitis. Four patients with granulomatous angiitis had normal arteriograms a few weeks before death even though arteritis and stenosis of one or more large vessels were observed at postmortem examination. Of 8 patients with granulomatous angiitis proved by brain biopsy,

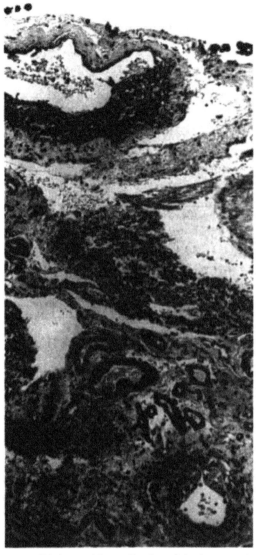

Fig. 1. Granulomatous angiitis located in small veins of the leptomeninges associated with a proliferation of epithelioid cells along the vascular walls in case 5. (*From* Calabrese HL, Mallek JA. Primary angiitis of the central nervous system: report of 8 new cases, review of the literature, and proposal for diagnostic criteria. Medicine 1988; 67:20–39; with permission.)

arteriographic findings were normal in 2, while 3 studies showed signs of an avascular mass suggesting brain tumor, with no 1 showing beading of vessels, and 2 nonspecific changes in vessels without frank beading. Beading of vessels considered diagnostic of granulomatous angiitis or IACNS was seen in only 3 patients and was not considered a reliable diagnostic sign.

To determine whether the "idiopathic" cases delineated a distinct disorder, Younger and colleagues[10] evaluated headache, hemiparesis, mental changes, abnormal cerebrospinal fluid (CSF) protein level, CSF pleocytosis, brain imaging, and cerebral

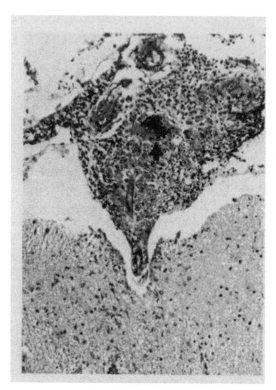

Fig. 2. Postmortem examination of a patient (case 3) with granulomatous angiitis of the brain in a patient with Hodgkin lymphoma. The photomicrograph on the left shows small leptomeningeal blood vessels of the left temporal lobe. A compact mass of epithelioid cells, multinucleated giant cell, and lymphocytes engulf several small blood vessels, one located in a depression of the cerebral cortical surface, in its path between leptomeninges and neural tissue. Mild astrocytosis is present in the molecular layer of cerebral cortex.

angiography. There was no difference in the frequency of these abnormalities in the idiopathic cases as compared with those with HZO, neurosarcoidosis, or lymphoma. There was no clear clinical syndrome that would mandate brain biopsy; nevertheless, biopsy of brain and overlying meninges would be warranted if there were no other cause to explain a clinical syndrome of encephalopathy (including confusion or alteration of consciousness), evolving over days or weeks and, especially, with focal "cerebral signs" or abnormal CSF with pleocytosis, high protein content (100 mg/dL), and normal glucose content. Signs of encephalopathy were dominant in 61 of 78 cases, including 10 of 12 patients who also had an acute stroke as well as all 7 with hemiparesis contralateral to skin lesions of HZO. In the absence of more diffuse encephalopathy, therefore, acute stroke with or without herpes zoster would not warrant biopsy.

Therapy for PCNSV is generally aimed at preventing infarction or hemorrhage from inflamed or scarred cerebral vessels. Seven of 10 patients with conditions diagnosed antemortem by CNS biopsy specimens were followed up prospectively for a mean of 7 months (range, 1 month to 1 year), including one each with HZO or lymphoma, and 5 with no associated disorder. All 7 improved taking corticosteroids alone (3 patients) or combined with cyclophosphamide or azathioprine (3 patients; or cyclophosphamide alone (1 patient).

In 1997, Younger and colleagues[12] conducted a historical review of pathologically confirmed cases of granulomatous angiitis, which still stands as the largest cohort of well-defined cases, presenting a balanced view of the merits of corticosteroids and other immunosuppressants, notwithstanding the selection bias due to the inclusion of cases of GAB.[10]

Altogether, 136 cases conformed to strict pathologic criteria. They included 78 patients described by Younger and colleagues[10] from 1922 to 1988; 57 additional literature patients, including 12 reported during the period surveyed by Younger and colleagues but not included in their analysis, and a new antemortem case. Overall, 35 of the 136 patients were diagnosed antemortem by brain and meningeal biopsy, and 100 were diagnosed postmortem. Fifty-one patients had granulomatous angiitis in association with other conditions, including 11 patients with temporal or systemic giant cell arteritis, 12 patients with herpes zoster virus (HZV) infection, 9 patients with lymphoma alone in 7 patients and together with HZV in 2 patients, 6 patients with sarcoidosis, 10 patients with amyloid angiopathy, 1 patient with systemic lupus, and 2 patients with human immunodeficiency virus (HIV) infection without AIDS.

Headaches, mental change, and gait disorder, that evolved over weeks to months or more followed by focal cerebral signs including seizure, aphasia, hemiparesis or tetraparesis, coma, and death, were noted in 77% (103/135) of patients overall. The neurologic disorder associated with temporal or systemic giant cell arteritis differed from other patients with granulomatous angiitis in the predilection for large intracranial vessels and the relentless progression despite corticosteroids. The neurologic disorder of granulomatous angiitis associated with HZV typically followed appearance of an ophthalmicus (V_1) rash by 2 to 3 weeks and was contralateral to the skin lesions and vasculitis involvement of the ipsilateral carotid, middle, or anterior cerebral artery, although several other patients had nonophthalmicus, spinal radicular dermatomal lesions, or disseminated HZV. Most patients with lymphoma-associated granulomatous angiitis had a subacute or chronic neurologic illness. One patient with a cavernous sinus syndrome had biopsy-proven granulomatous angiitis and occult primary lymphoma of the midbrain at autopsy. A second patient had a successfully treated malignant lymphoma of the parotid gland. At autopsy, there was evidence of granulomatous angiitis affecting spinal and cerebral leptomeningeal vessels, and a malignant lymphoma of the parotid gland. A third patient had headaches and progressive spastic paraparesis that prompted brain biopsy and discovery of granulomatous angiitis; reevaluation of a submandibular mass showed Hodgkin lymphoma. Treatment of the tumor with combination chemotherapy resulted in remission of the cancer and stabilization of the neurologic disorder. The neurologic disease in the 6 patients with sarcoidosis was essentially similar to other cases without sarcoid. Two patients had known systemic disease and were being treated with corticosteroids when neurologic symptoms developed. Asymptomatic systemic involvement was present in 3 of 4 others diagnosed at autopsy. The 10 patients with amyloid angiopathy were clinically and pathologically inseparable from other cases of granulomatous angiitis.

The pathologic heterogeneity of granulomatous angiitis was exemplified in the predilection of lesions for vessels of variable caliber, regardless of the presenting clinical syndrome or associated disorder. Of 50 cases studied postmortem, 6 had predominant involvement of small arteries and veins; 11 involved small and large vessels; 28 involved small and medium-sized arteries; and 5 had large cerebral vessel involvement alone. Isolated microscopic foci of vascular inflammation were seen in heart, lungs, and kidney specimens at general autopsy in 19 patients with otherwise typical granulomatous angiitis that were deemed to be of insufficient evidence for systemic vasculitis.

The diagnosis of granulomatous angiitis begins with a high index of suspicion based on the symptoms, signs, and laboratory studies at presentation and during the course of the illness. Screening blood studies, such as the white blood cells count, hematocrit, erythrocyte sedimentation rate, and serologic studies, are of little use in the diagnosis of granulomatous angiitis, but may be useful in suggesting the presence of an underlying systemic illness, serologically distinct connective tissue disorder, or systemic vasculitis. CSF should be analyzed in all suspected cases because pleocytosis of greater than 10 white blood cells/mm^3 and protein elevation of greater than 100 mg/dL lend strong support to the diagnosis of granulomatous angiitis. However, a normal profile does not exclude the diagnosis, because a quarter of proven cases had a normal cell count, and a third of proven cases showed a normal protein content. Oligoclonal bands were present in 3 of 6 patients with cerebral vasculitis so studied. It is important to culture CSF for obvious infectious organisms because mycobacteria, spirochetes, fungi, and herpes viruses can cause latent infection and cerebral vasculitis. Noninvasive imaging studies are of limited usefulness. MRI of the brain is generally more sensitive than computed tomography (CT), but both lack specificity. Brain CT was normal or showed nonspecific atrophy in 20 of 41 (49%) patients so studied; MRI was normal in none of 16 cases. The most common MRI findings were abnormal T_2 signal foci in the subcortical white matter, meningeal enhancement, and mass lesions, seen altogether in 75% of patients. Although these findings may be helpful in suggesting the need for further evaluation, magnetic resonance angiography (MRA), PET with [18]fluorodeoxyglucose, and single-photon emission CT (SPECT) provide useful complementary information to conventional MRI; however, the observed defects in cerebral blood flow do not always correlate with, or predict, neurologic symptoms and do not distinguish vasculitis from other forms of occlusive vascular disease. One patient with histologically proven granulomatous angiitis had abnormality of SPECT imaging. Fundic fluorescence angiography combined with slit-lamp microscopy has been advocated to estimate erythrocyte flow and cerebral perfusion in CNS vasculitis.

Cerebral angiography was normal in 23 of 49 (47%) patients. In 26% of patients, there were suggestive features of vasculitis, including segmental narrowing in 6 patients (12%), microaneurysms in 3 patients (6%), and beading in 4 patients (8%), but these too can be seen in nonvasculitic arteriopathy, intracranial atherosclerosis, vasospasm, mycotic aneurysm, infection, emboli, and tumor. Brain and meningeal biopsy is the gold standard for the diagnosis of cerebral vasculitis because it is the only way to identify the underlying histopathology and to exclude other causes. The preferred site for brain and meningeal biopsy is the temporal tip of the nondominant hemisphere in an area with a longitudinally oriented surface vessel. An infratentorial approach is considered in patients with sarcoidosis or tuberculosis because the basilar meninges are preferentially involved. A normal or nondiagnostic biopsy was noted in 9 of 43 (26%) histologically confirmed cases, reflecting the low sensitivity of the test. Six of 9 nondiagnostic biopsies contained brain tissue alone, compared with 2 of 35 diagnostic biopsies that combined brain and leptomeninges, indicating the importance of sampling the meninges to increase the likelihood of a diagnostic specimen. Tissue samples should be stained and cultured for bacterial, fungal, spirochetal, and viral organisms and preserved frozen for later investigations. It is difficult to know when to proceed with brain biopsy.

The outcome of treatment in 54 pathologically proven cases of granulomatous angiitis is summarized in **Table 1**. Among 30 patients diagnosed antemortem by meningeal and brain biopsy, 28 were treated with corticosteroids alone (in 11 patients) or with oral cyclophosphamide (in 16 patients), or azathioprine (in 1 patient), and followed for up to 1 year, of whom 18 (64%) improved, 7 (25%) remained unchanged, and 3 (11%) died

Table 1
Outcome of 54 patients with granulomatous angiitis of the nervous system

Outcome	CS	CS + CYC	CS + AZA	None	Total
Improved	8/0[a]	9/0	1/0	0	10/0
Same	3/0	4/0	0	1/0	8/0
Died	0/6	3/1	0	1/17	4/24

Abbreviations: AZA, azathioprine; CS, corticosteroids; CYC, cyclophosphamide.
[a] Patients diagnosed antemortem in the numerator, and patients diagnosed postmortem in the denominator.
From Younger DS, Calabrese LH, Hays AP. Granulomatous angiitis of the nervous system. Neurol Clin 1997;15:821–34; with permission.

with roughly equally satisfactory outcomes after treatment with corticosteroids with or without cyclophosphamide. Three patients diagnosed antemortem died while taking corticosteroids and cyclophosphamide; 2 patients suffered serious sequelae of the therapy, including fatal lymphoma, immunosuppression and opportunistic infection, or pneumonia and leukopenia. Of 24 patients diagnosed postmortem, 7 (29%) received treatment with corticosteroids alone (in 6 patients) or with cyclophosphamide (in 1 patient), and 17 (71%) were untreated. Thus, 17 of 18 (94%) untreated patients died, indicating that without therapy the disease was usually fatal. Treatment with corticosteroids, alone or in combination with cyclophosphamide, was associated with a considerable reduction in mortality; 24 of 34 (70%) so treated survived as either improved (50%) or clinically unchanged. Thus, there was no appreciable benefit in the addition of cyclophosphamide; however, the numbers were small, unmatched for age, disease activity, or other factors, and follow-up was not uniform. Cyclophosphamide should be reserved for histologically confirmed cases, especially those who continue to progress or fail to improve on corticosteroids alone, and those who can be monitored closely for serious medication side effects.

MODERN COHORTS

Commensurate with the refinement in clinical trials methods, adult patients with CNS vasculitis are reported in large retrospective cohorts at the Mayo Clinic[13] and in observational cohorts from the French Vasculitis Study Group, French NeuroVascular Society, and the French Internal Medicine Society consortia,[14] stratifying cases based on clinical, neuroradiographic, and histopathologic laboratory features, and offering additional insights into the management of CNS vasculitis. Patients included in each cohort based on tissue biopsy according to the original criteria of Calabrese and Mallek[9] continue to be a minority, attesting to the reliance of angiographic criteria for the diagnosis of cerebral vasculitis, a fact that adds selection bias to the frequency of granulomatous angiitis, and the assessment of the natural outcome or that of a given therapy.

In 2007, Salvarani and colleagues[15] diagnosed primary PCNSV from 1983 to 2003, 70 (69%) by angiography and 31 (31%) by histopathology, 18 of which were granulomatous, 8 of which were lymphocytic, and 5 of which were acute necrotizing among thirty–one patients diagnosed by histopathology, and 70 patients by angiography, of whom 18 had a granulomatous inflammatory pattern, 8 had a lymphocytic pattern, and 5 had an acute necrotizing pattern. Headache was the commonest symptoms so noted overall in 63% of patients, followed by abnormal cognition, hemiparesis, and persistent neurologic deficit. A granulomatous pattern of inflammation was seen most often in those with altered cognition and at an older age. There were no significant differences in survival when patients were stratified by treatment (prednisone alone vs prednisone and cyclophosphamide) or method of diagnosis (angiography or biopsy). Four manifestations at presentation were associated with increased mortality, including focal neurologic deficit, cognitive impairment, cerebral infarction, and large cerebral vessel involvement.

Between 2004 and 2011, Salvarani and collaborators[13] enrolled 105 patients, of whom (64%) met inclusion criteria for the diagnosis of probable CNS vasculitis based on cerebral angiography manifesting areas of smooth-wall segmental narrowing or dilatation, and occlusions that affected multiple cerebral arteries without the proximal vessel changes of atherosclerosis or other causes; 58 patients (36%) who met the definite diagnosis based on a CNS tissue biopsy showed transmural vascular inflammation involving leptomeningeal or parenchymal vessels. The latter histopathology was granulomatous in 35 (60.3%), lymphocytic in 13 (22.4%), and necrotizing alone in 10 (17.2%) patients. These histologic patterns appeared to identify subsets of disease rather than different stages of the same process because no individual patient had histologic evidence of more than 1 pattern. A favorable response to therapy, including corticosteroids (prednisone) alone or in association with cyclophosphamide, was observed in 85% of patients. Three patients treated with biological agents, including rituximab (1 patient) and a tumor necrosis factor-α inhibitor (2 patients) for treatment of refractory disease, were also improved. Relapses were observed in 27% of patients, and 25% of patients had discontinued therapy by the time of the last follow-up visit. Although response to treatment was not associated with any histologic pattern of the biopsy specimen, treatment with corticosteroids alone was associated with more frequent relapses (odds ratio [OR], 2.90), whereas large named vessel involvement (OR, 6.14) and cerebral infarcts at the time of diagnosis (OR, 3.32) were associated with a poor response to treatment. Among the patients diagnosed exclusively by angiography alone, relapses were more frequent when there was large-vessel involvement (30%) than only small-vessel changes (9%), with an increased mortality due to fatal neurovascular problems caused by PCNSV. Subsets of patients with PCNSV showed equally interesting insights.

Salvarani and coworkers[16] noted granulomatous vasculitis in all 8 (100%) cerebral biopsies of patients with lymphoma and PCNSV, 2 of whom had concomitant cerebral amyloid angiopathy. Among 131 consecutive patients with PCNSV, 11 (8.4%) had a rapidly progressive course that was resistant to immunosuppressive therapy, resulting in severe disability or death. Such patients had bilateral cortical and subcortical infarction on initial brain MRI and large named cerebral vessel involvement on cerebral angiography with granulomatous and necrotizing vasculitis in brain tissue biopsies. All 11 patients failed to respond to aggressive immunosuppressive therapy, only one of whom survived with major fixed neurologic deficits.

In 2018, De Boysson and colleagues[14] described the treatment and long-term outcomes of an observational cohort of 112 patients with PCNSV derived from 3 main networks: the French Vasculitis Study Group, French Neurovascular Society, and the French Internal Medicine Society. The criteria inclusion were (1) involvement of CNS vessels evidenced by biopsy or based or imaging (on digital subtraction angiography or MRA), showing intracranial arterial stenoses, occlusions, or fusiform dilations; (2) a complete workup performed, including infectious and immunologic serologies (HIV, hepatitis B virus, hepatitis C virus, syphilis, tuberculosis, antinuclear and antineutrophil cytoplasmic antibodies, echocardiography, and whole body imaging), to exclude alternative conditions than PCNSV affecting CNS vessels; and (3) a 6-month or more follow-up (unless the patient died before 6 months of biopsy-proven PCNSV) to prevent the inclusion of other vasculopathies, such as reversible cerebral vasoconstriction syndrome, where vascular lesions reverse within the first months.[17] The rate of prolonged remission was defined by the absence of relapse at ≥12 months after diagnosis; as was the functional status at last follow-up in accordance with 3 main groups of treatments administered: corticosteroids (group 1); induction treatment with corticosteroids and an immunosuppressant, but no maintenance (group 2); and combined treatment with corticosteroids and an immunosuppressant for induction followed by maintenance therapy (group 3). Good functional status was defined as a modified Rankin Scale score ≤2 at the last follow-up.

Among the 112 patients reported by De Boysson and colleagues,[14] 33 (29%) patients were included with a diagnostic CNS tissue biopsy, and 68 (61%) and 11 (10%), respectively, had digital subtraction angiography or MRA consistent with PCNSV. Remission was achieved with the initial induction treatment in 106 (95%) of the 112 patients. Prolonged remission without relapse was observed in 70 (66%) patients after a mean of 57 months (range 12–198) of follow-up. A good functional status at last follow-up (ie, modified Rankin Scale score ≤2) was observed in 63 (56%) patients. The overall mortality was 8%. More prolonged remissions (P = .003) and a better functional status at the last follow-up (P = .0004) were observed in group 3. In multivariate analysis, the use of maintenance therapy was associated with prolonged remission (OR, 4.32 [1.67–12.19]; P = .002) and better functional status (OR, 8.09 [3.24–22.38]; P<.0001). These findings suggest that maintenance therapy with an immunosuppressant combined with corticosteroids leads to the best long-term clinical and functional outcomes in patients with PCNSV after having achieved remission with either corticosteroids alone or in combination with another immunosuppressant. In that regards, cyclophosphamide in combination with corticosteroids for induction and azathioprine for maintenance were the 2 main immunosuppressants used in this registry. Whether other combinations or sequences can achieve better results remained to be ascertained.

The PedVas Initiative, a Canadian and United Kingdom collaborative study (ARChiVe Investigators Network within the PedVas Initiative [ARChiVe registry], BrainWorks, and Diagnostic and Classification Criteria in Vasculitis Study [DCCVS]) of pediatric and adult cases of antineutrophil cytoplasmic antibody-associated vasculitis (AAV) and PACNS (NIH identifier, NCT02006134), has been prospectively collecting clinical and biobank data since January 2013 of registered cases, within 12 months of study entry, with an expected completion in December 2019. The approach to the diagnosis and classification of childhood PACNS (cPACNS) is to start with inflammatory brain disease as the common denominator and to exclude mimics of angiography-positive cPACNS, and angiography-negative, brain biopsy-positive small vessel (SV)-cPACNS before initiating cytotoxic therapy for presumed cPACNS.[18] Children with angiographically negative SV-cPACNS[19] have persistent headache, cognitive decline, mood disorder, focal seizures, and abnormal brain neuroimaging. Among 13 such children in whom detailed brain biopsy findings were available,[20] the inflammatory cell infiltrate was located in intramural arterioles, capillaries, or venules in 11 patients so studied, consisting predominantly of a mixture of lymphocytes and macrophages, with occasional plasma cells, polymorphonuclear cells, and eosinophils. Granulomatous inflammation and multinucleated giant cells were characteristically absent. Affected blood vessels were found in leptomeninges, cortex, and subcortical white matter in 7 of 9 specimens. The remaining 2 patients without definable vasculitis exhibited nonspecific perivascular lymphocytic inflammation. A similar pathologic condition was noted in the distribution of large named cerebral vessels and single stenosis on cerebral angiography in a child with focal seizures and large arterial ischemic lesions.[21] It has been difficult to reconcile the early outcome of empiric cytotoxic therapy for any subtype cPACNS especially when the PedVas Initiative using corticosteroids, cyclophosphamide, methotrexate, or rituximab for remission-induction of childhood granulomatosis with polyangitiis[22] for AAV found a disappointing rate of remission status (42%) and visceral organ damage (63%) in its study cohort.

The aim of treatment in cPACNS is to rapidly control the underlying inflammatory response and stabilize the blood-brain barrier while protecting the brain from further insults. Methylprednisolone has been the first-line agent administered intravenously at a dose of 30 mg/kg/d to a maximum of 1 g per day for 3 to 5 days[23] followed by 1 to 2 mg/kg/d of oral CS to a maximum of 60 mg/d of prednisone.[24,25] After stabilization, immunosuppressive treatment is directed at the likeliest inflammatory pathways involved in the primary vasculitic process. Induction therapy with corticosteroids and pulse cyclophosphamide followed by maintenance therapy with azathioprine or mycophenolate mofetil has been recommended in cPACNS.[26] Children with SV-cPACNS treated in an open-label study[26] with cyclophosphamide in doses of 500 to 750 mg/m² monthly infusions for 6 months, and followed with maintenance treatment of azathioprine of 1 mg/kg/d and a target dose of 2 to 3 mg/kg/d, and mycophenolate mofetil at titrated doses of 800 to 1200 mg/m²/d were followed for up to 24 months using pediatric stroke outcome measures (PSOM). Among 19 such patients, 13 completed 24 months of follow-up, of whom 9 had a good neurologic outcome by Pediatric Stroke Outcome Measure (PSOM) scoring, 8 experienced disease flares, and 4 achieved remission of disease; mycophenolate mofetil was more effective than azathioprine. Rituximab, which may be appropriate therapy at doses of 375 mg/m² for 4 consecutive weeks or 500 mg/m² weekly for 2 weeks in cPACNS, was recently reported in SV-cPACNS.[27]

SUMMARY

It has been 2 decades since the seminal publication of Younger and colleagues[12] on granulomatous angiitis in the *Neurologic Clinics*. There has been a wealth of insight into the management of affected children and adults and overwhelming progress in observational and prospective cohorts. The future brings uncertainty in the current lack of postmortem-proven cases and diminished rates of CNS tissue biopsies in forming observational and prospective case cohorts, when it is still thought that the disease is imminently fatal if not promptly recognized and aggressively treated.

REFERENCES

1. Harbitz F. Unknown forms of arteritis with special reference to their relation to syphilitic arteritis and periarteritis nodosa. Am J Med Sci 1922;163:250–72.
2. Neuman W, Wolf A. Noninfectious granulomatous angiitis involving the central nervous system. Trans Am Neurol Assoc 1952;77:114–7.
3. McCormack H, Neuberger K. Giant cell arteritis involving small meningeal and intracerebral vessels. J Neuropathol Exp Neurol 1958;17:471–8.
4. Meyer J, Foley J, Campagna-Pinto D. Granulomatous angiitis of the meninges in sarcoidosis. Arch Neurol 1953;69:587–600.
5. Cravioto H, Fegin I. Noninfectious granulomatous angiitis with a predilection for the nervous system. Neurology 1959;9:599–607.
6. Hinck V, Carter C, Rippey C. Giant cell (cranial) arteritis. A case with angiographic abnormalities. Am J Roentgenol Radium Ther Nucl Med 1964;92:769–75.
7. Cupps T, Fauci A. Central nervous system vasculitis. Major Probl Intern Med 1981;21:123–32.

8. Cupps TR, Moore PM, Fauci AS. Isolated angiitis of the central nervous system. Prospsective diagnostic and therapeutic experience. Am J Med 1983;74:97–105.

9. Calabrese HL, Mallek JA. Primary angiitis of the central nervous system: report of 8 new cases, review of the literature, and proposal for diagnostic criteria. Medicine 1988;67:20–39.

10. Younger DS, Hays AP, Brust JCM, et al. Granulomatous angiitis of the brain. An inflammatory reaction of diverse etiology. Arch Neurol 1988;45:514–8.

11. Ferris E, Levine H. Cerebral arteritis: classification. Neuroradiology 1973;41: 327–41.

12. Younger DS, Calabrese LH, Hays AP. Granulomatous angiitis of the nervous system. Neurol Clin 1997;15:821–34.

13. Salvarani C, Brown RD Jr, Christianson TJH, et al. Adult primary central nervous system vasculitis: treatment and course. Arthritis Rheum 2015;67:1637–45.

14. De Boysson H, Arquizan C, Touze E, et al. Treatment and long-term outcomes of primary central nervous system vasculitis. Stroke 2018;49:1946–52.

15. Salvarani C, Brown RD Jr, Calamia KT, et al. Primary central nervous system vasculitis: analysis of 101 patients. Ann Neurol 2007;62:442–51.

16. Salvarani C, Brown RD Jr, Christianson TJH, et al. Primary central nervous system vasculitis associated with lymphoma. Neurology 2018;90:e847–55.

17. Ducros A, Boukobza M, Porcher R, et al. The clinical and radiological spectrum of reversible cerebral vasoconstriction syndrome. A prospective series of 67 patients. Brain 2007;130:3091–101.

18. Twilt M, Benseler SM. Childhood inflammatory brain diseases: pathogenesis, diagnosis and therapy. Rheumatology (Oxford) 2014;53:1359–68.

19. Benseler SM, deVeber G, Hawkins C, et al. Angiography-negative primary central nervous system vasculitis in children. Arthritis Rheum 2005;52:2159–67.

20. Elbers J, Halliday W, Hawkins C, et al. Brain biopsy in children with primary small-vessel central nervous system vasculitis. Ann Neurol 2010;68:602–10.

21. Lanthier S, Lortie A, Michaud J, et al. Isolated angiitis of the CNS in children. Neurology 2001;56:837–42.

22. Morishita KA, Moorthy LN, Lubieniecka JM, et al. Early outcomes in children with antineutrophil cytoplasmic antibody-associated vasculitis. Arthritis Rheum 2017; 69:1470–9.

23. Cellucci T, Benseler SM. Central nervous system vasculitis in children. Curr Opin Rheumatol 2010;22:590–7.

24. Twilt M, Benseler SM. The spectrum of CNS vasculitis in children and adults. Nat Rev Rheumatol 2012;8:97–107.

25. Golumbek P. Pharmacologic agents for pediatric neuroimmune disorders. Semin Pediatr Neurol 2010;17:245–53.

26. Hutchinson C, Elbers J, Halliday W, et al. Treatment of small vessel primary CNS vasculitis in children: an open-label cohort study. Lancet Neurol 2010;9:1078–84.

27. Deng J, Fang G, Wang XH, et al. Small vessel-childhood primary angiitis of the central nervous system: a case report and literature review. Zhonghua Er Ke Za Zhi 2018;56:142–7.

Stroke due to Vasculitis in Children and Adults

David S. Younger, MD, MPH, MS[a,b,*]

KEYWORDS

- Stroke • Vasculitis • Central nervous system

KEY POINTS

- The vasculitides are diseases characterized by inflammation of blood vessels and inflammatory leukocytes in vessel walls.
- There is an increased propensity for ischemic stroke resulting from thrombosis and compromise of vascular lumina.
- This results in distal tissue ischemia with hemorrhagic or nonhemorrhagic stroke and aneurysmal bleeding due to loss of vessel integrity.
- Vascular inflammation is the leading cause of stroke in children but the pathophysiology of childhood vasculitis is poorly understood. Moreover, it is rarely proven histologically.
- Small-vessel or large-vessel arteriopathy as useful models of primary central nervous system vasculitides of childhood are based on predictive clinical, neuroradiographic, and histopathologic features.

INTRODUCTION

The vasculitides are diseases characterized by inflammation of blood vessels and inflammatory leukocytes in vessel walls. There is an increased propensity for ischemic stroke because of the compromise of vessel lumina and distal tissue ischemia, and hemorrhagic stroke and aneurysmal bleeding due to loss of vessel integrity. The revised 2012 Chapel Hill Consensus Conference (CHCC)[1] provides a systematic nosology and categorization of primary and secondary vasculitides. Central nervous system (CNS) vasculitides leads to stroke as a result of a single-organ vasculitic syndrome, variably termed primary CNS vasculitis (PCNSV),[2] granulomatous angiitis of the brain,[3] and adult primary angiitis of the CNS (PACNS) or childhood PACNS (cPACNS)[4]; and as a secondary consequence of systemic vasculitides. Although applicable to pediatric patients, the CHCC nosology[1] was not specifically designed

The author has nothing to disclose or declare.
[a] Department of Neurology, Division of Neuro-Epidemiology, New York University School of Medicine, New York, NY, USA; [b] School of Public Health, City University of New York, New York, NY, USA
* 333 East 34th Street, Suite 1J, New York, NY 10016.
E-mail address: youngd01@nyu.edu
Website: http://www.davidsyounger.com

for this population. The European League Against Rheumatism and the Pediatric Rheumatology European Society[5] developed consensus criteria for the classification of the childhood forms of adult vasculitis disorders, including childhood polyarteritis nodosa (cPAN), granulomatosis with polyangiitis (GPA) as childhood GPA (cGPA), and microscopic polyangiitis (MPA) as childhood MPA (cMPA). Others are not specifically abbreviated with the childhood designation because of their common pediatric occurrence, including Takayasu arteritis (TAK) and Kawasaki disease (KD). The subtypes of childhood PACNS[6] are distinguished by vessel size, angiographic and pathologic findings, and the presence or absence of long-term progression.

Stroke Patterns and Classification

Patterns of stroke identified by the region of brain supplied by the affected vessel, and the size of the vessels and infarctions that ensue, are referred to as large-vessel or small-vessel (SV) lesions. Large-vessel infarcts typically result in wedge-shaped parenchymal lesions that occur secondary to occlusion of branches of the major arteries of the circle of Willis. SV diseases result in smaller, often multifocal or diffuse parenchymal infarcts with highly variable imaging appearances. Large-vessel infarcts present with sudden onset focal neurologic deficits, such as contralateral hemiparesis when the middle cerebral artery (MCA) is occluded. In contrast, strokes in SV territories present with subacute, nonlocalizing neurologic complaints, such as headache, behavioral changes, seizures, or cognitive decline.

Adult strokes classified according to Trial of Org 10172 in Acute Stroke Treatment (TOAST) criteria[7] (into large-artery atherosclerotic, cardioembolic, SV lacunar, other, determined, and undetermined cause) have not been widely applicable to pediatric stroke patients owing to often underdetermined causes.[8] The International Pediatric Stroke Study (IPSS), applying standardized classification and diagnostic evaluations to childhood arterial ischemic stroke (AIS), developed the Childhood AIS Standardized Classification and Diagnostic Evaluation (CASCADE) criteria.[9] Vascular inflammatory mechanisms incorporated into the CASCADE system recognize SV arteriopathy of childhood, unilateral focal cerebral arteriopathy (FCA) of childhood, bilateral cerebral arteriopathy of childhood, aortic or cervical arteriopathy, cardioembolic, other, and multifactorial causes of AIS, making it a useful starting point with the potential for ongoing modification as new information about childhood AIS is learned. However, there were limitations to the CASCADE. First, it did not recognize all of risk factors potentially related to structural disease of the heart or blood vessels. Second, future modifications of the CASCADE criteria need to unify and elaborate classification of these factors in a secondary classification system. Third, additional revisions need to address the recurrences beyond the acute period of childhood AIS.[10]

The Vascular effects of Infection in Pediatric Stroke (VIPS)[11] study prospectively enrolled 355 children with AIS between 2010 and 2014 to diagnose childhood arteriopathy and classify subtypes, including arterial dissection, FCA-inflammatory type (FCA-i), which included transient cerebral arteriopathy, moyamoya, and diffuse or multifocal vasculitis. The most common childhood arteriopathies in the cohort of children presenting with acute AIS were moyamoya, arterial dissection (intracranial and extracranial), and FCA-i but not primary SV-PACNS, which typically presents only with headache or cognitive decline, and less so with focal signs or symptoms.

Primary Central Nervous System Vasculitis

Adults

With several proposed diagnostic schemes for PCNSV over the years,[12] the combination of clinical, neuroradiographic, and histopathological findings remains the recommended method for reliable diagnosis and facilitates the identification of clinico-pathologic subtypes, including those with persistent focal deficits, stroke, and intra-cranial hemorrhage. Persistent neurologic deficits, including stroke and headache, were the commonest initial symptoms affecting 68% of 101 studied subjects with PCNSV,[13] as defined by diagnostic criteria of Calabrese and Mallek[4] and modified by Birnbaum and Hellmann.[14] Infarctions were the commonest type of lesion noted with MRI of the brain, among 53% of 90 subjects so studied, and were multiple in ap-pearances in 85% and bilateral in 83%, with cortical and subcortical involvement in 63% overall, suggesting larger artery, branch-artery, and small-artery distributions (**Fig. 1**). Intracranial hemorrhage was noted in 8% of subjects.

In a retrospective cohort of 163 patients with PCNSV from 1983 to 2011 at the Mayo Clinic,[2] 105 patients (64%) showed angiographic changes supporting the diagnosis of PCNSV (manifesting areas of smooth-wall segmental narrowing or dilatation, and oc-clusions that affected multiple cerebral arteries without the proximal vessel changes of atherosclerosis or other causes) and 58 patients (36%) showed CNS tissue changes of vasculitis (demonstrating transmural vascular inflammation involving leptomeningeal or parenchymal vessels). The histopathology was granulomatous in 35 (60.3%), lym-phocytic in 13(22.4%), and necrotizing alone in 10 (17.2%). These histologic patterns seem to identify subsets of disease rather than different stages of the same process because no individual subject had histologic evidence of more than 1 pattern. Comparatively, among the 112 subjects reported by De Boysson and colleagues,[15] 68 (61%) and 11 (10%) had digital subtraction angiography or magnetic resonance angiography (MRA) consistent with PCNSV, respectively, whereas 33 (29%) subjects had CNS tissue diagnosis of vasculitis.

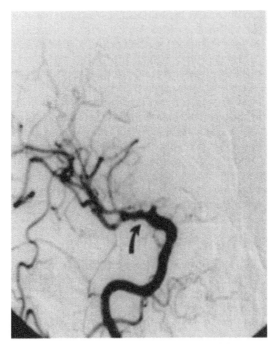

Fig. 1. Radiographic features of cerebral Vasculitis. Ectasia and beading in the M1 segment and lack of flow in the A1 segment of the right anterior cerebral artery (*arrow*). (*From* Younger DS. Adult and childhood vasculitis of the nervous system. In: Younger DS, editor. Motor Disor-ders. Third edition. Brookfield, CT: Rothstein Publishing; 2015. p. 242; with permission.)

Children

Advances in the understanding of childhood AIS occurred independent of pediatric inflammatory brain disease (IBrainD) and cPACNS,[6] with inconsistencies between the adult PACNS and cPACNS, making the latter problematic for several reasons.

First, unlike antemortem pediatric cases of cerebral vasculitis that show angiographic evidence of large named vessel involvement, children with SV-cPACNS can only be conclusively diagnosed by CNS biopsy tissues that show transmural inflammation of small meningeal and penetrating cortical vessels. Affected patients present with focal symptoms suggesting an association with stroke but are more likely to develop subacute, nonlocalizing, neurologic complaints, such as headache, behavioral changes, seizures, school failure, or cognitive decline. Moreover, childhood strokes may be highly variable in character and distribution.

Second, compared with their adult counterparts, the estimated incidence of hemorrhagic lesions in children is minimal, making up less than 10% of all strokes.[16]

Third, neuroimaging is far less specific in cPACNS. Noninvasive arterial imaging using computed tomography (CT) angiography and MRA show typically normal findings even when parenchymal MRI imaging ranges from normal to diffusely abnormal across a wide array of lesion characteristics.

Fourth, childhood AIS associated with conventional angiography that fails to show radiographic changes consistent with SV-cPACNS are placed in the category of angiography-negative SV-cPACNS,[17] typically with unsubstantiated histopathology, yet suggesting a corresponding caliber of vessel involvement.

Fifth, despite the similarities to adult forms of PACNS, recent cPACNS series[6] fail to mention prototypical granulomatous pathologic conditions, suggesting a bias of selection, making clinicopathological comparisons further problematic.

Sixth, while awaiting the results of the Pediatric Vasculitis Initiative, a Canadian and United Kingdom collaborative study of pediatric and adult cases of antineutrophil cytoplasmic antibody (ANCA)-associated vasculitides (AAV) such as GPA and PACNS, the approach of cPACNS has been to lump them into the broader category of inflammatory brain disease (IBrainD)[18] and systematically exclude angiography-positive mimics of cPACNS and angiography-negative, brain biopsy–positive true SV-cPACNS.

Seventh, because the approach to management of SV-cPACNS is patterned after SV vasculitides (SVV), including antineutrophil AAV, it is difficult to reconcile the disappointing results of the PedVas Initiative,[19] which showed a remission status of 42%, and visceral organ damage in 63% of cases following treatment with corticosteroids, cyclophosphamide, methotrexate, or rituximab for remission induction; plasma exchange in conjunction with cyclophosphamide and/or rituximab; and azathioprine, methotrexate, rituximab, mycophenolate mofetil, and cyclophosphamide for up to 12 months for remission maintenance.

LARGE-VESSEL SYSTEMIC VASCULITIDES

Giant cell arteritis (GCA) and TAK are prototypical large-vessel granulomatous vasculitides that involve the aorta and its major branches; however, any size artery can be affected. Kermani and colleagues[20] reported a population-based incident cohort of 204 patients with GCA seen between 1950 and 2004 at the Mayo Clinic, noting a mean age of diagnosis of 76 years, and a female to male ratio of 1.5:1. It is the most common vasculitis in populations with predominantly Northern European ancestry, with an annual incidence of 15 to 33 cases per 100,000 age 50 years and older.[21] GCA is a polygenic disease in which multiple environmental and genetic factors influence susceptibility and severity.[22]

Neuroimaging studies using ultrasonography, high-resolution MRI, and [18]flurodeoxyglucose ([18]FDG) PET are useful imaging modalities to identify superficial cranial and extracranial, and large-vessel subclavian artery and aortic involvement in GCA and TAK.[23] CNS involvement in GCA results from thrombosis of the carotid and vertebral arteries rather than intracranial arteritis, affects vessels that contain elastin, more specifically the internal elastic lamina that is absent from intracranial vessels more than 5 mm beyond the point of dural perforation. Hollenhorst and colleagues[24] noted CNS events, including stroke in 7.4% of 175 subjects with confirmed GCA, including 1 with massive cerebral hemorrhage, 2 with stroke, and 6 with occlusive disease of the aortic arch. Caselli and colleagues[25] noted transient ischemic attacks or stroke in 7% of 166 subjects with biopsy-proven GCA, among whom 4 had events in the vertebrobasilar system and 8 were affected in the carotid arterial system. Approximately 30% of subjects manifested neurologic findings, the commonest of which were neuropathies of the arms and legs, according to Caselli and colleagues.[25] Salvarani and colleagues[22] observed that transient ischemic attacks or stroke in the territory of the carotid or vertebrobasilar arteries were less common neurologic findings. Gonzalez-Gay and colleagues[26] studied GCA among 239 patients in a multicenter retrospective, noting stroke occurrence in only 8 patients (3%), equally divided between the vertebrobasilar and carotid territories. Other symptoms of arteritis preceded ischemic events by a median of 1.5 months, and were more frequent in those with visual involvement, especially permanent visual loss. Two patients with vertebrobasilar stroke died within a month despite aggressive corticosteroid therapy. Stepwise logistical regression analysis revealed visual loss and jaw claudication as the predictors of stroke.

The reported mean annual incidence of TAK was .4 per million in a population study in eastern Denmark between 1990 and 2009.[27] Stroke occurrence was noted in 17% of 230 reported children with TAK between 1994 and 2008.[28] There is risk of both focal AIS from thromboembolism, and hypoperfusion-induced brain infarction secondary to proximal arterial stenosis. Although the pediatric presentation of TAK includes hypertension similar to adults,[29] affected children more commonly manifest fever, weight loss, abdominal pain, and headaches.[28] Kerr and colleagues[30] summarized the clinical, laboratory, and treatment responses of 60 subjects with TAK based on the presence of symptoms and signs of ischemic, inflammatory large-vessel disease, as well as supportive arteriography findings, so noted in 10 (17%) subjects with either transient ischemic attacks or stroke, and carotid or vertebral artery disease. Riehl[31] and Riehl and Brown[32] reported the clinical and pathologic features of 6 cases of TAK, noting widespread arteritis that involved not only the aortic arch and its tributaries by clinical and angiographic, studies but also many other medium-size and large-size vessels, including the cerebral arteries, by granulomatous panarteritis in 1 patient studied at postmortem examination. That patient, a 43-year-old woman who presented with rapidly disappearing blood pressure and complained of spells of progressively worsening dizziness and dimness of vision, died of severe congestive heart failure. At postmortem examination, there was severe stenosis of the distal aorta and thrombosis of an aortic arch graft, with nearly complete obstruction of all the great vessels. Vascular thromboses were noted along proximal portions of the left MCA, both posterior cerebral arteries, and the anterior third of the basilar artery. There was massive infarction of the left temporoparietal region, the left half of the midbrain, brain stem, and cerebellum.

Although arterial biopsy is impractical given the restriction of lesions to the aorta and its branches, MRA and conventional angiography demonstrate vessel irregularities, stenosis, poststenotic dilatations, aneurysmal formation, occlusions, and increased collateralization. There are strong similarities and subtle differences in the distribution of arterial disease on cerebral arteriography between GCA and TAK that suggest that the two disorders may nonetheless exist on a spectrum of a similar disease.[33] Ishikawa[34] reported the natural history of TAK among 54 Japanese subjects from 1957 to 1975, classified as uncomplicated (group I), monocomplicated (group II), and multicomplicated (group III). The 5-year survival rate after the established diagnosis in the 54 subjects was 83%. The major factors related to death among the 8 subjects so studied included fatal cerebral events in 3, cardiac events in 3, and events related to aortic reconstruction surgery or steroid withdrawal in another. Ohigashi and colleagues[35] ascertained an improved prognosis among 106 consecutive subjects with TAK in those with onset before 1999 compared with those diagnosed after 2000 (4.2% vs 0%, respectively). This was attributed to reduction in the time from onset to diagnosis; replacement of digital subtraction angiography (79% vs 9%) with ultrasound (6% vs 34%), CT angiography (24% vs 77%), MRA (21% vs 57%), and ^{18}FDG PET (0% vs 20%); less frequent complications of moderate or severe aortic regurgitation; increase in the use and maximal dose of corticosteroids (70% vs 97%); and the use of first-line and second-line immunosuppressant agents (7% vs 42%). Surgical treatment of TAK was similar between those with onset before 1999 and after 2000 (22.5% vs 22.8%, respectively).

MEDIUM-VESSEL SYSTEMIC VASCULITIDES

Watts and colleagues[36] used the 2012 revised CHCC[1] and American College of Rheumatology (ACR) criteria for PAN,[37] noting its incidence in the United Kingdom compared with Spain, varying from 9.7 versus 6.2 per million, respectively. KD is common in childhood, with the highest incidence in Japan where it exceeds 120 per 100,000, with 80% of these children younger than 5 years of age and a boy to girl ratio of 1.5:2.[38,39] Both are prototypical medium-vessel vasculitides, although arteries of any size may be affected. PAN is associated with necrotizing arteritis of medium or small arteries without glomerulonephritis or vasculitis in arterioles, capillaries, or venules. Such are not features of AAV. By contrast, KD is an infantile or childhood disorder associated with the mucocutaneous lymph node syndrome, predominantly affecting medium and small arteries, occasionally coronary, the aorta, and other large arteries (1).

Kernohan and Woltman[40] summarized the clinicopathological aspects of adult PAN in 6 subjects studied at postmortem examination, estimating CNS involvement, including stroke, to be about 8% of cases, and noting a combination of acute and chronic lesions that correlated with known exacerbations. According to Guillevin and colleagues,[41] CNS involvement was uncommon but motor deficits, stroke, and brain hemorrhage occur, the cause of which was generally multifactorial. Cases with cognitive disturbances, such as abrupt memory loss in which MRI shows scattered T_2-weighted hyperintensities suggestive of brain vasculitis, have generally not been demonstrated as such histopathologically. CNS involvement, including stroke, was noted in 9.6% (26) of 115 subjects registered in the French Vasculitis Study Group (FVSG) with hepatitis B virus (HBV)-PAN. These cases were seen between 1972 and 2002, and had biopsy-proven PAN or demonstration of microaneurysms and multiple stenoses by abdominal or renal angiography. There were associated clinical symptoms of vasculitis with concomitant hepatitis B surface antigen (HBsAg) antigenemia and demonstration of viral replication supported by hepatitis B e antigen, viral DNA, or DNA polymerase. A retrospective study of 348 adult subjects registered in the FVSG[42] who satisfied criteria for the diagnosis of PAN between 1963 and 2005 noted CNS involvement, including stroke, in 4.6% of subjects overall, with relatively equivalent frequency in those with and without HBV-related illness.

cPAN is rare, and the classification criteria for cPAN requires histologic evidence of necrotizing vasculitis in medium-sized or small-sized arteries or angiographic abnormalities demonstrating aneurysm formation or vascular occlusions as a mandatory criterion, plus 2 of 5 features: myalgia, skin involvement, hypertension, neuropathy, or abnormal urinalysis, or impaired renal function.[43] Disease manifestations range from a benign cutaneous form with clinical, laboratory, and molecular characteristics of familial Mediterranean fever[44,45] to severe disseminated multisystemic disease. Ozen and colleagues[46] studied 110 children of mean age 9 years, from 21 pediatric centers worldwide, diagnosed with cPAN, dividing them into 4 groups, including systemic PAN (57%), cutaneous PAN (30%), and classic PAN with HBsAg (4.6%) as well as 8% manifesting ANCA seropositivity, so qualifying for MPA. Cutaneous cPAN was confined to the skin and musculoskeletal system. There are reported children with serologic and microbiologic evidence of preceding streptococcal infection.[47]

The diagnosis of KD requires the presence of fever for at least 5 days and 4 of the following criteria: desquamation of extremities or perineum, polymorphous exanthema, bilateral conjunctiva injection, injection of oral or pharyngeal mucosa, and cervical lymphadenopathy.[5] The disease affects the coronary arteries and stroke as a complication has only rarely been reported, predominantly large-vessel cardioembolic stroke but also cerebral microhemorrhages.[48–50] Evaluation of 24 subjects with KD using MRI revealed 1 cryptogenic cardioembolic posterior inferior cerebellar artery infarct.[51] Risk is potentially higher in patients with ventricular dysfunction secondary to myocardial infarction or arrhythmia. Stroke should be considered in children with signs or histories of medium-vessel vasculitis and neurologic symptoms, particularly acute focal neurologic deficits.

SMALL-VESSEL SYSTEMIC VASCULITIS

SVV predominantly affects SVs, defined as small intraparenchymal arteries, arterioles, capillaries, and venules; however, medium-sized vessels and veins may be affected. Two major categories of SVV include AAV characterized by necrotizing vasculitis with few or no immune deposits predominantly affecting small arteries, arterioles, capillaries, and venules associated with myeloperoxidase (MPO) ANCA or proteinase 3 (PR3), whereas immune complex vasculitis is characterized by marked vessel wall deposits of immunoglobulin (Ig) and/or complement. GPA (Wegener granulomatosis type), eosinophilic GPA (EGPA; Churg-Strauss syndrome), and MPA (microscopic polyarteritis) are prototypical AAV, whereas cryoglobulinemic vasculitis (CV), IgA vasculitis, and hypocomplementemic urticarial vasculitis (HUV) associated with C1q antibodies comprise the immune complex vasculitides.

The classification of AAV has been controversial,[52] with existing systems developed by the ACR,[53,54] the CHCC,[1] and the European Medicines Agency algorithm,[55] to provide a standardized method for their application in epidemiologic studies, each with separate deficiencies, especially when applied to unselected patients. These systems were developed as classification criteria and not as diagnostic criteria. Because there were no validated diagnostic criteria for AAV, the Diagnostic and Classification Criteria for Vasculitis Study (DCVAS), developed by Watts and colleagues,[55] led to the consensus development and validation of diagnostic criteria by an algorithm to avoid inclusion of patients with other conditions. In incident cases of primary systemic vasculitis identified in Seine-St. Denis County, Paris, France, Mahr and colleagues[56] estimated the prevalence of GPA at 23.7, MPA at 25.1, and EGPA at 10.7 per million adults in a population of 1,093,515, 28% of whom were of non-European ancestry, with an overall prevalence that was 2-fold higher for those of European ancestry

(104.7 5 per million) compared with others of non-European ancestry (52.5 per million). Mohammad and colleagues[57] estimated incident cases of GPA, MPA, and EGPA in southern Sweden 9.8, 10.1, and 0.9 per million, respectively, in a total population of 641,000 between 1997 and 2006, with a progressive increase in age-specific incidence rates over the study period.

Antineutrophil Cytoplasmic Antibody–Associated Vasculitides

Granulomatosis and polyangiitis

GPA is characterized by necrotizing granulomatous inflammation of the upper and lower respiratory tracts and necrotizing AAV affecting small to medium arteries, arterioles, capillaries, veins, and venules, together with glomerulonephritis. Drachman[58] described a patient with 1 month of headache that awakened him from sleep followed by rhinitis, nasal obstruction, epistaxis, mononeuropathy multiplex, confusion, and hypertension. Active arteritis and necrotizing granulomata were found in the brain, not in peripheral nerves. Based on his observations in a single postmortem case, cerebral involvement stroke resulted from a combination of 4 separate entities, including frank vasculitis of larger arterial branches, particularly over the surface of the brain as demonstrated in his patient report, with evidence of ischemia in portions of the territory supplied by the affected vessels; subarachnoid hemorrhage, hypertensive encephalopathy evidenced by microscopic infarcts in close relation to arteries with fibrinoid impregnation of their walls; and meningeal infiltration by mononuclear cells.

Nishino and colleagues[59] described neurologic involvement in 34% of 324 consecutive patients with GPA at the Mayo Clinic between 1973 and 1991, classified according to the ACR,[53] that included peripheral neuropathy in 16% compared with cerebrovascular events in 4% at some time in the course of illness, rarely, if ever, at presentation. Of 5 patients with presumed clinical vasculitis, cerebral angiography was negative in 2; and of 12 patients studied at postmortem examination, findings of vasculitis were detected in only 2 patients.

Fauci and colleagues[60] noted nervous system involvement in 22% of 85 subjects, 10 subjects (12%) of whom had CNS involvement, including strokes, at some point in the illness, although not ever specifically mentioned at presentation. Moore and Cupps[61] estimated the frequency of neurologic abnormalities of GPA to be 23% to 50%, with commonly encountered focal deficits due to CNS involvement, citing the mechanism of neural dysfunction to be inflammation from primary sites, remote granuloma formation, and vasculitis. The opinion of Drachman[58] was that contiguous extension of necrotizing granulomas might account for up to 24% of all neurologic complications, including those of the CNS. Extensive cerebral infarction in the territory of bilateral anterior cerebral arteries was ascertained in a 67-year-old man with frontal headache that preceded detection of a large midline frontal mass lesion on CT and known biopsy-proven GPA and granulomatous vasculitis of the nasal cavity, liver, and kidney. Postmortem examination showed cerebral infarction in the areas supplied by A2 branches of both ACAs, with occlusion of large-sized ACA vessels by organized mural thrombi, fibrinoid necrosis in the arterial branches, and similar vasculitis, with multinucleated giant cells involving small arteries and veins diffusely in the frontal region of the brain, suggesting contiguous spread from granulomatous nasal cavity lesions.

Hoffman and colleagues[62] ascertained nervous system involvement in 23% of 110 subjects, with GPA noted in 15% of subjects and CNS involvement, including strokes, in 8% of subjects. de Groot and colleagues[63] performed a prospective analysis of 128 GPA subjects, noting CNS involvement, including stroke, in 7% of subjects. The latter included granulomatous infiltration of frontobasal cortex arising from adjacent paranasal sinus granulomas, cerebral vasculitis, vascular myelopathy, and meningeal granulomatosis.

CNS involvement in cGPA is not common and often appears at a later stage in the disease. The criteria for cGPA requires the presence of 3 of the following 6 criteria: abnormal urinalysis; granulomatous inflammatory on tissue biopsy; nasal-sinus-oral inflammation; subglottic, tracheal, or endobronchial stenosis; abnormal chest radiograph or CT; and positive ANCA staining.[43] Single large or multifocal insults involving 1 or more lobes consistent with the distribution of cerebral arteries are typical childhood presentations and respond to high-dose corticosteroid and intravenous immune globulin therapy.[64]

Microscopic polyangiitis

MPA is a necrotizing AAV vasculitis with few or no immune complex deposits and is commonly associated glomerulonephritis without granulomatous inflammation. From 1934 to 1947, Davson and colleagues[65] separated 14 reported postmortem subjects with MPA into 2 groups based on the presence of severe widespread glomerular damage. Wainwright and Davson,[66] who described MPA among 6 studied postmortem subjects from 1947 to 1948, failed to note CNS or stroke-onset, or histopathologic changes in the brain. Savage and colleagues,[67] who studied 34 subjects with MPA, all of whom presented with clinical evidence of a systemic SVV predominantly affecting the skin and musculoskeletal system associated with focal necrotizing glomerulonephritis, cited CNS involvement at presentation in 18% of subjects without specific mention of stroke. Serra and colleagues,[68] who reported the presentation, histopathology, and long-term outcome of 53 subjects with MPO from 1965 to 1981, cited CNS involvement at presentation in 15% of subjects that included stroke, convulsions, headache, confusion, and drowsiness, providing further breakdown of the individual frequencies thereof. Guillevin and colleagues,[69] who reported the clinical and laboratory findings in 85 subjects from the FVSG with MPA from 1969 to 1995, noted CNS involvement in 11.8% of subjects at presentation and in 3% of 29 subjects who experienced a relapse; however, there was no specific mention of stroke. Gayraud and colleagues,[70] who analyzed 4 prospective trials that included 278 subjects with PAN, MPA, and EGPA from 1980 to 1993, reported stroke occurrence among 85 deaths. Villiger and Guillevin,[71] who reviewed several retrospective European subject cohorts, cited CNS involvement that was described in a few subjects that included subarachnoid hemorrhage, cerebrovascular disease, meningitis, and diffuse brain injury. Ben Sassi and colleagues[72] described intracerebral hemorrhage secondary to necrotizing vasculitis that similarly involved the nerves and muscles, and citing 3 additional subjects with hemorrhagic stroke due to MPA.[73–75] Ahn and colleagues,[76] who studied 55 subjects with MPA, 69% of whom demonstrated perinuclear ANCA by immunofluorescence or MPO ANCA-seropositivity, noted neurologic involvement at diagnosis in 43.6% of subjects, and CNS involvement in 5 (9.1%), none of whom developed endstage renal disease and 1 of whom was dead at follow-up.

cMPA is uncommon and the criteria for diagnosis includes 3 of the following features to be present: abnormal urinalysis, granulomatous inflammation on tissue biopsy, nasal sinus inflammation, subglottic, tracheal, or endobronchial stenosis; abnormal chest radiograph or CT scan; and PR3 ANCA staining.[43] Those with cMPA accounted for 4 of the first 32 children in the United States-Canadian: A Registry for Childhood Vasculitis (ARChiVe) registry.[77] Treatment of cMPA does not significantly differ from that of adults or other forms of AAV. An analysis of 4 prospective trials of 278 subjects comparing PAN, MPA, and EGPA[70] observed excess deaths during follow-up of MPA subjects, with survival probability trends adjusted to the

Five-Factor Score[78] and the Birmingham Vasculitis Activity Score,[79] which suggested increased mortality in MPA subjects compared with the other forms of vasculitis. Of 53 subjects studied by Serra and colleagues,[68] all 10 oliguric and untreated subjects at presentation died. Among the remaining 43 subjects treated with varying immunosuppressive regimens, including corticosteroids, cyclophosphamide, and azathioprine, in varying combination, 33 (77%) survived the acute stage of disease, 30 of whom made up a long-term analysis that showed stable vasculitis in 12 (40%), smoldering disease in 16 (53%), and recurrent vasculitis in 2 (7%) subjects. Savage and colleagues[67] noted an overall survival rate of 65%, and an actuarial survival rate of 70% at 1 year and 65% at 5 years following treatment with prednisolone, azathioprine, and cyclophosphamide or plasma exchange in varying combinations.

Eosinophilic granulomatosis with polyangiitis

EGPA is a necrotizing vasculitis involving small to medium vessels that differs from GPA by the presence of eosinophil-rich necrotizing granulomatous inflammation of the respiratory tract in association with asthma and eosinophilia, and ANCA seropositivity when glomerulonephritis is present. Churg and Strauss[80] described the clinical and postmortem findings of 13 subjects with asthma, fever, and hypereosinophilia. This was accompanied by eosinophilic exudation, fibrinoid change, and granulomatous proliferation that constituted the so-called allergic granuloma. The latter were found within vessels walls and extravascular connective tissue of major organ systems. CNS organ manifestations were described in 8 (61.5%) subjects and in the cause of death in 3 subjects who sustained cerebral hemorrhage (2 subjects) or subarachnoid hemorrhage.

Chumbley and colleagues[81] described 30 asthmatic patients from the Mayo Clinic over the period 1950 to 1974 with necrotizing vasculitis of small arteries and veins, with extravascular granulomas and infiltration of vessels and perivascular tissue with eosinophilia. Neurologic involvement, so noted in 19 (63%) patients, was consistent with mononeuritis multiplex. Lanham and colleagues,[82] who emphasized that the combination of necrotizing vasculitis, tissue infiltration by eosinophils, and extravascular granulomas similar to Churg and Strauss,[80] found them contemporaneously in only a minority of subjects. Such histologic findings, which could be encountered in other granulomatous, vasculitic, and eosinophilic disorders, even in the absence of clinical asthma, allergic rhinitis, sinusitis, pulmonary infiltrates, and cardiac involvement (pathognomonic of EGPA), was accompanied by CNS involvement in up to 25% of cases. Moreover, cerebral hemorrhage or infarction as a consequence of vasculitis or hypertension was a major cause of morbidity and mortality, accounting for 16% of deaths in their series of 16 subjects combined with 34 subjects reported in the literature.

Sehgal and colleagues[83] noted neurologic involvement among 14 subjects with the clinical diagnosis of EGPA. Three subjects had cerebral infarction 2 to 15 years after initial diagnosis, including a 68-year-old woman with a stroke involving the territory of the MCA manifested as hemiparesis and aphasia. A 34-year-old man with a right parietal lobe infarction pursuant to embolization of a left ventricular thrombus manifested incoordination and hemisensory loss of the arm, as did a 62-year-old woman with a thalamic infarction, who developed hemibody sensory loss. Guillevin and colleagues[84] studied 96 subjects with EGPA between 1963 and 1995, noting ischemic stroke in 6 (6%) as assessed by brain CT at presentation and none during follow-up, 1 of whom had clinically asymptomatic brain lesions, another who had cognitive disturbances related to vasculitis that improved with corticosteroid therapy, and focal deficits in the other 4. Mouthon and colleagues[85] reported 38 subjects with EGPA from

1978 to 1998, citing CNS involvement in 3 (7.9%) elderly subjects that suggested CNS vasculitis on MRI of the brain in only 1 subject so studied. Among 383 subjects with EGPA enrolled in the French FVSG Cohort (58), CNS involvement was noted in 20 (5.2%) of subjects at onset, with 2-fold greater frequency with ANCA-seropositive status than ANCA-seronegative but no specific mention of stroke frequency.

Immune Complex Vasculitis

Cryoglobulinemic vasculitis
Cryoglobulinemic vasculitis (CryoVas) is typified by cryoglobulinemic immune complexes deposited along SVs, predominantly arterioles, capillaries, veins, and venules in association with serum cryoglobulins that typically have associated rheumatoid factor activity consisting of IgM and polyclonal IgG, so-called mixed cryoglobulinemia (MC) and hepatitis C virus (HCV) infection.[86] Purpura, among the commonest features of cryoglobulinemia, was noted in 24% of subjects at presentation[60] and in 15% to 33% during disease evolution, in whom skin biopsy typically showed leukocytoclastic vasculitis. Neurologic manifestations noted in 23% of cases included peripheral neuropathy in 17% and CNS involvement in 6%. HCV infection is a main etiologic factor noted overall in 75% of subjects; antibodies to HCV and human immunodeficiency virus are noted in 75% and 19%, respectively, followed by HBsAg in 3%. A concomitant autoimmune disorder was noted in 24%, with frank hematologic disease in 7%, and essential cryoglobulinemia in 11% of subjects.

Historically, the patient described by Lerner and Watson,[87] a 56-year-old man who presented with chest pain, purpuric rash, and a cold precipitating serum protein, did not have symptoms or postmortem findings referable to the nervous system. Marshall and Malone[88] noted widespread cerebral purpura with hemorrhage ascribed to occlusion of small blood vessels by eosinophilic protein precipitates that correlated with the clinical presentation of progressively fatal coma. Abramsky and Slavin[89] described MC in a 55-year-old woman with anarthria, hyperreflexia, bilateral Babinski signs, and progressively fatal coma, who was later found to have multiple thrombotic occlusions of small intracerebral blood vessels with adjacent foci of ischemia and marked demyelination at postmortem examination. A second patient, a 50-year-old woman, who presented with a Wallenberg syndrome, had MC and angiographically demonstrable occlusion of the left posterior inferior artery. A third patient, a 50-year-old woman who presented with right hemiparesis and pyramidal signs, had a cryoprecipitate with occlusion of the left MCA.

Gorevic and colleagues[90] summarized the clinical aspects of long-term follow-up of 40 subjects with MC, noting incidental CNS involvement at postmortem examination; and a fatal stroke in another subject. Petty and colleagues[91] described a 35-year-old woman with type II cryoglobulinemia, headache, purpura, and seizures who was found to have multiple areas of T_2 and proton density signal abnormalities in the cerebral and cerebellar hemispheres, with a gyral pattern of enhancement in the cerebral cortex and a nodular pattern of enhancement in the cerebellum, and early cortical infarction on right frontal brain biopsy, without vasculitis. Cerebral angiography was normal. HCV RNA was detected by polymerase chain reaction (PCR) assay.

Ince and colleagues[92] described a subject with paranoid psychosis and MC who was later found to have right basal ganglia hemorrhage and multifocal SV occlusions by amorphous bland protein plugs, and abundant Russel bodies present in arterioles and venules, with relative sparing of capillaries.

Cacoub and colleagues[93] compared the features of subjects with HCV examined for systemic vasculitis manifestations of PAN or MC, noting 2 subjects with cerebral vasculitis in the former versus none in the latter. Cacoub and colleagues[94] described 3 subjects with CNS involvement with HCV infection and MC, 1 of whom was found to have a hemorrhagic lesion of the external capsule in association with pontine T_2 hyperintensities and parietal lobe infarcts. A second subject had a hemorrhagic occipital lobe lesion in association with cerebellar infarction and abnormal periventricular hyperintensities. A third subject had abnormal white matter hyperintensities.

Ferri and colleagues[95] studied the demographic, clinical, and serologic features and survival of 231 subjects with MC seen between 1972 and 2001. There was widespread vasculitis involving small-sized to medium-sized arteries, capillaries, and venules with greater than 2 or more visceral organs, including the CNS, kidney, gut, and lung, in a small percentage of subjects, with the exception of focal dystonia in 1 subject during interferon treatment. The investigators[95] found no other manifestations of CNS involvement related to MC.

Filipini and colleagues[96] reported a 63-year-old woman with acute severe encephalopathy HCV-related MC, dysarthria, and hemiplegia. Fragoso and colleagues[97] reported a 35-year-old woman with dysarthria, left facial and left limb hemiparesis, and hemisensory loss with MC in whom MRI showed ischemic lesions in the tail of the right caudate nucleus, corona radiate, and posteromedial putamen. Casato and colleagues[98] reported the CNS findings in 40 subjects with HCV-related CV in a multicenter case-control study using MRI and neuropsychological testing. Although none evidenced cerebral infarction, small white matter lesions were found in all HCV-related MC subjects, a higher mean number of white matter intensities compared with HCV and healthy controls. Terrier and colleagues[99] analyzed the data of 242 subjects registered in the CryoVas survey, ascertaining CNS involvement in 5 (2%) subjects without specifying whether stroke was encountered. Terrier and Cacoub[100] reviewed CNS findings in HCV-seronegative and seropositive MC in CryoVas, noting 2 (.7%) subjects among the former with CNS involvement, compared with 9 (5%) subjects among the latter group evidencing CNS involvement but without further mention as to presence of stroke in any of the subjects.

Cryoglobulinemia is rarely reported in the pediatric literature. One comparison cohort[101] showed a significantly higher prevalence of prolonged fever, arthralgia, arthritis, and cutaneous involvement in children compared with adults. There are no prospective controlled trials of treatment in children to assess relative efficacy of the various available agents; however, Giménez-Roca and colleagues[102] described successful treatment of pediatric CV with rituximab.

Hypocomplementemic urticarial vasculitis–C1q

HUV-C1q is an uncommon immune complex–mediated entity characterized by urticaria with persistent acquired hypocomplementemia.[103] It is associated with several systemic findings, including leukocytoclastic vasculitis, severe angioedema, laryngeal edema, pulmonary involvement, arthritis, arthralgia, glomerulonephritis, and uveitis. These manifestations should be present for at least 6 months. Laboratory findings include low complement levels of classical pathway, namely C1q, C2, C3, and C4. The disease marker is the serum presence of anti-C1q antibodies.

The disorder presents with recurrent attacks of erythematous, urticarial, and hemorrhagic skin lesions lasting up to 24 hours at a time, associated with recurrent attacks of fever; joint swelling; and variable abdominal distress. Circulating hypocomplementemia and C1q antibodies are associated with necrotizing SVV in skin biopsy tissue, affecting arterioles, capillaries, and venules. Apart from orbital pseudotumor with ptosis, diplopia, and headache in 1 subject with HUV syndrome, there was no mention of CNS involvement or stroke in a review of 18 subjects with HUV-C1q.[104] Nor was stroke mentioned in a review of 4 subjects studied at postmortem examination with HUV-C1q.[105]

Buck and colleagues[106] cited rare CNS manifestations in HUV-C1q, including aseptic meningitis, pseudotumor cerebri, transverse myelitis but not stroke or cerebral vasculitis. Grotz and colleagues[107] did not mention stroke or CNS vasculitis in HUV-C1q in a case report and review of the literature of HUV-C1q. In a review of urticarial vasculitis and HUV syndrome, Davies and Brewer[108] attributed development of pseudotumor cerebri to vasculitis of the venous sinus system. Ludivico and colleagues[109] suggested that chronic pseudotumor cerebri, as in their subjects, was a diagnosis of exclusion, possibly related to chronic corticosteroid use, and did not cite subjects with cerebral vasculitis or stroke.

The diagnosis and management of HUV-C1q was reviewed in 3 children by Pasini and colleagues[110] emphasizing the need for prompt diagnosis and treatment for concomitant renal involvement.

Variable Vessel Vasculitides

Behçet disease
Behçet disease (BD) is a rare disease encountered along the Silk Road in 20 to 420 per 100,000 in Turkey, 80 per 100,000 in Iran, and 0.64 per 100,000 in the United Kingom.[111] The disorder is characterized by relapsing aphthous ulcers of the mouth, eye, and genitalia.[112] The most widely used diagnostic criteria of BD were formulated by the International Study Group (ISG)[113] that included recurrent oral ulcerations plus any 2 of genital ulceration, typically defined eye lesions, typical skin lesions, or a positive pathergy. Recurrent oral ulcerations were categorized as minor aphthous, major aphthous, and herpetiform ulcerations that recurred at least 3 times in a 12-month period. Recurrent genital ulcerations were defined as aphthous ulceration and scarring. Eye lesions were defined as anterior uveitis, posterior uveitis, or cells in the vitreous on slit lamp examination; and retinal vasculitis. Compatible skin lesions included erythema nodosum, pseudofolliculitis, papulopustular lesions, and acneiform nodules in postadolescent subjects not receiving corticosteroids. A positive pathergy test of cutaneous hypersensitivity was defined as positive when a sterile pustule developed after 24 to 48 hours at the site of a needle prick to the skin.[114] Although the usual onset of BD is in the third or fourth decade of life, pediatric onset patients have been described.[115]

Two population-based studies, both fulfilling ISG criteria, studied prevalence data for BD, including 1 from France[116] and another from the United States.[117] The overall prevalence in France was 7.1 per 100,000, with immigrants of North African and Asian ancestry manifesting significantly higher prevalence rates of BD than those of European ancestry (17.5 per 100,000 compared with 2.4 per 100,000), comparable with those of North Africa and Asia. This suggested that BD risk was not related to age at immigration but has a primarily hereditary basis. The point prevalence of BD in the United States was 5.2 per 100,000. Genetic studies that focused on molecules related to innate immune responses identified an association with the endothelial nitric oxide (eNOS) gene located on chromosome 7q35-36, a variant of which causes deficient NOS, contributes to the pathogenesis of endothelial abnormalities, and increases thrombotic tendency in BD.

Uluduz and colleagues[118] studied 2 large Istanbul BD cohorts totaling 728 subjects, ascertaining and comparing pediatric-onset (26 subjects) and adult-onset (702 subjects) neuro-BD (NBD). The mean age of pediatric-onset of BD and NBD onset were 13 and 13.5 years, respectively, compared with adult-onset BD and NBD of 26 and 32 years, respectively. The commonest initial neurologic symptom in the pediatric-onset subjects was headache in 92%, followed by seizures in 11.5%, compared with adult-onset BD that manifested corticospinal tract signs in 59% followed by headache in 58% and dysarthria in 23%. Significant differences in neurologic involvement consisted of a higher frequency of cerebral venous sinus thrombosis (CVST) so noted in 88.5% of children and 17% of adults, whereas parenchymal involvement was noted in 74.8% of adults compared with 11.6% of children. None of the children had associated cortical venous infarcts. Oral ulcers were noted in 100% of both groups, and there were no significant statistical differences in the occurrence of skin lesion, uveitis, or arthralgia; however, genital ulcers were less common in children compared with adults (54% compared with 84%).

Headache may be due to migraine, tension-type headache, uveitis, or the direct consequence of NBD. A case-control study of headache in BD reported by Haghighi and colleagues[119] found that 65% of subjects suffered from chronic headache due to migraine with aura in 1.7%, migraine without aura in 25%, tension headache in 24%, NBD in 8%, uveitis in 3%, and the remainder were due to other factors. Frontal and occipital headache and deep-seated pain around the eyes were presenting symptoms in several subjects with imminent florid involvement later studied at postmortem examination,[120–123] or as a clue to silent neurologic involvement in other cohorts so studied.[124] Cognitive impairment involving mainly memory functions occurs in BD without overt NBD, so noted in 46% of BD subjects compared with none in control subjects, with high disease activity and prednisone dosage independently associated with cognitive impairment.[125]

Siva and Saip[126] classified neurologic involvement into 2 major primary types: a primarily vascular-inflammatory mechanism with focal or multifocal parenchymal involvement, presenting most often as a subacute brainstem syndrome; and an unrelated vasculitis type with few symptoms and more favorable prognosis, due to isolated CVST and intracranial hypertension. A secondary form results instead from CNS involvement, such as cerebral emboli from cardiac disease, intracranial hypertension from superior vena cava syndrome, and neurotoxicity of specific mediations used in treatment. Mortality among neurologically complicated, clinicopathologically confirmed approaches 41%, with 59% occurring within 1 year of onset of neurologic involvement. Among nonfatal cases, residual neurologic signs are common. The neuropathological findings in BD in brain biopsies and postmortem examination have been remarkably consistent among patients over the past several decades, evidencing perivascular cuffing of small meningovascular and parenchymal arteries and veins[120,121,123,127,128]; rarely, medium-sized arteries displaying fibrinoid degeneration and recanalization; and examples of venous thrombosis, generally with frank necrotizing vasculitis. The inflammatory cell infiltrates were generally composed of lymphocytes, both T-cells and B-cells; macrophages; rarely, plasma cells; and eosinophils, with reactive astrocytosis and microscopic gliosis in neighboring cerebral, cerebellar, and brainstem white matter.

Matsumoto and colleagues[129] noted large-vessel lesions in 7 of 8 subjects aged 31 to 56 years with BD, including saccular aneurysms of the sinus of Valsalva or aortic arch; thoracic and abdominal aorta; pulmonary, femoral, and iliac arteries; and thrombotic occlusions in the pulmonary vein and superior and inferior vena. Aortitis, noted histologically in 6 of the 8 subjects, was active in 1, scarred in 6, and intermixed in another. Active aortitis was characterized by intense infiltration of inflammatory cells in the media and adventitia more frequently than in the interim with occasional giant cell formation. The scar stage was characterized by fibrous thickening of the intima and adventitia with condensation of the elastic lamina and proliferation of vasa vasorum with slight perivascular lymphocytic and plasma cell infiltrates. The subjects with large venous occlusions had thrombophlebitis with luminal obstruction by organized thrombi.

CVST in BD presents with subacute or chronic onset of symptoms of isolated intracranial hypertension accompanied by headache, blurred vision, and diplopia[130] compared with those without BD in whom the onset is typically acute and associated with headache, hemiparesis, aphasia, and seizure. Venous infarcts occur in up to 63% of those with CVST of other causes, and in only 6% of subjects with BD. The rarity of venous infarcts, long delay to diagnosis, and clinical signs of isolated intracranial hypertension are more typical of BD-related CVST in which prothrombosis is presumed to commence as an endothelial dysfunction that takes longer to develop. Although anticoagulation would not be recommended for BD-related CVST, it might be considered in association with arterial occlusions, with both venous and arterial occlusive episodes warranting prompt consideration of corticosteroids alone or in association with another immunosuppressant agent.

Cogan syndrome

Cogan syndrome (CS) is a rare multisystem inflammatory vascular disease, characterized by nonsyphilitic interstitial keratitis (IK) and vestibuloauditory symptoms. A review of 79 cases of CS by Bicknell and Holland[131] found that more than half had nervous system involvement, including electroencephalographic or spinal fluid abnormality, headache, psychosis, coma, convulsion, neuropathy, and stroke. CS should be considered when neurologic deficits are accompanied by eye, ear, and systemic symptoms.

Gluth and colleagues[132] reviewed a cohort of CS patients seen at the Mayo Clinic between 1940 and 2002. The commonest symptoms at presentation were sudden hearing loss (50%), balance disturbance (40%), ocular irritation (32%), photophobia (23%), tinnitus (13%), and blurred vision (10%). Systemic symptoms noted alone at presentation included headache (40%), arthralgia (35%), fever (27%), myalgia (23%), abdominal pain (22%), rash (12%), peripheral neuropathy (10%), hematuria (7%), meningismus (5%), encephalitis (5%), and cerebral infarction. Otolaryngologic symptoms noted in the course of the disease included hearing loss (100%), vertigo or dizziness (90%), tinnitus (80%), ataxia (53%), oscillopsia (25%); similarly, those related to inflammatory eye involvement included interstitial keratitis (77%), iritis or uveitis (37%), scleritis or episcleritis (23%), and conjunctivitis (10%). Laboratory evidence of elevated ANCA antibodies was detected in 2 of 21 patients (10%), both in a perinuclear pattern.

There is ample literature to attest to the variable caliber of vessels affected by the underlying vasculitic process. Pathologically proven necrotizing vasculitis in association with CS was confirmed at postmortem examination alone in 3 patients,[133–135] by examination of subcutaneous nodular tissue and amputated limbs in life, and confirmed at postmortem examination in another patient[136]; and by examination of biopsy tissue alone in 10 living patients.[133,134,137–141]

Crawford[133] observed 3 patients with systemic necrotizing vasculitis, both whom had headache at onset of CS. Postmortem examination in the first patient (case 1) with frontal headaches and IK before onset of vestibuloauditory symptoms showed necrotizing arteritis involving small arteries and arterioles of the brain, gastrointestinal tract, and kidneys, in addition to cerebral edema and petechial hemorrhages.

Eisenstein and Taubenhaus[134] reported a second postmortem description of CS and systemic vasculitis without preceding headache, in association with terminal heart failure (case 1), in which fibrinoid necrosis of an affected aortic valve extended to the endocardium and intimal surface of the aorta. There was marked intimal thickening and fibrosis of several small intramural branches of the coronary arteries combined with dense perivascular infiltration by lymphocytes and polymorphonuclear cells.

Fisher and Hellstrom[136] described a third subject with CS and systemic vasculitis, also without obvious headache, in whom initial biopsy of a subcutaneous nodule showed marked infiltration by polymorphonuclear cells throughout all coats and into the surrounding tissue of a large vein and artery, as well as in smaller arteries by a severe lymphocytic infiltrate. The amputated extremities of the same subject showed intense inflammatory cell infiltration and necrosis of the media of the distal tibial and smaller muscular arteries, with focal fibrous intimal thickening; and, rarely, organized thrombi reminiscent of thromboangiitis obliterans or Buerger disease. Postmortem examination of the eyes and ears demonstrated IK, degeneration of the vestibular and spiral ganglia, edema of the cochlea and semicircular canals, and inflammation of the ligamentum spirale, without vascular changes. Vasculitic lesions noted in the amputated extremities were seen in some viscera.

Cogan and Dickerson[135] described a subject with CS and fatal aortitis, also without preceding headache, noting severe thickening of small arteries of the aortic wall with reduplication of the elastica, destruction of smooth and elastic tissue of the media, and infiltration of the intima and media by polymorphonuclear and mononuclear inflammatory cells. Vollertsen and colleagues[142] noted generalized aortic dilatation of the aorta at postmortem examination in 1 subject without mention of necrotizing vasculitis. In an analysis of vessels other than the aorta in 5 subjects, 2 had vasculitis in biopsy tissue of small muscular femoral arteries at the time of femoral arterial thrombosis, 1 had chronic venous inflammation at the site of thrombosis of the right arm, 1 had intimal fibrosis suggestive of resolved vasculitis, and 1 had a normal temporal artery biopsy.

Darougar and colleagues[143] described a child with CS, antibodies to *Chlamydia psittaci*, and sudden cardiac arrest in whom postmortem examination showed destructive atrial and coronary artery, and aortic lesions in association with lymphocytic inflammation of the intima but without frank vasculitis.

Lunardi and colleagues[144] used pooled IgG from 8 subjects with CS to screen a random peptide library to identify possible autoantibodies in CS in a peptide library. One isolated immunodominant peptide, which showed similarly with the autoantigens Systemic Sjögren's SAntibody (SSA), also called anti-Ro, and reovirus III major core protein lambda 1, and the peptide sequence of tyrosine phosphatase-1 (CD148 [clusters of differentiation]), expressed on the sensory epithelia of the inner ear and on endothelial cells. IgG antibodies against the peptide purified from patient sera recognized CD148 protein, bound human cochlea, and inhibited proliferation of cells expressing CD148. The same antibodies bound connexin 26, gene mutations of which lead to congenital inner-ear deafness, and were able to induce the feature of CD in mice.

Early recognition of the diagnosis of childhood CS is important in instituting corticosteroid therapy to preserve hearing, especially when hearing loss is a later occurrence. A combination of oral and intravenous corticosteroids may be considered in children who partly but not fully improve. Chaudhuri and colleagues[145] described a 7-year-old boy who was promptly diagnosed after concomitant headache, IK, and sensorineural hearing loss occurred, leading to commencement of prednisone 1 mg per kilogram per day and prednisolone acetate ophthalmic 1% solution, leading to resolution of IK. The addition of pulse intravenous methylprednisolone at 30 mg per kilogram per day for 5 doses in conjunction with a 1-month course of prednisone, however, led to marked improvement in hearing loss.

Chronic auditory and ophthalmologic childhood disease may occur before recognition of CS, similarly warranting aggressive management. Orsoni and colleagues[146] described 2 children with chronic ocular inflammation and hearing loss prompting consideration of CS. A 6-year-old boy had recurrent bilateral keratoconjunctivitis, followed at age 13 years by sudden hearing loss, headache, asthenia, and recurrent arthralgia, leading to the diagnosis of CS. A 3-year-old boy had chronic bilateral uveitis from age 6 months, followed by sudden hearing loss at age 5 years, accompanied by headaches and arthralgia, prompting consideration of CS. Both children were treated with combination (noncorticosteroid) immunosuppressant for 6 months, leading to resolution first of headache and arthralgia in the first 2 months in both children, followed by improvement in ocular inflammation and auditory symptoms in the first child but not in the other.

REFERENCES

1. Jennette JC, Falk RJ, Bacon PA, et al. 2012 revised International Chapel Hill Consensus Conference Nomenclature of Vasculitides. Arthritis Rheum 2013; 65:1–11.
2. Salvarani C, Brown RD Jr, Christianson TJH, et al. Adult primary central nervous system vasculitis: treatment and course. Arthritis Rheum 2015;67:1637–45.
3. Younger DS, Hays AP, Brust JCM, et al. Granulomatous angiitis of the brain. An inflammatory reaction of diverse etiology. Arch Neurol 1988;45:514–8.
4. Calabrese HL, Mallek JA. Primary angiitis of the central nervous system: report of 8 new cases, review of the literature, and proposal for diagnostic criteria. Medicine 1988;67:20–39.
5. Ozen S, Ruperto N, Dillon MJ, et al. EULAR/PReS endorsed consensus criteria for the classification of childhood vasculitides. Ann Rheum Dis 2006;65:936–41.
6. Twilt M, Benseler SM. Central nervous system vasculitis in adults and children. Handb Clin Neurol 2016;133:283–300.
7. Adams HP Jr, Bendixen BH, Kappelle LJ, et al. Classification of subtype of acute ischemic stroke. Definitions for use in a multicenter clinical trial. TOAST. Trial of Org 10172 in Acute Stroke Treatment. Stroke 1993;24:35–41.
8. Putaala J, Metso AJ, Metso TM, et al. Analysis of 1008 consecutive patients aged 15 to 49 with first-ever ischemic stroke: the Helsinki young stroke registry. Stroke 2009;40:1195–203.
9. Bernard TJ, Manco-Johnson MJ, Lo W, et al. Towards a consensus-based classification of childhood arterial ischemic stroke. Stroke 2012;43:371–7.
10. Bernard TJ, Beslow LA, Manco-Johnson MJ, et al. Inter-rater reliability of the CASCADE criteria: challenges in classifying arteriopathies. Stroke 2016; 47(10):2443–9.
11. Wintermark M, Hills NK, DeVeber GA, et al. Clinical and imaging characteristics of arteriopathy subtypes in children with arterial ischemic stroke: results of the VIPS study. AJNR Am J Neuroradiol 2017;38:2172–9.
12. Younger DS. Vasculitis of the nervous system. Curr Opin Neurol 2004;17: 317–36.
13. Salvarani C, Brown RD Jr, Calamia KT, et al. Primary central nervous system vasculitis of 101 patients. Ann Neurol 2007;62:442–51.
14. Birnbaum J, Hellmann DB. Primary angiitis of the central nervous system. Arch Neurol 2009;66:704–9.
15. De Boysson H, Arquizan C, Touze E, et al. Treatment and long-term outcomes of primary central nervous system vasculitis. Stroke 2018;49:1946–52.

16. Pistracher K, Gellner V, Riegler S, et al. Cerebral haemorrhage in the presence of primary childhood central nervous system vasculitis–a review. Childs Nerv Syst 2012;28:1141–8.

17. Benseler SM, deVeber G, Hawkins C, et al. Angiography-negative primary central nervous system vasculitis in children: a newly recognized inflammatory central nervous system disease. Arthritis Rheum 2005;52:2159–67.

18. Twilt M, Benseler SM. Childhood inflammatory brain diseases: pathogenesis, diagnosis and therapy. Rheumatology (Oxford) 2014;53:1359–68.

19. Morishita KA, Moorthy LN, Lubieniecka JM, et al. Early outcomes in children with antineutrophil cytoplasmic antibody-associated vasculitis. Arthritis Rheum 2017; 69:1470–9.

20. Kermani TA, Warrington KJ, Crowson CS, et al. Large-vessel involvement in giant cell arteritis: a population based cohort study of the incidence-trends and prognosis. Ann Rheum Dis 2012;72(12):1989–94.

21. Nuenninghoff DM, Hunder GG, Christianson TJH, et al. Incidence and predictors of large-artery complication (aortic aneurysm, aortic dissection, and/or large artery stenosis) in patients with giant cell arteritis. Arthritis Rheum 2003; 48:3522–31.

22. Salvarani C, Cantini F, Boiardi L, et al. Polymyalgia rheumatic and giant cell arteritis. N Engl J Med 2002;347:261–71.

23. Blockman D, Bley T, Schmidt W. Imaging for large-vessel vasculitis. Curr Opin Rheumatol 2009;21:19–28.

24. Hollenhorst RW, Brown JR, Wagener HP, et al. Neurologic aspects of temporal arteritis. Neurology 1960;10:490–8.

25. Caselli RJ, Hudner GG, Whisnant JP. Neurologic disease in biopsy-proven giant cell (temporal) arteritis. Neurology 1988;38:352–9.

26. Gonzalez-Gay MA, Blanco R, Rodriguez-Valverde V, et al. Permanent visual loss and cerebrovascular attacks in giant cell arteritis. Predictors and response to treatment. Arthritis Rheum 1998;41:1497–504.

27. Dreyer L, Faurschou M, Baslund B. A population-based study of Takayasu's arteritis in eastern Denmark. Clin Exp Rheumatol 2011;29(Suppl 64):S40–2.

28. Brunner J, Feldman BM, Tyrrell PN, et al. Takayasu arteritis in children and adolescents. Rheumatology (Oxford) 2010;49:1806–14.

29. Jain S, Sharma N, Singh S, et al. Takayasu arteritis in children and young Indians. Int J Cardiol 2000;75(Suppl 1):S153–7.

30. Kerr GS, Hallahan CW, Giordano J, et al. Takayasu arteritis. Ann Intern Med 1994;120:919–29.

31. Riehl J-L. Idiopathic arteritis of Takayasu. Neurology 1963;13:873–84.

32. Riehl J-L, Brown WJ. Takayasu's arteritis. Arch Neurol 1965;12:92–7.

33. Grayson PC, Maksimowicz-McKinnon K, Clark TM, et al. Distribution of arterial lesions in Takayasu's arteritis and giant cell arteritis. Ann Rheum Dis 2012;71: 1329–34.

34. Ishikawa K. Natural history and classification of occlusive thromboaortopathy (Takayasu's disease). Circulation 1978;57:27–35.

35. Ohigashi H, Haraguchi G, Konishi M, et al. Improved prognosis of Takayasu arteritis over the past decade. Circ J 2012;76:1004–11.

36. Watts RA, Gonzalez-Gay MA, Lane SE, et al. Geoepidemiology of systemic vasculitis: comparison of the incidence in two regions of Europe. Ann Rheum Dis 2001;60:170–2.

37. Lightfoot RW Jr, Michel BA, Bloch DA, et al. The American College of Rheumatology 1990 criteria for the classification of polyarteritis nodosa. Arthritis Rheum 1990;33:1088–93.
38. Nakamura Y, Yashiro M, Uehara R, et al. Epidemiologic features of Kawasaki disease in Japan: results from the nationwide survey in 2005-2006. J Epidemiol 2008;18:167–72.
39. Shulman ST, Rowley AH. Advances in Kawasaki disease. Eur J Pediatr 2004; 163:285–91.
40. Kernohan JW, Woltman HW. Periarteritis nodosa: a clinicopathologic study with special reference to the nervous system. Arch Neurol 1938;39:655–86.
41. Guillevin L, Lhote F, Gherardi R. Polyarteritis nodosa, microscopic polyangiitis and Churg-Strauss syndrome: clinical aspects, neurologic manifestations, and treatment. Neurol Clin 1997;15:865–86.
42. Pagnoux C, Seror R, Henegar C, et al. Clinical features and outcomes in 348 patients with polyarteritis nodosa. Arthritis Rheum 2010;62:616–26.
43. Ozen S, Pistorio A, Iusan SM, et al. EULAR/PRINTO/PReS criteria for Henoch-Schönlein purpura, childhood polyarteritis nodosa, childhood Wegener granulomatosis and childhood Takayasu arteritis. Ankara 2008. Part II: Final Classification. Ann Rheum Dis 2010;69:798–806.
44. Tekin M, Yalcinkaya F, Turner N, et al. Clinical, laboratory and molecular characteristics of children with familial Mediterranean fever-associated vasculitis. Acta Paediatr 2000;89:177–82.
45. Rogalski C, Sticherling M. Panarteritis cutanea benigna-an entity limited to the skin or cutaneous presentation of a systemic necrotizing vasculitis? Report of seven cases and review of the literature. Int J Dermatol 2007;46:817–21.
46. Ozen S, Anton J, Arisoy N, et al. Juvenile polyarteritis: results of a multicenter survey of 110 children. J Pediatr 2004;145:517–22.
47. David J, Ansell BM, Woo P. Polyarteritis nodosa associated with streptococcus. Arch Dis Child 1993;69:685–8.
48. Gitiaux C, Kossorotoff M, Bergounioux J, et al. Cerebral vasculitis in severe Kawasaki disease: early detection by magnetic resonance imaging and good outcome after intensive treatment. Dev Med Child Neurol 2012;54:1160–3.
49. Templeton PA, Dunne MG. Kawasaki syndrome: cerebral and cardiovascular complications. J Clin Ultrasound 1987;15:483–5.
50. Laxer RM, Dunn HG, Flodmark O. Acute hemiplegia in Kawasaki disease and infantile polyarteritis nodosa. Dev Med Child Neurol 1984;26:814–8.
51. Muneuchi J, Kusuhara K, Kanaya Y, et al. Magnetic resonance studies of brain lesions in patients with Kawasaki disease. Brain Dev 2006;28:30–3.
52. Khan II, Watts RA. Classification of ANCA-associated vasculitis. Curr Rheumatol Rep 2013;15:383.
53. Leavitt RY, Fauci AS, Bloch DA, et al. The American College of Rheumatology 1990 criteria for the classification of Wegener's granulomatosis. Arthritis Rheum 1990;33:1101–7.
54. Masi AT, Hunder GG, Lie JT, et al. The American College of Rheumatology 1990 criteria for the classification of Churg-Strauss syndrome (allergic granulomatosis and angiitis). Arthritis Rheum 1990;33:1094–100.
55. Watts RA, Lane S, Hanslik T, et al. Development and validation of a consensus methodology for the classification of the ANCA-associated vasculitides and polyarteritis nodosa for epidemiological studies. Ann Rheum Dis 2007;66:222–7.
56. Mahr A, Guillevin L, Poissonnet M, et al. Prevalences of polyarteritis nodosa, microscopic polyangiitis, Wegener's granulomatosis, and Churg-Strauss

syndrome in a French urban multiethnic population in 2000: a capture –recapture estimate. Arthritis Rheum 2004;51:92–9.

57. Mohammad AJ, Jacobsson LTH, Westman KWA, et al. Incidence and survival rates in Wegener's granulomatosis, microscopic polyangiitis, Churg-Strauss syndrome and polyarteritis nodosa. Rheumatology 2009;48:1560–5.

58. Drachman DA. Neurological complications of Wegener's granulomatosis. Arch Neurol 1963;8:45–55.

59. Nishino H, Rubino FA, DeRemee RA, et al. Neurological involvement in Wegener's granulomatosis: an analysis of 324 consecutive patients at the Mayo Clinic. Ann Neurol 1993;33:4–9.

60. Fauci AS, Haynes BF, Katz P, et al. Wegener's granulomatosis: Prospective clinical and therapeutic experience with 85 patients over 21 years. Ann Intern Med 1983;98:76–85.

61. Moore PM, Cupps TR. Neurological complications of vasculitis. Ann Neurol 1983;14:155–67.

62. Hoffman GS, Kerr GS, Leavitt RY, et al. Wegener granulomatosis: an analysis of 158 patients. Ann Intern Med 1992;116:488–98.

63. de Groot K, Schmidt DK, Arlt AC, et al. Standardized neurologic evaluations of 128 patients with Wegener's granulomatosis. Arch Neurol 2001;58:1215–21.

64. Lu T, Bao J, Lin D, et al. Pediatric granulomatosis with polyangiitis exhibiting prominent central nervous system symptoms. Childs Nerv Syst 2016;32:1517–21.

65. Davson J, Ball M, Platt R. The kidney in periarteritis nodosa. QJM 1948;17:175–202.

66. Wainwright, Davson J. The renal appearance in the microscopic form of periarteritis nodosa. J Pathol Bacteriol 1950;62:189–96.

67. Savage COS, Winearls CG, Evans DJ, et al. Microscopic polyarteritis: presentation, pathology and prognosis. QJM 1985;220:467–83.

68. Serra A, Cameron JS, Turner DR, et al. Vasculitis affecting the kidney: presentation, histopathology and long-term outcome. QJM 1984;201:181–207.

69. Guillevin L, Durand-Gasselin B, Cevallos R, et al. Microscopic polyangiitis. Arthritis Rheum 1999;42:421–30.

70. Gayraud M, Guillevin L, le Toumelin P, et al, and the French Vasculitis Study Group. Long-term followup of polyarteritis nodosa, microscopic polyangiitis, and Churg-Strauss syndrome. Arthritis Rheum 2001;44:666–75.

71. Villiger PM, Guillevin L. Microscopic polyangiitis: clinical presentation. Autoimmun Rev 2010;9:812–9.

72. Ben Sassi S, Ben Ghorbel I, Mizouni H, et al. Microscopic polyangiitis presenting with peripheral and central neurological manifestations. Neurol Sci 2011;32:727–9.

73. Honda H, Hasegawa T, Morokawa N, et al. A case of MPO-ANCA related vasculitis with transient leukoencephalopathy and multiple cerebral haemorrhages. Rinsho Shinkeigaku 1996;36:1089–94.

74. Han S, Rehman HU, Jayaratne PS, et al. Microscopic polyangiitis complicated by cerebral haemorrhage. Rheumatol Int 2006;26:1057–60.

75. Ito Y, Suzuki K, Yamazaki T, et al. ANCA-associated vasculitis (AAV) causing bilateral cerebral infarction and subsequent intracerebral haemorrhage without renal and respiratory dysfunction. J Neurol Sci 2006;240:99–101.

76. Ahn JK, Hwang J-W, Lee J, et al. Clinical features and outcome of microscopic polyangiitis under a new consensus algorithm of ANCA-associated vasculitides in Korea. Rheumatol Int 2012;32:2979–86.

77. Cabral DA, Uribe AG, Benseler S, et al, for the ARChiVe (A Registry for Childhood Vasculitis: e-entry) Investigators Network. Classification, presentation, and initial treatment of Wegener's granulomatosis in childhood. Arthritis Rheum 2009;60:3413–24.

78. Guillevin L, Lhote F, Gayraud M, et al. Prognostic factors in polyarteritis nodosa and Churg-Strauss syndrome: a prospective study of 342 patients. Medicine 1996;75:17–28.

79. Luqmani RA, Bacon PA, Moots RJ, et al. Birmingham Vasculitis Activity Score (BVAS) in systemic necrotizing vasculitis. QJM 1994;87:671–8.

80. Churg J, Strauss L. Allergic granulomatosis, allergic angiitis, and periarteritis nodosa. Am J Pathol 1951;27:277–301.

81. Chumbley LC, Harrison EG, DeRemee RA. Allergic granulomatosis and angiitis (Churg-Strauss syndrome). Report and analysis of 30 cases. Mayo Clin Proc 1977;52:477–84.

82. Lanham JG, Elkon KB, Pussey CD, et al. Systemic vasculitis with asthma and eosinophilia: a clinical approach to the Churg-Strauss syndrome. Medicine 1984;63:65–81.

83. Sehgal M, Swanson JW, DeRemee RA, et al. Neurologic manifestations of Churg-Strauss syndrome. Mayo Clin Proc 1995;70:337–41.

84. Guillevin L, Cohen P, Gayraud M, et al. Churg-Strauss syndrome. Medicine 1999;78:26–37.

85. Mouthon L, Le Toumelin P, Andre MH, et al. Polyarteritis nodosa and Churg-Strauss angiitis. Characteristics and outcome in 38 patients over 65 years. Medicine 2002;81:27–40.

86. Comarmond C, Pagnoux C, Khellaf M, et al, for the French Vasculitis Study Group. Eosinophilic granulomatosis with polyangiitis (Churg-Strauss). Arthritis Rheum 2013;65:270–81.

87. Lerner AB, Watson CJ. Studies of cryoglobulins. II. The spontaneous precipitation of protein from serum at 5°C in various disease states. Am J Med Sci 1947; 214:416–21.

88. Marshall RJ, Malone RGS. Cryoglobulinemia with cerebral purpura. BMJ 1954; 2:279–80.

89. Abramsky O, Slavin S. Neurologic manifestations in patients with mixed cryoglobulinemia. Neurology 1974;24:245–9.

90. Gorevic PD, Kassab HJ, Levo Y, et al. Mixed cryoglobulinemia: clinical aspects and long-term follow-up of 40 patients. Am J Med 1980;69:287–308.

91. Petty GW, Duffy J, Huston J. Cerebral ischemia in patients with hepatitis C virus infection and mixed cryogloblinemia. Mayo Clin Proc 1996;71:671–8.

92. Ince PG, Duffey P, Cochrane HR, et al. Relapsing ischemic encephalopathy and cryoglobulinemia. Neurology 2000;55:1579–81.

93. Cacoub P, Costedoat-Chalumeau N, Lidove O, et al. Cryoglobulinemia vasculitis. Curr Opin Rheumatol 2002;14:29–35.

94. Cacoub P, Sbai A, Hausfater P, et al. Atteinte neurologique central et infection par le virus de l'hèpatite. Gastroenterol Clin Biol 1998;22:631–3.

95. Ferri G, Antonelli A, Puccini R, et al. Mixed cryoglobulinemia: demographic, clinical, and serologic features and survival in 231 patients. Semin Arthritis Rheum 2004;33:355–74.

96. Filipini D, Colombo F, Jann S, et al. Central nervous system manifestations of HCV-related MC: review of the literature. Reumatismo 2002;54:150–5 [in Italian].

97. Fragoso M, Carneado J, Tuduri I, et al. Essential mixed cryoglobulinemia as the cause of ischemic cerebrovascular accident. Rev Neurol 2000;30:444–6 [in Spanish].

98. Casato M, Sasdoun D, Marchetti A, et al. Central nervous system involvement in hepatitis C virus cryoglobulinemia vasculitis: a multicentre case-control study using magnetic resonance imaging and neuropsychological tests. J Rheumatol 2005;32:484–8.

99. Terrier B, Krasinova E, Marie I, et al. Management of non-infectious mixed cryoglobulinemia vasculitis: data from 242 cases included in the CryoVas survey. Blood 2012;119:5996–6004.

100. Terrier B, Cacoub P. Cryoglobulinemia vasculitis: an update. Curr Opin Rheumatol 2013;25:10–8.

101. Liou YT, Huang JL, Ou LS, et al. Comparison of cryoglobulinemia in children and adults. J Microbiol Immunol Infect 2013;46:59–64.

102. Giménez-Roca C, Iglesias E, Vicente MA, et al. Pediatric cryoglobulinemic vasculitis successfully managed with rituximab. Dermatol Ther 2017;30(2):1–3.

103. Jara LJ, Navarro C, Medina G, et al. Hypocomplementemic urticarial vasculitis syndrome. Curr Rheumatol Rev 2009;11:410–5.

104. Wisnieski JJ, Baer AN, Christensen J, et al. Hypocomplementemic urticarial vasculitis syndrome. Medicine 1995;74:24–41.

105. McDuffie FC, Sams WM, Maldonado PH, et al. Hypocomplementemia with cutaneous vasculitis and arthritis. Mayo Clin Proc 1973;48:340–8.

106. Buck A, Christensen J, McCarty M. Hypocomplementemic urticarial vasculitis syndrome. A case report and literature review. J Clin Aesthet Dermatol 2012; 5:36–46.

107. Grotz W, Baba HA, Becker JU, et al. Hypocomplementemic urticarial vasculitis syndrome. Dtsch Arztebl Int 2009;106:756–63.

108. Davies MDP, Brewer JD. Urticarial vasculitis and hypocomplementemic urticarial vasculitis syndrome. Immunol Allergy Clin N Am 2004;24:183–213.

109. Ludivico CL, Myers AR, Maurer K. Hypocomplementemic urticarial vasculitis with glomerulonephritis and pseudotumor cerebri. Arthritis Rheum 1979;22: 1024–8.

110. Pasini A, Bracaglia C, Aceti A, et al. Renal involvement in hypocomplementemic urticarial vasculitis syndrome: a report of three paediatric cases. Rheumatology (Oxford) 2014;53:1409–13.

111. Davatchi F, Chams-Davatchi C, Shams H, et al. Behcet's disease: epidemiology, clinical manifestations, and diagnosis. Expert Rev Clin Immunol 2017;13:57–65.

112. Behcet H, Matteson EL. On relapsing, aphthous ulcers of the mouth, eye and genitalia caused by a virus. 1937. Clin Exp Rheumatol 2010;28(Suppl 60):S2–5.

113. Criteria for diagnosis of Behçet's disease. International Study Group for Behçet's Disease. Lancet 1990;335:1078–80.

114. Sobel JD, Haim S, Shafrir A, et al. Cutaneous hyper-reactivity in Behçet disease. Dermatologica 1973;146:350–6.

115. Özen S. Pediatric onset Behcet disease. Curr Opin Rheumatol 2010;22:585–9.

116. Mahr A, Belarbi L, Wechsler B, et al. Population-based prevalence study of Behçet disease. Differences by ethnic origin and low variation by age at immigration. Arthritis Rheum 2008;58:3951–9.

117. Calamia KT, Wilson FC, Icen M, et al. Epidemiology and clinical characteristics of Behcet's disease in the US: a population-based study. Arthritis Rheum 2009; 61:600–4.

118. Uluduz D, Kürtüncü M, Yapici Z, et al. Clinical characteristics of pediatric-onset neuro-Behçet disease. Neurology 2011;77:1900–5.
119. Haghighi AB, Aflaki E, Ketabchi L. The prevalence and characteristics of different types of headache in patients with Behcet's disease, a case-control study. Headache 2008;48:424–9.
120. McMenemey WH, Lawrence BJ. Encephalomyelopathy in Behcet's disease. Report of necropsy findings in two cases. Lancet 1957;2:353–8.
121. Rubinstein LJ, Urich H. Meningo-encephalitis of Behçet's disease. Case report with pathological findings. Brain 1963;86:151–60.
122. Kawakita H, Nishimura M, Satoh Y, et al. Neurological aspects of Behçet's disease. A case report and clinico-pathological review of the literature in Japan. J Neurol Sci 1967;5:417–39.
123. Arai Y, Kohno S, Takahashi Y, et al. Autopsy case of neuro-Behcet's disease with multifocal neutrophilic perivascular inflammation. Neuropathology 2006;26:579–85.
124. Koseoglu E, Yildirim A, Borlu M. Is headache in Behcet's disease related to silent neurologic involvement? Clin Exp Rheumatol 2011;29(Suppl 67):S32–7.
125. Monastero R, Camarda C, Pipia C, et al. Cognitive impairment in Behcet's disease without overt neurological involvement. J Neurol Sci 2004;220:99–104.
126. Siva A, Saip S. The spectrum of nervous system involvement in Behcet's syndrome and its differential diagnosis. J Neurol 2009;256:513–29.
127. Wolf SM, Schotland DL, Phillips LL. Involvement of nervous system in Behçet's syndrome. Arch Neurol 1965;12:315–25.
128. Hadfield MG, Aydin F, Lippman HR, et al. Neuro-Behçet's disease. Clin Neuropathol 1997;16:55–60.
129. Matsumoto T, Uekusa T, Fukuda Y. Vasculo-Behcet's disease: a pathologic study of eight cases. Hum Pathol 1991;22:45–51.
130. Yesilot N, Bahar S, Yilmazer S, et al. Cerebral venous thrombosis in Behcet's disease compared to those associated with other etiologies. J Neurol 2009;256:1134–42.
131. Bicknell JM, Holland JV. Neurologic manifestations of Cogan syndrome. Neurology 1978;28:278–81.
132. Gluth MB, Baratz KH, Matteson EL, et al. Cogan syndrome: a retrospective review of 60 patients throughout a half century. Mayo Clin Proc 2006;81:483–8.
133. Crawford WJ. Cogan's syndrome associated with polyarteritis nodosa. A report of three cases. Pa Med J 1957;60:835–8.
134. Eisenstein B, Taubenhaus M. Nonsyphilitic interstitial keratitis and bilateral deafness (Cogan's syndrome) associated with cardiovascular disease. N Engl J Med 1958;258:1074–9.
135. Cogan DG, Dickerson GR. Nonsyphilitic interstitial keratitis with vestibuloauditory symptoms. A case with fatal aortitis. Arch Ophthalmol 1964;71:172–5.
136. Fisher ER, Hellstrom HR. Cogan's syndrome and systemic vascular disease. Analysis of pathological features with reference to its relationship to thromboangiitis obliterans (Buerger). Arch Pathol 1961;72:572–92.
137. Oliner L, Taubenhaus M, Shapira TM, et al. Nonsyphilitic interstitial keratitis and bilateral deafness (Cogan's syndrome) associated with essential polyangiitis (periarteritis nodosa). A review of the syndrome with consideration of a possible pathogenic mechanism. N Engl J Med 1953;248:1001–8.
138. Gelfand ML, Kantor T, Gorstein F. Cogan's syndrome with cardiovascular involvement: aortic insufficiency. Bull NY Acad Med 1972;48:647–60.

139. Cheson BD, Bluming AZ, Alroy J. Cogan's syndrome: a systemic vasculitis. Am J Med 1976;60:549–55.

140. Del Caprio J, Espinozea LR, Osterland SK. Cogan's syndrome in HLA Bw 17 [letter to the editor]. N Engl J Med 1976;295:1262–3.

141. Pinals RS. Cogan's syndrome with arthritis and aortic insufficiency. J Rheumatol 1978;5:294–8.

142. Vollertsen RS, McDonald TJ, Younge BR, et al. Cogan's syndrome: 18 cases and a review of the literature. Mayo Clin Proc 1986;61:344–61.

143. Darougar S, John AC, Viswalingam M, et al. Isolation of Chlamydia psittaci from a patient with interstitial keratitis and uveitis associated with otological and cardiovascular lesions. Br J Ophthalmol 1978;62:709–14.

144. Lunardi C, Bason C, Leandri M, et al. Autoantibodies to inner ear and endothelial antigens in Cogan's syndrome. Lancet 2002;360:915–21.

145. Chaudhuri K, Das RR, Chinnakkannan S. Reversible severe sensorineural hearing loss in a 7-year-old child. Acta Paediatr 2011;100:322–3.

146. Orsoni JG, Zavota L, Vincenti V, et al. Cogan syndrome in children: early diagnosis and treatment is critical to prognosis. Am J Ophthalmol 2004;137:757–8.

Peripheral Nerve Vasculitis
Classification and Disease Associations

Kelly G. Gwathmey, MD[a], Jennifer A. Tracy, MD[b],
P. James B. Dyck, MD[b],*

KEYWORDS

- Vasculitis • Vasculitic neuropathy • Nonsystemic vasculitic neuropathy • ANCA
- Radiculoplexus neuropathy • Microvasculitis • Nerve large arteriole vasculitis

KEY POINTS

- Vasculitic neuropathies result from inflammation and ischemic injury to the vasa nervorum and are typically divided into systemic and nonsystemic types.
- Classically, patients with vasculitic neuropathies will present with multiple mononeuropathies (ie, multifocal neuropathy) manifesting as painful, stepwise progression of mixed sensory and motor deficits.
- Vasculitic neuropathies may be associated with primary systemic vasculitis, secondary to other etiologies, or may be nonsystemic, which is localized only to the peripheral nerves.
- Vasculitic neuropathies can be divided into 2 categories based on the size of blood vessel involvement: large arteriole vasculitis (usually systemic) and microvasculitis (usually nonsystemic).

INTRODUCTION

When vasculitis affects the peripheral nerves, inflammatory cells infiltrate the vasa nervorum (blood vessels of the peripheral nerves) and subsequently causes ischemic injury. The resulting vasculitic neuropathies may occur in the setting of systemic vasculitis or may be exclusively localized to the peripheral nervous system (ie, nonsystemic vasculitic neuropathy [NSVN]). Systemic vasculitis can be further subdivided into primary systemic vasculitis, in which there is no known cause, and secondary systemic vasculitis, which may be associated with connective tissue diseases, viral infections, drugs, or paraneoplastic syndromes. All peripheral nerve vasculitides involve small blood vessels, and these small blood vessel vasculitides can be further subdivided into large arteriole vasculitis and microvasculitis. In general, the nerve large arteriole vasculitis of are more likely to be part of a systemic vasculitis, whereas

Disclosure Statement: The authors have nothing to disclose.
[a] Department of Neurology, Virginia Commonwealth University, 1101 East Marshall Street, PO Box 980599, 6th Floor, Room 6-013, Richmond, VA 23298, USA; [b] Department of Neurology, Mayo Clinic, 200 1st Street SW, Rochester, MN 55905, USA
* Corresponding author.
E-mail address: Dyck.pjames@mayo.edu

the nerve microvasculitis is more likely to be nonsystemic vasculitis. Although vasculitic neuropathy classification schemes are constantly redefined, the radiculoplexus neuropathies (RPNs), including diabetic lumbosacral RPN (DLRPN), nondiabetic lumbosacral RPN (LRPN), painless diabetic motor neuropathy (PDMN), diabetic cervical radiculoplexus neuropathy (DCRPN), and neuralgic amyotrophy (NA), are best categorized as NSVN variants characterized by the histopathological finding of microvasculitis. These, and NSVN, differ from most systemic vasculitic neuropathies, which are histopathologically classified as nerve large arteriole vasculitis and portend a worse prognosis. The purpose of this review is to bring the neurologist up to date on the classification, clinical presentation, diagnosis, etiologies, and treatment of the vasculitic neuropathies.

CLASSIFICATION

The size of the involved blood vessels directs the organizational framework for the vasculitides. The 2012 revised Chapel Hill Consensus Conference classification of the vasculitides remains the most current, categorizing vasculitis by the size of the affected vessel (large vessel, medium vessel, small vessel) and by etiology.[1] This version updates the nomenclature and eliminates eponyms (eg, Churg-Strauss syndrome is now eosinophilic granulomatosis with polyangiitis [EGPA] and Wegener granulomatosis is now granulomatosis with polyangiitis [GPA]). In this revised version, the small vessel vasculitides are further subdivided into those with minimal immune-complex deposition, the antineutrophil cytoplasmic antibody (ANCA)-associated vasculitides (AAVs), and immune-complex small vessel vasculitis. The systemic vasculitides most commonly associated with vasculitic neuropathies include the medium vessel vasculitis polyarteritis nodosa (PAN, which also affects small vessels); the AAVs, including microscopic polyangiitis (MPA), GPA, and EGPA; and the immune-complex associated cryoglobulinemic vasculitis. In this classification scheme, NSVN would be classified as a single-organ vasculitis. The secondary vasculitic neuropathies, such as those associated with connective tissue diseases, drugs, viral infections and paraneoplastic syndromes, would be classified as "vasculitis associated with probable etiology" or "vasculitis associated with systemic disease."

In 2010, the Peripheral Nerve Society Task Force developed a vasculitic neuropathy-specific classification that is widely accepted.[2] It subdivides systemic vasculitic neuropathy into primary and secondary forms, NSVN, and other localized forms (**Box 1**). An update of this classification, in accordance with the Chapel Hill Consensus Conference in 2012 was recently proposed in 2017.[3]

An easy classification of vasculitic neuropathies can be categorized based on their histopathologic features. Although all vasculitis in nerve involves small vessels, these can be separated into nerve large arteriole vasculitis or nerve microvasculitis. Nerve large arteriole vasculitis affects blood vessels that range from 75 to 300 μm in diameter, including small arteries, large arterioles, and smaller vessels. Nerve microvasculitis affects blood vessels measuring less than 40 μm in diameter and includes small arterioles, endoneurial microvessels, capillaries, and venules. This binary system may occasionally oversimplify the classification, as many vasculitic neuropathies lie on a spectrum affecting vessels of varying sizes. For example, NSVN, classically considered nerve microvasculitis, in some cases is a localized form of MPA[4] and in some series has the histopathological features of nerve large arteriole vasculitis.[5–7] The NSVN variants, the RPNs and NA, however, more clearly fall in the nerve microvasculitis category and most secondary systemic vasculidities are clearly large arteriole vasculitis.

Box 1
Classification of vasculitides associated with neuropathy according to the Peripheral Nerve Society Guideline of 2010

I. Primary systemic vasculitides
  a. Predominantly small vessel vasculitis
    i. Microscopic polyangiitis[a]
    ii. Churg-Strauss syndrome[a]
    iii. Wegener granulomatosis[a]
    iv. Essential mixed cryoglobulinemia (non-HCV)
    v. Henoch-Schölein purpura
  b. Predominantly medium vessel vasculitis
    i. Polyarteritis nodosa
  c. Predominantly large vessel vasculitis
    i. Giant cell vasculitis

II. Secondary systemic vasculitides associated with 1 of the following:
  a. Connective tissue diseases
    i. Rheumatoid arthritis
    ii. Systemic lupus erythematosus
    iii. Sjögren syndrome
    iv. Systemic sclerosis
    v. Dermatomyositis
    vi. Mixed connective tissue disease
  b. Sarcoidosis
  c. Behcet disease
  d. Infection (such as HBV, HCV, HIV, CMV, leprosy, Lyme disease, HTLV-1)
  e. Drugs
  f. Malignancy
  g. Inflammatory bowel disease
  h. Hypocomplementemic urticarial vasculitis syndrome

III. Nonsystemic/localized vasculitis
  a. Nonsystemic vasculitic neuropathy (includes nondiabetic radiculoplexus neuropathy and some cases of Wartenberg migrant sensory neuritis)
  b. Diabetic radiculoplexus neuropathy
  c. Localized cutaneous/neuropathic vasculitis
    i. Cutaneous polyarteritis nodosa
    ii. Others

Abbreviations: CMV, cytomegalovirus; HBV, hepatitis B virus; HCV, hepatitis C virus; HIV, human immunodeficiency virus; HTLV, human T-lymphotrophic virus.

[a] Antineutrophil cytoplasmic antibody (ANCA)-associated vasculitides.

Adapted from Collins MP, Dyck PJB, Gronseth GS, et al. Peripheral Nerve Society Guideline on the classification, diagnosis, investigation, and immunosuppressive therapy of non-systemic vasculitic neuropathy: executive summary. J Peripher Nerv Syst 2010;15(3):176–84.

CASE DEFINITIONS

The diagnostic gold standard of vasculitis is the demonstration of histopathological evidence of definite vasculitis. The 2010 Peripheral Nerve Society Task Force published consensus definitions of histopathologically definite, probable, and possible vasculitic neuropathies (**Boxes 2–4**).[2] For those patients without features of definite vasculitis, clinically probable vasculitic neuropathy relies on the presentation including symptoms, signs, supportive laboratory, and histopathological findings. The 2010 Peripheral Nerve Society Task Force also generated diagnostic criteria for NSVN including 2 new exclusionary criteria both with greater than 95% specificity for systemic vasculitic neuropathy (SVN) including ANCAs and erythrocyte sedimentation rate (ESR) >/100 mm/h.

Box 2

Diagnostic criteria for pathologically definite

I. *Active lesion:* Nerve biopsy showing collection of inflammatory cells in vessel wall AND 1 or more signs of acute vascular damage:
   a. Fibrinoid necrosis
   b. Loss/disruption of endothelium
   c. Loss/fragmentation of internal elastic lamina
   d. Loss/fragmentation/separation of smooth muscle cells in media (can be highlighted with anti–smooth muscle actin staining)
   e. Acute thrombosis
   f. Vascular/perivascular hemorrhage OR
   g. Leukocytoclasia

II. *Chronic lesion with signs of healing/repair:* Nerve biopsy showing collection of mononuclear inflammatory cells in vessel wall AND 1 or more signs of chronic vascular damage with repair:
   a. Intimal hyperplasia
   b. Fibrosis of media
   c. Adventitial/periadventitial fibrosis OR
   d. Chronic thrombosis with recanalization

III. No evidence of another primary disease process that can mimic vasculitis pathologically, such as lymphoma, lymphomatoid granulomatosis, or amyloidosis.

Presence of a chronic lesion does not exclude active vasculitis (vasculitides are usually segmental and multifocal, producing lesions of different ages in the same tissue or end-organ).

From Collins MP, Dyck PJB, Gronseth GS, et al. Peripheral Nerve Society Guideline on the classification, diagnosis, investigation, and immunosuppressive therapy of non-systemic vasculitic neuropathy: executive summary. J Peripher Nerv Syst 2010;15(3):176–84; with permission.

Box 3

Diagnostic criteria for pathologically probable vasculitic neuropathy

I. Pathologic criteria for definite vasculitic neuropathy not satisfied (see **Box 2**) AND

II. Predominantly axonal changes AND

III. Perivascular inflammation accompanied by signs of active or chronic vascular damage (as defined in **Box 2**) OR perivascular/vascular inflammation plus at least 1 additional class II or III pathologic predictor of definite vasculitic neuropathy[a]:
   a. Vascular deposition of complement, immunoglobulin M, or fibrinogen by direct immunofluorescence
   b. Hemosiderin deposits (Perls' stain for iron)
   c. Asymmetric/multifocal nerve fiber loss or degeneration
   d. Prominent active axonal degeneration or
   e. Myofiber necrosis, regeneration, or infarcts in concomitant peroneus brevis muscle biopsy (not explained by underlying myopathy)

[a] Additional alterations used by some investigators as supportive of vasculitis but lacking in adequate evidence (more study required): (1) neovascularization (class II/III evidence suggests that this finding is probably not a predictor of vasculitis); (2) endoneurial hemorrhage (1 negative class II study; 1 positive class III study); (3) focal perineurial inflammation, degeneration, thickening (only class IV evidence); (4) injury neuroma, microfasciculation (only class IV evidence); and (5) swollen axons filled with organelles (1 negative but nonconvincing class II study) and other experimentally demonstrated axonal changes of acute ischemia, such as attenuated axons, flattened myelin profiles, tubular profiles, and axonal cytolysis.

From Collins MP, Dyck PJB, Gronseth GS, et al. Peripheral Nerve Society Guideline on the classification, diagnosis, investigation, and immunosuppressive therapy of non-systemic vasculitic neuropathy: executive summary. J Peripher Nerv Syst 2010;15(3):176–84; with permission.

Box 4
Diagnostic criteria for pathologically possible vasculitic neuropathy

I. Pathologic criteria for definite and probable vasculitic neuropathy not satisfied AND

II. Predominantly axonal changes AND

III. Inflammation in vessel wall without other signs of definite vasculitic neuropathy OR one or more signs of *active/chronic vascular damage* (as defined in **Box 2**) or *pathologic predictors* of definite vasculitic neuropathy (see **Box 3**), without vessel wall or perivascular inflammation.

From Collins MP, Dyck PJB, Gronseth GS, et al. Peripheral Nerve Society Guideline on the classification, diagnosis, investigation, and immunosuppressive therapy of non-systemic vasculitic neuropathy: executive summary. J Peripher Nerv Syst 2010;15(3):176–84; with permission.

In 2015, the Brighton Criteria revisited the diagnostic criteria for vasculitic neuropathies and adopted the same criteria for histopathologically definite vasculitis (Level 1, "gold standard" case definition) as the Peripheral Nerve Society Task Force criteria.[8] Regarding the Level 2 case definition, clinical features of vasculitic neuropathy must be present in addition to evidence of vasculitis with peripheral nerve biopsy meeting histopathologically probable vasculitic neuropathy criteria, or other organ biopsy in systemic vasculitis, or muscle or skin biopsy meeting histopathologically definite vasculitis criteria. The Level 3 case definition of vasculitic neuropathy, which includes a nerve biopsy that fails to meet definite or probable criteria, or which was not performed, requires clinical features consistent with vasculitic neuropathy. These clinical features were substantially modified from the Peripheral Nerve Society Task Force guideline and are available as **Box 5**.

CLINICAL AND DIAGNOSTIC FEATURES OF VASCULITIC NEUROPATHIES
Clinical Features

Acute to subacute onset of painful sensory or mixed sensory and motor deficits is the typical presentation of the vasculitic neuropathies.[9,10] When individual peripheral nerves are sequentially affected, it results in the multifocal neuropathy (ie, mononeuritis multiplex or multiple mononeuropathy) pattern. Recently this multifocal neuropathy pattern has been defined as "an anatomic pattern of peripheral neuropathy that affects 2 or more noncontiguous individual, named, somatic, sensory, motor or sensorimotor peripheral or cranial nerves simultaneously or sequentially."[3] Overlapping mononeuropathies may appear more confluent, and result in a length-dependent symmetric or asymmetrical pattern.[2,11–13] Some patients, particularly those with systemic vasculitis, have a fulminant presentation, whereas others, such as patients with NSVN, may have a gradually progressive form that can go on for a decade or longer without diagnosis.[3,14,15] A minority of patients with NSVN will have acute, rapidly progressive deficits.[3] Vasculitis has a predilection for the distal extremity nerves, including the common fibular nerve, the fibular division of the sciatic nerve, and the ulnar nerve of the arm.[16,17] In the RPNs, the proximal extremity nerves, in addition to the nerve roots and plexuses, are targeted. Cranial nerve involvement has been reported in NSVN, EGPA, and GPA.[18–21]

Patients with systemic vasculitis will often have multiorgan involvement, including rash, gastrointestinal symptoms, respiratory impairment, and hematuria, that eclipses the peripheral neuropathy.[12,22–24] In these patients, constitutional symptoms, such as fever, chills, night sweats, and weight loss, are common. In contrast, NSVN is localized solely to the peripheral nervous system and extraneural manifestations will not occur

---

Box 5
Clinical features suggestive of vasculitic neuropathy modified by the 2015 Brighton Criteria

I. Evidence of peripheral neuropathy
   a. Electrodiagnostic evidence of an axonal neuropathy (symmetric or asymmetric)
      OR
   b. Clinical examination signs of peripheral neuropathy
      AND

II. Clinical presentation typical for vasculitic neuropathy
   a. Sensory-motor or sensory (*not pure motor*)
      AND
   b. Multifocal or asymmetric pattern at any time, AND this is not attributable to compression or entrapment of peripheral nerves or roots
      AND
   c. Either
      i. Further clinical features:
         1. Lower limb predominant
            AND
         2. Painful
            AND
         3. One or more acute attacks, or variable speed of progression, or improvement of motor or sensory deficit
            OR
      ii. Biopsy of nerve shows histopathologically probable vasculitis

Adapted from Collins MP, Dyck PJ, Gronseth L, et al. Peripheral Nerve Society Guideline on the classification, diagnosis, investigation, and immunosuppressive therapy of non-systemic vasculitic neuropathy: executive summary. J Peripher Nerv Syst, 15 (2010), pp. 176–84. In Hadden RDM, Collins MP, Živković SA, et al. Vasculitic peripheral neuropathy: Case definition and guidelines for collection, analysis, and presentation of immunisation safety data.Vaccine. 2017 Mar 13;35(11):1567–78; with permission.

---

or be very minor. A minority of patients will experience mild constitutional symptoms, such as weight loss, fatigue, arthralgia, and myalgia.[2,3]

Electrodiagnostic Features

Electrodiagnostic studies can further define the specific pattern of the polyneuropathy, be it sensory or sensorimotor, multifocal, symmetric length-dependent, or asymmetric length-dependent. These studies can also identify affected nerves and muscles that would be appropriate targets for biopsy. The typical electrodiagnostic approach is to sample multiple nerves and muscles, distal and proximal, with side-to-side comparisons. The electrodiagnostic study needs to be designed with clinical correlation, so that the appropriate nerves are tested; otherwise the focality or multifocality of the process may be overlooked. Although vasculitic neuropathies are axonopathies, in the acute setting, pseudoconduction block has been reported.[25,26] This finding is the result of focal axonal conduction failure at the site of infarction. With subsequent Wallerian degeneration, the nerve conduction studies develop the expected axonal changes. A large retrospective review of electrodiagnostic studies in vasculitic neuropathies found that 27.5% of patients had the multifocal neuropathy pattern and 50% had an axonal sensorimotor polyneuropathy with side-to-side asymmetry of amplitudes defined as a twofold amplitude difference (50%).[27]

Laboratory Studies

All patients suspected to have a vasculitic neuropathy will require laboratory studies to evaluate for multiorgan involvement, systemic inflammation, and disease-specific serologic studies. Published guidelines exist to guide physicians regarding the highest yield studies.[2] The following standard laboratory studies are necessary: ESR, C-reactive protein (CRP), antinuclear antibody (ANA), rheumatoid factor (RF), hepatitis B and C panel, cryoglobulins, complete blood count, and comprehensive metabolic panel.[28] Spinal fluid analysis is not typically indicated in the vasculitic neuropathies, although can characteristically demonstrate elevated protein in the RPNs.

ANCAs, which should be tested in all patients with vasculitic neuropathy, are auto-antibodies that react against antigens present on polymorphonuclear cells. There is an International Consensus Statement suggesting that ANCAs should be tested by screening via immunofluorescence testing (IFT) and reflex to antigen-specific enzyme-linked immunosorbent assay testing for any positive IFT tests.[29,30] Cytoplasmic ANCA (c-ANCA) occurs often with active generalized GPA. Perinuclear ANCA (p-ANCA) occurs in patients with MPA and EGPA. Autoantibodies with specificity for myeloperoxidase are called MPO-ANCA and those against proteinase 3 are PR3-ANCA. Most often, the C-ANCA staining pattern is associated with PR-3 antibodies and P-ANCA staining pattern is less specific but is often associated with MPO antibodies.[31]

Specific biomarkers, including serum neurofilament light chain levels, may serve as a marker of peripheral nervous system involvement in those with systemic vasculitis and a marker of disease activity.[32] Vascular endothelial growth factor (VEGF) is a potent cytokine derived from endothelial cells and pericytes in response to hypoxia. As VEGF is activated in response to hypoxia and induces angiogenesis, the hypoxia that occurs due to vascular ischemia may account for the elevated VEGF levels in vasculitic neuropathies.[33]

Nerve Biopsy

Biopsy of a cutaneous sensory nerve, often with accompanying neighboring muscle, is mandatory in all cases of suspected NSVN (except RPN) and in patients with suspected SVN without histopathological confirmation of vasculitis from another organ. In RPN, a biopsy may not be necessary in straightforward cases. In those with atypical features or progressive symptoms, a biopsy demonstrating ongoing active inflammation may change management and should be considered. In the lower extremity, the sural and superficial fibular nerves are most commonly sampled, and in the arm, the superficial radial nerve.[11] When a sensory nerve is biopsied, a whole nerve biopsy rather than a fascicular nerve biopsy is preferred, because the main potential diagnostic findings of vasculitis are in the interstitium. When selecting a nerve to biopsy, it is imperative to select a nerve that is affected based on clinical and/or electrodiagnostic findings. The addition of a muscle biopsy from the same incision site may increase the yield of the nerve biopsy by up to 15% to 25%, resulting in an overall sensitivity of 50% to 60% in some series.[6,11,34]

Histopathological Features

Certain histopathological features may be present in vasculitic neuropathy regardless of the size of the involved vessels. These include multifocal nerve fiber loss with varying degrees of axonal degeneration, hemosiderin-laden macrophages, immune-complex deposition, neovascularization, perivascular inflammation, and fibrinogen in epineurial vessel walls.[2,35–39] Nerve large arteriole vasculitic neuropathy is differentiated from microvasculitis, by size of involved vessels as well as the presence of fibrinoid necrosis of the tunica media and intima (**Figs. 1** and **2**). In the 2010 Peripheral Nerve Society Task Force criteria, inflammatory changes in the microvessels without associated vascular damage or associated ischemic

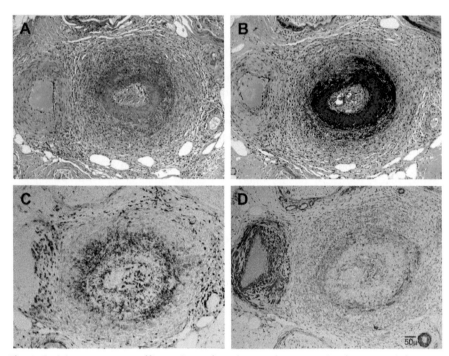

Fig. 1. Serial transverse paraffin sections of sural nerve demonstrating large arteriole necrotizing vasculitis with fibrinoid degeneration. (*A*) The vessel structure is markedly altered with cellular, almost complete occlusion of the lumen; necrosis of the muscle cells of the tunica media; fibrinoid degeneration of the inner portions of the media; and necrosis of the outer tunica media and perivascular inflammation (hematoxylin and eosin). (*B*) Red fibrinoid degeneration (trichrome). Immunohistochemical reactions to (*C*) CD45 (lymphocytes) and (*D*) to smooth muscle actin. These sections illustrate the inflammatory cell involvement in necrotizing vasculitis and the separation, fragmentation, and disappearance of muscle cells.

injury, such as may be seen in microvasculitis, may be considered nonspecific.[2] In general, most of the primary and secondary forms of vasculitis are due to large arteriole necrotizing vasculitis, and cannot be further differentiated based on nerve biopsy findings, whereas most of the nonsystemic forms of vasculitis are due to microvasculitis and also cannot be separated based on pathology. Consequently, from a pathologic perspective, it is often best to separate them into 2 forms: large arteriole vasculitis and microvasculitis.

ETIOLOGIES
Primary Systemic Vasculitic Neuropathies

Polyarteritis nodosa (nerve large arteriole vasculitis)
PAN, a small and medium vessel necrotizing vasculitis, spares the microscopic vessels including the arterioles, venules, or capillaries, which distinguishes it from MPA.[40] The annual incidence of PAN, which affects patients in their fifth and sixth decades, ranges from 0 to 16 per million and prevalence from 2 to 33 per million.[41,42] PAN does not result in glomerulonephritis, a finding common in MPA. Patients with PAN will lack ANCAs and pulmonary involvement, setting it apart from the AAVs.[43] Up to three-quarters of patients will have peripheral neuropathy, which is typically

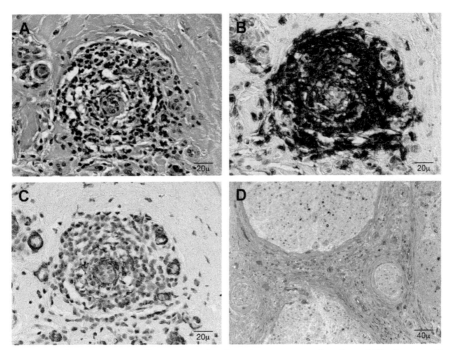

Fig. 2. Serial transverse paraffin sections (*A–C*) and an epoxy section (panel *D*) of a superficial peroneal nerve demonstrating nerve microvasculitis. (*A*) Inflammation involving the vessel walls (hematoxylin and eosin), (*B*) the transmural inflammation is mostly leukocytes (CD45), (*C*) disruption and fragmentation of the vessel walls' muscular layers (smooth muscle actin), (*D*) the nerve fascicles demonstrate multifocal fiber loss and perineurial thickening consistent with ischemic changes (methylene blue).

vasculitic.[41] The skin is the other most commonly affected organ in PAN.[41] Palpable purpura, livedo reticularis and nodules are the most common manifestations.[44] Microaneurysms of the kidneys and mesentery may also occur.[45,46] Subphenotypes of PAN include hepatitis B virus (HBV), hepatitis C virus (HCV), and human immunodeficiency virus (HIV)-associated PAN and will be discussed as secondary systemic vasculitic neuropathies.[47]

Antineutrophil cytoplasmic antibody–associated vasculitis

Microscopic polyangiitis (nerve large arteriole vasculitis) MPA is a small vessel vasculitis that is associated with p-ANCA (MPO-ANCA) in up to 70% of patients and c-ANCA (PR3-ANCA) in 20% to 30%.[48] In contrast to the other AAVs, there is no granuloma formation. The incidence in Europe ranges from 3 to 15 per million and the usual age of onset is 60 to 70 years.[49–51] Half of patients with MPA will develop a vasculitic neuropathy.[13,52,53] Nearly 100% of patients will have renal involvement with rapidly progressive glomerulonephritis.[52] Pulmonary capillaritis resulting in pulmonary hemorrhage is a classic manifestation and is reported in up to 55%.[54,55] Lung involvement overall, and including pulmonary fibrosis, in present in up to 92% of patients.[56,57] The skin is affected in 30% to 60% of patients. most often in the form of palpable purpura.[52,58–60] Nodules, livedo reticularis, ulcers, and urticaria are also encountered.[60] Gastrointestinal involvement is quite rare and is characterized by abdominal pain and gastrointestinal bleeding.[61] Relapses are less common than other AAVs, which raises the question of whether or not long-term immunosuppression is required.[62]

Eosinophilic granulomatosis with polyangiitis (nerve large arteriole vasculitis) EGPA (previously known as Churg-Strauss syndrome) is a rare systemic vasculitis with incidence of 0.5 to 6.8 cases per million per year.[63] It affects younger people, with an average age of onset of 48 to 52 years.[64,65] Asthma, eosinophilia, and granulomatous inflammation distinguish EGPA. The American College of Rheumatology 1990 Criteria requires 4 of 6 of the following: asthma, eosinophilia, allergy, pulmonary infiltrates, extravascular eosinophils, and paranasal sinus abnormalities.[66] Although it is classified as an AAV, most patients are ANCA-negative.[1] Thirty percent to 40% of patients are positive for MPO-ANCA, and PR3-ANCA is infrequently reported. ANCA positivity is associated with more renal and peripheral nerve involvement but less cardiac involvement than ANCA-negative EGPA.[22,31,65,67] There are 3 sequential phases: allergic, eosinophilic, and vasculitic.[68] The allergic phase is associated with allergic rhinitis, sinusitis, and asthma, whereas the eosinophilic phase is characterized by peripheral eosinophilia and eosinophilic tissue infiltration. The systemic vasculitic phase is defined by peripheral neuropathy and cutaneous involvement with palpable purpura and petechiae.[69] Neuropathy occurs in 60% to 70% of patients and cranial neuropathies have been reported.[18,53,65,68,70–72] Cardiac manifestations are highly variable, and may occur in up to 47% of patients and include pericarditis and cardiomyopathy.[22,67,69,72] The kidneys are involved less frequently than in other AAVs. The nerve biopsies show large arteriole necrotizing vasculitis often associated with eosinophilia.

Granulomatosis with polyangiitis (nerve large arteriole vasculitis) The annual incidence of GPA (previously known as Wegner granulomatosis) is 5 to 10 cases per million with the peak incidence between the ages of 45 and 60.[73,74] GPA affects many different organs, such as the skin (including ulcers, livedo reticularis, and palpable purpura),[63] oral ulcers, orbital involvement,[75] sensorineural and conductive hearing loss, nasal involvement (epistaxis, nasal ulceration, sinus inflammation),[76] pulmonary involvement (pulmonary hemorrhage, pulmonary infiltrates, pleural effusions),[77] cardiac involvement (vascular disease, pericarditis, pericardial effusions, cardiomyopathy, valvular disease), peritonitis or bowel ischemia perhaps due to mesenteric vasculitis,[78] and diffuse pauci-immune crescentic necrotizing glomerulonephritis. The disease presents in 2 stages: first localized granulomatous inflammation of the respiratory tracts and then the generalized vasculitis phase with other organ involvement.[13,79] Neuropathy occurs in a minority at approximately 25% of patients[80,81] and cranial neuropathies have been reported.[19,23,82,83] Nearly half of patients with GPA will experience a clinical relapse rate of 50%.[84,85] The nerve biopsies often show large arteriole vasculitis with granuloma involving the blood vessels.

Secondary Systemic Vasculitic Neuropathies

Rheumatoid vasculitis (nerve large arteriole vasculitis)
Rheumatoid vasculitis is typically a complication of long-standing, severe rheumatoid arthritis in seropositive patients with poor control.[86] Given the emergence of biologic therapy, rheumatoid vasculitis has become relatively rare.[87] Despite this, recognition and immediate initiation of treatment for rheumatoid vasculitis is imperative, as it causes significant morbidity and even mortality in up to 25%.[86] Blood vessels of many sizes can be affected, including the small, medium, and large vessels.[87] Men and older patients are at highest risk.[88,89] Coexisting vascular disease and smoking may also increase the risk of rheumatoid vasculitis.[86] Many organ systems may be affected. Ninety percent of patients with rheumatoid vasculitis will have skin changes, including digital ischemia, ulceration, and palpable purpura.[87] The eyes,

gastrointestinal tract, kidneys, lungs, or brain are very rarely affected,[87,88] and the peripheral nervous system is affected in 40%.[87] The 3-dimensional pathologic description of vasculitic neuropathy being caused by infarcts at the watershed zones of vascular territories within nerve was first described in a case of rheumatoid vasculitis.[16]

Sjögren syndrome (nerve large arteriole vasculitis and microvasculitis)

Sjögren syndrome–associated vasculitic neuropathy is quite rare,[90–92] although the overall estimates of peripheral nervous system involvement is likely 5% to 15%.[93] Other forms of polyneuropathies include autonomic neuropathies, small and large fiber sensory neuropathies, and distal sensorimotor polyneuropathies, as well as trigeminal sensory neuropathies. Vasculitic neuropathy is reported in 0% to 5% of cohort studies and is associated with a higher likelihood of extraglandular disease.[93] Patients with Sjögren-associated vasculitic neuropathy should be tested for cryoglobulins.[94] If a patient with Sjögren-associated vasculitis has low complement C4 levels, they are at increased risk of developing non-Hodgkin lymphoma and should be promptly evaluated should any constitutional symptoms develop.[95] The size of the vessel involved in Sjögren vasculitis is often smaller than other systemic vasculidities and can be large arteriole vasculitis or microvasculitis.

Viral infections

Viral polyarteritis nodosa (nerve large arteriole vasculitis) Certain viruses have been clearly associated with vasculitic neuropathies, including HBV, HCV, HIV and parvovirus B19.[96–98] The incidence of HBV-associated PAN is declining due to widespread vaccination. HBV-associated PAN occurs in younger individuals and is more highly associated with orchitis, gastrointestinal involvement, renal infarction, and peripheral neuropathy.[41,47,99] Hepatitis C is less commonly associated with PAN, although has been reported in 7.6% of patients with HCV in one series.[100] Hepatitis C–associated PAN has a higher incidence of constitutional symptoms, polyneuropathy, hypertension, livedo reticularis, and gastrointestinal tract involvement.[101] Hepatitis may be undiagnosed at the time of onset of PAN.

Cryoglobulinemic vasculitis (nerve large arteriole vasculitis) Cryoglobulinemia, especially in the setting of chronic HCV, is associated with vasculitic neuropathy in 65% of patients.[102] Additional systemic features include glomerulonephritis, palpable purpura, skin ulceration, and arthritis. Cryoglobulinemic vasculitis causes complement-dependent immune-complex–mediated inflammation of small blood vessels resulting in tissue ischemia. Although cryoglobulinemic neuropathy is relatively common, one large series of 71 patients identified only 9% of patients had vasculitic neuropathies.[103]

HIV-associated vasculitis (nerve large arteriole vasculitis) HIV-associated vasculitic neuropathy is rare compared with the distal symmetric neuropathy associated with HIV.[104] Histopathologically there is marked inflammatory infiltration of the endoneurium and capillaries.[11] Immune complexes and cytokines enhance HIV replication and ultimately result in vascular injury.[105] HIV causes a PAN-like vasculitis that is unlikely to relapse.[106]

Drug-induced vasculitic neuropathy (nerve large arteriole vasculitis)

Drug-induced vasculitis has been defined as "any case of inflammatory vasculitis in which a specific drug (including toxins) is established as a causal agent of disease when other forms of vasculitis are excluded."[107] Numerous drugs have been associated with vasculitis, including tumor necrosis factor (TNF) inhibitors, cocaine/levamisole, minocycline, and checkpoint inhibitors.[108] On nerve biopsy, patients with TNF inhibitor–associated vasculitic neuropathy will have perivascular epineural inflammation and perivascular inflammation.[109] Discontinuation of the drug typically results in discontinuation of the symptoms.

Cocaine may trigger a form of pseudovasculitis with atypical ANCA patterns.[110,111] Palpable purpura, erosive sinus involvement, and inflammatory arthritis have been reported in addition to vasculitic neuropathy. ANCA positivity may be c-ANCA or p-ANCA.[110] Corticosteroids, methotrexate, co-trimoxazole, and cyclophosphamide have been used for treatment.[110]

Minocycline, an antibiotic commonly used for acne vulgaris, has been reported to cause PAN-like vasculitis. There are several case reports of vasculitic neuropathy, some with skin involvement, in the literature.[112–114] Treatment includes withdrawal of the offending agent and corticosteroids. The time course between the initiation of the minocycline and the onset of the vasculitic neuropathy varies.

Vasculitic neuropathies are emerging as a complication of immune checkpoint inhibitor therapy. These monoclonal antibody cancer drugs that block programmed cell death protein 1 (PD-1), programmed cell death protein-ligand 1 (PDL-1) and cytotoxic T lymphocyte–associated antigen 4 (CTLA-4) have been linked to large and medium vessel vasculitis.[115] Several cases of nivolumab-associated and pembrolizumab-associated vasculitic neuropathy have been reported.[115–117] Discontinuation of the drug and initiation of corticosteroids can result in improvement.[115,116]

Paraneoplastic vasculitic neuropathy (nerve large arteriole vasculitis)

Paraneoplastic vasculitic neuropathy, although reported with numerous types of cancer, including hematologic tumors, thymoma, small cell lung, gastric, colon, and breast cancer, remains the subject of case reports.[118–122] In 2007, Živković and colleagues[27] reported that 6 (15%) of 40 patients with vasculitic neuropathy developed a malignancy within 2 years, suggesting an association. Anti-Hu or serum antineuronal nuclear antigen-2 (ANNA-2) autoantibodies have been reported with these paraneoplastic vasculitic neuropathies.[123] Like other paraneoplastic syndromes, there may be concomitant sensory ataxia and autonomic dysfunction in those with anti-Hu antibodies.

Localized Vasculitis (Nerve Large Arteriole Vasculitis and Microvasculitis)

NSVN is a single-organ vasculitis localized to the peripheral nerves and is likely the most commonly diagnosed vasculitic neuropathy.[3] Although classification is evolving, NSVN likely encompasses the subtypes of Wartenberg migratory sensory neuropathy and postsurgical inflammatory neuropathy, as well as variants including the RPN (DLRPN, LRPN, PDMN, DCRPN) and NA.

Nonsystemic vasculitic neuropathy (nerve large arteriole vasculitis and microvasculitis)

Although in the past NSVN has been clinicopathologically associated with MPA, recent studies by Takahashi and colleagues[124] demonstrate a distinct pathogenesis in NSVN and MPA. In NSVN, C3d deposition is noted in epineurial small vessels, whereas neutrophils attach to vascular endothelial cells in MPA. NSVN contrasts systemic vasculitic neuropathy by its slower progression and nonfatal outcome.[70] Based on pooled data from the 10 largest series of NSVN, the average age of onset is 60 years old with men and women equally affected.[3] Extraneural involvement is absent, although constitutional symptoms such as fever and weight loss occur in a minority.[3] Opposed to the systemic vasculitic neuropathies, most cases of NSVN progress subacutely or chronically. Ten percent, however, will present with acute, rapidly progressive deficits.[15,125–127] Delays in diagnosis of a decade or longer have been reported in most larger series.[14,15,126] Deficits in NSVN are typically distal, although proximal involvement may occur. Although classically NSVN is characterized by an axonal, mixed sensory, and motor polyneuropathy, it is of note that 15% of patients with NSVN will have pure sensory signs and symptoms and 20% will have a painless presentation.[3] Collins and Hadden reviewed 5 NSVN series and found that the most commonly involved peripheral motor nerves, in descending order, are the common fibular (or fibular division of sciatic), tibial (or tibial division of sciatic), ulnar, femoral, superior gluteal, median, radial, axillary, and musculocutaneous.[3,125,126,128,129] Continued monitoring of NSVN is recommended, as up to 10% of patients will evolve to SVN. The vessel size involved in NSVN tends to be smaller than in systemic vasculitis and involves large arterioles and microvessels.

Wartenberg migratory sensory neuropathy (microvasculitis)
Wartenberg migratory sensory neuropathy is a rare, benign sensory subtype of NSVN, which is characterized by chronic, relapsing, multifocal sensory neuropathy.[2] Patients experience loss of sensation, often with neuropathic pain and paresthesia, in cutaneous nerve distributions.[130] Involvement of the trigeminal nerve has also been reported.[130] In some patients, an episode of stretching may precede the sensory complaints. Most patients will have persistent numbness, although deficits may be reversible in a minority.[130,131] Electrodiagnostic studies support low amplitude or absent sensory nerve action potentials of the clinically affected nerves.[132] On nerve biopsy, perivascular inflammatory changes have been described.[130,133] The pathology probably best fits with a microvasculitis.

Postsurgical inflammatory neuropathy
Postsurgical inflammatory neuropathy is a self-limited NSVN subtype that emerges within 30 days of a surgical procedure.[134] The median delay between surgery and symptoms was 2 days in a large series of 21 patients.[135] Patients are identified because of involvement of nerves remote from the surgical sites and continued neurologic worsening in the postoperative period. Proximal lower extremity nerves and the lumbosacral and brachial plexuses are the primary targets. Nerve biopsy demonstrates ischemic injury and perivascular inflammatory collections and findings consistent with microvasculitis.[134,135] Recovery following corticosteroids, with and without additional immunosuppressant therapy, has been reported.[3,134]

Radiculoplexus neuropathies and other nonsystemic vasculitic neuropathy variants
One important group of stereotypically presenting NSVNs are the RPNs that can involve the cervical (CRPN, including NA), thoracic, and lumbosacral (LRPN) levels, either singly or in combination. These conditions can occur in people with and without diabetes mellitus.[136–138] These conditions occur commonly and have diabetes mellitus as a risk factor for developing them and generally have associated weight loss (often substantial). These monophasic disorders have a typical presentation of acute to subacute onset of pain followed by sensory loss and weakness usually beginning focally and then progressing to be more widespread in an extremity with involvement of proximal and distal segments and becomes bilateral in most patients. The PDMN variant differs considerably, as it is painless, relatively symmetric, involves the upper limbs frequently, and is mostly a motor presentation.[139] Both the diabetic and nondiabetic RPN may affect the lumbosacral, thoracic, and cervical regions with variable clinical overlap. Diabetic LRPN is more recognized than the nondiabetic LRPN, but the clinical, laboratory, electrophysiological, and pathologic features are similar.

NA (otherwise known as brachial plexus neuritis, or Parsonage-Turner syndrome) is sporadic or hereditary, affects motor predominant peripheral nerves in the cervical region, and may be considered as a self-limited variant of NSVN.[140] A diabetic cervical RPN has been described that has other associated RPN and more lower trunk involvement than typical NA.[138] Biopsies from diabetic and nondiabetic LRPN, from diabetic cervical RPN, and from PDMN have all shown evidence of ischemic nerve injury (perineurial thickening, injury neuroma, neovascularization, and multifocal fiber loss) and perivascular inflammatory infiltrates and microvasculitis.[136–139,141] Please refer to **Table 1** for the specific clinical features of these NSVN variants.

TREATMENT
Induction Therapy

The treatment approach in vasculitic neuropathies is dictated by the underlying etiology. In general, as neurologists we find it useful to work in conjunction with rheumatologists when caring for patients with necrotizing vasculitis. The neurologists are often better at ascertaining when a symptom represents new ischemic infarcts of nerve and the rheumatologists are better at managing the non-neurological manifestations of vasculitis, cytotoxic drugs, and their complications. Primary systemic vasculitis, if untreated, carries a 1-year mortality rate of nearly 90%.[2,142] Therefore, rapid diagnosis, induction of remission, and continued maintenance therapy for 18 to 24 months is mandatory in this patient population.[143–147] Most treatment evidence is based on disease-specific guidelines. For example, several guidelines exist to direct the treatment of the AAVs, including the European League Against Rheumatism guideline published in 2016,[148] the British Society for Rheumatology guideline published in 2014,[149] and the 2017 clinical practice guidelines of the Japan Research Committee of the Ministry of Health, Labor, and Welfare.[150] The conventional treatment approach for both SVN and NSVN is the initiation of high-dose corticosteroids. Prednisone is started at a dosage of 1.0 mg/kg per day, sometimes preceded by methylprednisolone (1000 mg daily for 3–5 days) and is then slowly tapered over months.[28,151,152] Given the high incidence of adverse effects with corticosteroids, in a recent study, 49 patients with AAV were treated with 2 doses of rituximab, 3 months of low-dose cyclophosphamide, and 1 to 2 weeks of oral glucocorticoids.[153] With this early withdrawal of glucocorticoids, patients had similar outcomes compared with 2 matched historical cohorts, ultimately had less exposure to corticosteroids and cyclophosphamide, less severe infections, and a lower incidence of diabetes.

High-dose corticosteroids are often combined with cyclophosphamide or rituximab for induction of remission in AAV. Pulse cyclophosphamide at a dose of 0.6 to 0.75 g/m^2 every 2 to 4 weeks is associated with fewer side effects than an oral regimen. Rituximab has recently emerged as first-line induction therapy for MPA and GPA vasculitis and can be used instead of cyclophosphamide.[148,149] Two large multicenter randomized controlled trials compared rituximab with cyclophosphamide combined with glucocorticoid therapy for induction therapy of GPA or MPA.[154,155] Rituximab and cyclophosphamide were similar with regard to remission rates and safety profiles. For relapses, rituximab was associated with higher remission rate. In EGPA, corticosteroids remain the mainstay of treatment, and cyclophosphamide is indicated in those with a poor prognosis.[156,157] Similarly, in PAN, corticosteroid monotherapy can be initiated and other steroid-sparing immunosuppressants added depending on response.[45,158] Plasma exchange is recommended as an alternative therapeutic option for patients with fulminant, life-threatening vasculitis.[148,149,159,160] Intravenous immune globulins have been used infrequently for refractory AAV SVN.[161–164] For

Table 1
The nonsystemic vasculitic neuropathy variants

Diagnosis	Clinical Presentation	Diagnostic Evaluation	Treatment	Prognosis
Diabetic lumbosacral radiculoplexus neuropathy (ie, Bruns Garland syndrome, diabetic amyotrophy, proximal diabetic neuropathy)	Subacute onset of asymmetrical, painful neuropathy with focal involvement of leg and thigh. Concomitant autonomic dysfunction and weight loss common. Concomitant thoracic and cervical radiculoplexus neuropathies may occur.	Laboratory studies: rare elevation of ESR, CRP, ANA, ENA, RF, or other markers of autoimmunity. Elevated fasting glucose, glycosylated hemoglobin expected. Elevated CSF protein. Electrodiagnostic studies: reduced CMAP and SNAP amplitudes in the leg, reduced recruitment of high amplitude, long duration MUPs in multiple muscles belonging to different lumbosacral myotomes. Paraspinal muscles typically involved. Quantitative sensory testing abnormal. MRI may demonstrate increased T2 signal in the plexus and roots, enlargement and contrast enhancement. Biopsy demonstrates ischemic injury and microvasculitis.	Likely a role for IVIg and IVMP early in the course of the disease or in the presence of progression. Neuropathic pain control. Bracing. Physical therapy.	Monophasic, with very gradual, often incomplete, recovery over months to years.

(continued on next page)

Table 1
(continued)

Diagnosis	Clinical Presentation	Diagnostic Evaluation	Treatment	Prognosis
Diabetic thoracic radiculopathy	Gradual, intermittent onset of severe neuropathic trunk pain with associated sensory deficits. Abdominal/thoracic muscle weakness. Anterior trunk typically involved, multiple dermatomes may be affected. Concomitant weight loss reported.	Electrodiagnostic studies: abnormal EMG of paraspinal muscles. Abdominal and intercostal muscle EMG abnormal in the same distribution as the symptoms.	Neuropathic pain control.	Spontaneous remission in most.
Diabetic cervical radiculoplexus neuropathy	Acute onset of unilateral arm pain followed by or simultaneously with weakness and sensory complaints. Commonly bilateral upper extremity with lower trunk involvement. Concomitant autonomic dysfunction and weight loss common.	Laboratory studies: rare elevation of ESR, CRP, ANA, ENA, RF, or other markers of autoimmunity. Elevated CSF protein. Electrodiagnostic studies: reduced CMAP and SNAP amplitudes in the arm, reduced recruitment of high amplitude, long duration MUPs in multiple muscles belonging to different cervical myotomes, often supporting pan-plexus involvement. Paraspinal muscles typically involved. Quantitative sensory testing abnormal. MRI may demonstrate increased T2 signal in the plexus, enlargement and contrast enhancement. Biopsy demonstrates ischemic injury and microvasculitis.	Potentially a role for IVIg and IVMP early in the course of the disease or in the presence of progression. Neuropathic pain control. Physical therapy.	Monophasic, with very gradual, often incomplete, recovery over months to years.

Painless diabetic motor neuropathy	Subacute onset of bilateral symmetric foot drop that progresses to proximal lower extremity. Lesser upper extremity involvement. Numbness and paresthesia common. Concomitant autonomic dysfunction and weight loss common.	Laboratory studies: rare elevation of ESR, CRP, ANA, ENA, RF, or other markers of autoimmunity. Elevated CSF protein. Electrodiagnostic studies: diminished CMAP and SNAP amplitudes in the leg, reduced recruitment of high amplitude, long duration MUPs in multiple muscles belonging to different lumbosacral myotomes, often supporting pan-plexus involvement. Paraspinal muscles typically involved. Quantitative sensory testing abnormal. Biopsy demonstrates ischemic injury and microvasculitis.	Likely a role for IVIg, IVMP, or TPE early in the course of the disease or in the presence of progression. Bracing. Physical therapy.	Monophasic, with very gradual, often incomplete, recovery over months to years.
Nonsystemic vasculitic neuropathy with proximal involvement (or nondiabetic lumbosacral radiculoplexus neuropathy)	Subacute onset of asymmetrical, painful neuropathy with focal involvement leg and thigh. Concomitant autonomic dysfunction and weight loss common. Concomitant thoracic and cervical radiculoplexus neuropathies may occur.	Laboratory studies: rare elevation of ESR, CRP, ANA, ENA, RF, or other markers of autoimmunity. Electrodiagnostic studies: reduced CMAP and SNAP amplitudes in the leg, reduced recruitment of high amplitude, long duration MUPs in multiple muscles belonging to different lumbosacral myotomes. Paraspinal muscles typically involved. Quantitative sensory testing abnormal. MRI may demonstrate increased T2 signal in the plexus and roots, enlargement and contrast enhancement. Biopsy demonstrates ischemic injury and microvasculitis.	Likely a role for IVIg and IVMP early in the course of the disease or in the presence of progression. Neuropathic pain control. Bracing.	Monophasic, with very gradual, often incomplete, recovery over months to years.

(continued on next page)

Table 1
(continued)

Diagnosis	Clinical Presentation	Diagnostic Evaluation	Treatment	Prognosis
Neuralgic amyotrophy (ie, Parsonage-Turner syndrome, brachial plexus neuritis)	Acute onset of typically unilateral upper extremity pain followed by weakness and atrophy. Often deficits concentrated in the upper brachial plexus, with extraplexal nerves affected including phrenic, recurrent laryngeal, and lumbosacral plexus. Sensory symptoms common. Concomitant autonomic dysfunction and weight loss in a minority. Sensory symptoms common. May recur, especially if hereditary.	Laboratory Studies: SEPT9 mutation testing if hereditary form suspected. Other laboratory studies typically normal. Elevated LFTs reported in a minority. Electrodiagnostic studies: diminished CMAP and SNAP amplitudes in the arm, reduced recruitment of high amplitude, long duration MUPs in multiple muscles belonging to different cervical myotomes, though abnormalities may be concentrated in the upper portion of the plexus. MRI brachial plexus may be obtained to exclude alternative diagnoses. May demonstrate increased T2 signal change in the plexus/motor nerves, enlargement and contrast enhancement. Biopsy typically not indicated.	Likely a role for corticosteroids early in the course of the disease. Neuropathic pain control. Physical therapy.	Monophasic, with very gradual, often incomplete, recovery over months to years.

Abbreviations: ANA, antinuclear antibodies; CMAP, compound motor action potential; CRP, C-reactive protein; CSF, cerebrospinal fluid; EMG, electromyography; ENA, extractable nuclear antigen; ESR, erythrocyte sedimentation rate; IVIg, intravenous immune globulins; IVMP, intravenous methylprednisolone; LFTs, liver function tests; MUP, motor unit potential; RF, rheumatoid factor; SNAP, sensory nerve action potential; TPE, therapeutic plasma exchange.

refractory PAN, infliximab has been reported to be helpful.[165,166] Mepolizumab, an anti–interleukin-5 monoclonal antibody, has recently been demonstrated in a large, double-blind, parallel-group, phase 3 trial to induce remission in EGPA and allow tapering of corticosteroids.[167]

NSVN, although typically not fatal, also requires urgent initiation of treatment to prevent the development of permanent deficits. Much of the treatment approach is inferred from the SVN literature given the paucity of high-quality treatment evidence.[3] Often the treatment approach is less aggressive given the nonsystemic nature of the disease. However, 2 retrospective cohort studies demonstrated that corticosteroids with a steroid-sparing immunosuppressant (cyclophosphamide, azathioprine, or methotrexate) are likely superior to corticosteroid monotherapy.[126,127] It is suspected that those who receive combination therapy from the outset may have fewer relapses and long-term sequelae. There is also some evidence to support that cyclophosphamide is superior to azathioprine for induction therapy.[3,15] NSVN experts have recently recommended that combination induction therapy be standard and that rituximab may be considered as a first-line alternative to cyclophosphamide for induction therapy.[3]

An exception in the management of NSVN is in cases of known monophasic microvasculitic processes (eg, DLRPN). In such cases, when presentation and clinical course is typical, long-term immunosuppression is not warranted. Short-term treatment with corticosteroids, such as intravenous (IV) methylprednisolone or IV immune globulins, without the additional use of oral steroid-sparing agents, is a common course of management in these patients, with some evidence for clinical improvement for improvements in DLRPN.[168–170] A large clinical trial of patients with DLRPN did not show a significant difference in the time to improve the lower limb neuropathy impairment score between treated and untreated patients, but did show some improvement in positive sensory symptoms and pain measures in the treated group.[171] There is still controversy in the literature regarding how significant the impact of immunotherapy is in these patients, particularly given the monophasic nature and partial recovery eventually typically experienced even without immunotherapy given.[172] It is the opinion of the authors that given the clear evidence of a microvasculitic etiology, the lack of significant response reported to immunotherapy in some patients may be due to a delay in onset of diagnosis and treatment in a monophasic illness and in general we favor treating these patients, usually with pulsed IV corticosteroids (often 1 g methylprednisolone weekly) for a 12-week course.

Maintenance Therapy

Methotrexate, occasionally used also for induction therapy in mild AAV SVN and NSVN, has been demonstrated to be noninferior to cyclophosphamide for remission maintenance in AAV.[28,173] It is typically given at a dosage of 20 to 25 mg/wk. Azathioprine, dosed at 1 to 2 mg/kg per day, has also been used for maintenance therapy.[174] The role of mycophenolate mofetil in the treatment of vasculitis is still under debate.[157] Rituximab also may be used as maintenance therapy.[175]

Treatment of Viral Vasculitis

Hepatitis C virus

The landscape of hepatitis C treatment has evolved rapidly in the past several years. Interferon therapy is less often used, and direct-acting antiviral agents (DAAs) directed against HCV have emerged. HCV has the following structural proteins, including core protein, envelope proteins (E1 and E2), and nonstructural proteins, such as NS2, NS3,

NS4A, NS4B, NS5A, and NS5B as well as P7.[176] Second-generation NS3/4A protease inhibitors, and NS5A and NS5B inhibitors are on the market and are highly effective in the treatment of HCV.[177] In HCV-associated cryoglobulinemic vasculitis, the DAAs have been less effective.[178] Rituximab has been especially beneficial in this patient population.[178–183] Plasma exchange, which removes circulating cryoglobulins, is recommended as an urgent treatment for patients with severe cryoglobulinemic vasculitis, especially with renal impairment.[184] Treatment of HCV-PAN requires the use of antiviral therapy. If severe, immunosuppressive therapy, such as corticosteroids, cyclophosphamide, or rituximab are used.[101]

Hepatitis B virus

In patients with mild PAN and HBV, antivirals (lamivudine or interferon alpha) should be used as first-line treatment. Some patients with moderate to severe PAN with HBV benefit from a short course of steroids and plasma exchange until the antiviral therapy is effective.[185] Prolonged corticosteroid treatment is not recommended, as it results in viral persistence and replication.[186] The French Vasculitis Study Group has a treatment protocol that recommends antiviral agents and plasma exchange, followed by 2 weeks of corticosteroids, which results in complete remission in 80% to 90% of patients.[97,187]

Assessing Treatment Response

Treatment response may be monitored in a variety of ways, including with the physical examination, electrodiagnostic studies, and specific instruments such as the neuropathy impairment score. The revised Five-Factor Score can assist with prognostication and treatment decision making in the primary systemic vasculitides.[156,188] Four factors: renal insufficiency, cardiomyopathy, gastrointestinal manifestations, and age older than 65, if present are allocated 1 point. The fifth factor, ear, nose or throat involvement, only used for EGPA and GPA, is protective if absent (allocated on point). Five-year mortality rates for scores of 0, 1, and >/2 are 9%, 21%, and 40%, respectively. Treatment should be escalated depending on patient response and if additional neurologic deficits develop. As most vasculitic neuropathies are extremely painful, aggressive management of pain should be a cornerstone of any treatment regimen. Many different types of neuropathic pain medications are used, including tricyclic antidepressants, gabapentin, pregabalin, duloxetine, venlafaxine, carbamazepine, tramadol, topical lidocaine, topical capsaicin, and narcotics, with the choice depending on multiple factors including coexisting organ system dysfunction, cost, efficacy, refractoriness to treatment, side effects, and concern for tolerance and addictive potential.

SUMMARY

Vasculitic neuropathy is easily divided into 2 main categories: systemic peripheral nerve vasculitis (both primary and secondary to connective tissue disorders) and nonsystemic peripheral nerve vasculitis. Systemic vasculitis is more likely to involve large arterioles, whereas nonsystemic vasculitis is more likely to involve microvessels. Prompt diagnosis of vasculitic neuropathy and immediate initiation of treatment is mandatory to prevent permanent neurologic deficits, significant morbidity, and even death. All neurologists and rheumatologists should be able to recognize the characteristic clinical pattern of painful multifocal neuropathy or asymmetric length-dependent neuropathy, consider the diagnosis, and begin the diagnostic evaluation. An understanding of the potential underlying etiologies will result in monitoring for extraneural involvement and disease-specific therapy. NSVN and its variants, mostly exemplified by histopathological evidence of microvasculitis, carry a more benign prognosis, although recognition and appropriate treatment remain important.

REFERENCES

1. Jennette JC, Falk RJ, Bacon PA, et al. 2012 revised International Chapel Hill Consensus Conference Nomenclature of Vasculitides. Arthritis Rheum 2013; 65(1):1–11.

2. Collins MP, Dyck PJB, Gronseth GS, et al. Peripheral Nerve Society Guideline on the classification, diagnosis, investigation, and immunosuppressive therapy of non-systemic vasculitic neuropathy: executive summary. J Peripher Nerv Syst 2010;15(3):176–84.

3. Collins MP, Hadden RD. The nonsystemic vasculitic neuropathies. Nat Rev Neurol 2017;13(5):302–16.

4. Sugiura M, Koike H, Iijima M, et al. Clinicopathologic features of nonsystemic vasculitic neuropathy and microscopic polyangiitis-associated neuropathy: a comparative study. J Neurol Sci 2006;241(1–2):31–7.

5. Kararizou E, Davaki P, Karandreas N, et al. Nonsystemic vasculitic neuropathy: a clinicopathological study of 22 cases. J Rheumatol 2005;32(5):853–8. Available at: http://www.ncbi.nlm.nih.gov/pubmed/15868621. Accessed April 30, 2013.

6. Vital C, Vital A, Canron M-H, et al. Combined nerve and muscle biopsy in the diagnosis of vasculitic neuropathy. A 16-year retrospective study of 202 cases. J Peripher Nerv Syst 2006;11(1):20–9.

7. de Luna G, Chauveau D, Aniort J, et al. Plasma exchanges for the treatment of severe systemic necrotizing vasculitides in clinical daily practice: Data from the French Vasculitis Study Group. J Autoimmun 2015;65:49–55.

8. Hadden RDM, Collins MP, Živković SA, et al. Vasculitic peripheral neuropathy: case definition and guidelines for collection, analysis, and presentation of immunisation safety data. Vaccine 2017;35(11):1567–78.

9. Schaublin GA, Michet CJ, Dyck PJB, et al. An update on the classification and treatment of vasculitic neuropathy. Lancet Neurol 2005;4(12):853–65.

10. Kissel JT, Mendell JR. Vasculitic neuropathy. Neurol Clin 1992;10(3):761–81. Available at: http://www.ncbi.nlm.nih.gov/pubmed/1323752. Accessed April 7, 2013.

11. Said G, Lacroix C. Primary and secondary vasculitic neuropathy. J Neurol 2005; 252(6):633–41.

12. Lacomis D, Zivković SA. Approach to vasculitic neuropathies. J Clin Neuromuscul Dis 2007;9(1):265–76.

13. Collins MP, Arnold WD, Kissel JT. The neuropathies of vasculitis. Neurol Clin 2013;31(2):557–95.

14. Cassereau J, Baguenier-Desormeaux C, Letournel F, et al. Necrotizing vasculitis revealed in a case of multiple mononeuropathy after a 14-year course of spontaneous remissions and relapses. Clin Neurol Neurosurg 2012;114(3):290–3.

15. Üçeyler N, Geng A, Reiners K, et al. Non-systemic vasculitic neuropathy: single-center follow-up of 60 patients. J Neurol 2015;262(9):2092–100.

16. Dyck PJ, Conn DL, Okazaki H. Necrotizing angiopathic neuropathy. Three-dimensional morphology of fiber degeneration related to sites of occluded vessels. Mayo Clin Proc 1972;47(7):461–75. Available at: http://www.ncbi.nlm.nih.gov/pubmed/4402730. Accessed April 7, 2013.

17. Collins M, Kissel JT. Vasculitic neuropathies and neuropathies of connective tissue diseases. In: Katirji B, Kaminski HJ, Ruff RL, et al, editors. Neuromuscular disorders in clinical practice. 2nd edition. New York: Springer; 2014. p. 733–85.
18. André R, Cottin V, Saraux J-L, et al. Central nervous system involvement in eosinophilic granulomatosis with polyangiitis (Churg-Strauss): report of 26 patients and review of the literature. Autoimmun Rev 2017;16(9):963–9.
19. Lee E, Park J, Choi SH, et al. Seronegative granulomatosis with polyangiitis presenting with multiple cranial nerve palsies. Neuropathology 2017. https://doi.org/10.1111/neup.12437.
20. Kim S-H, Park J, Bae JH, et al. ANCA-negative Wegener's granulomatosis with multiple lower cranial nerve palsies. J Korean Med Sci 2013;28(11):1690–6.
21. Kim JY, Kim DS, Ku BD, et al. A case of nonsystemic vasculitic neuropathy presenting with multiple cranial neuropathies. Neurol India 2012;60(6):653–5.
22. Comarmond C, Pagnoux C, Khellaf M, et al. Eosinophilic granulomatosis with polyangiitis (Churg-Strauss): clinical characteristics and long-term followup of the 383 patients enrolled in the French Vasculitis Study Group cohort. Arthritis Rheum 2013;65(1):270–81.
23. Nishino H, Rubino FA, DeRemee RA, et al. Neurological involvement in Wegener's granulomatosis: an analysis of 324 consecutive patients at the Mayo Clinic. Ann Neurol 1993;33(1):4–9.
24. Guillevin L, Le Thi Huong DU, Godeau P, et al. Clinical findings and prognosis of polyarteritis nodosa and Churg-Strauss angiitis: a study in 165 patients. Br J Rheumatol 1988;27(4):258–64. Available at: http://www.ncbi.nlm.nih.gov/pubmed/2900659. Accessed April 7, 2013.
25. McCluskey L, Feinberg D, Cantor C, et al. "Pseudo-conduction block" in vasculitic neuropathy. Muscle Nerve 1999;22(10):1361–6. Available at: http://www.ncbi.nlm.nih.gov/pubmed/10487901.
26. Sandbrink F, Klion AD, Floeter MK. "Pseudo-conduction block" in a patient with vasculitic neuropathy. Electromyogr Clin Neurophysiol 2001;41(4):195–202. Available at: http://www.ncbi.nlm.nih.gov/pubmed/11441636.
27. Zivković SA, Ascherman D, Lacomis D. Vasculitic neuropathy–electrodiagnostic findings and association with malignancies. Acta Neurol Scand 2007;115(6):432–6.
28. Burns TM, Schaublin GA, Dyck PJB. Vasculitic neuropathies. Neurol Clin 2007;25(1):89–113.
29. Savige J, Gillis D, Benson E, et al. International consensus statement on testing and reporting of antineutrophil cytoplasmic antibodies (ANCA). Am J Clin Pathol 1999;111(4):507–13. Available at: http://www.ncbi.nlm.nih.gov/pubmed/10191771.
30. Csernok E, Holle JU. Twenty-eight years with antineutrophil cytoplasmic antibodies (ANCA): how to test for ANCA—evidence-based immunology? Auto Immun Highlights 2010;1(1):39–43.
31. Weiner M, Segelmark M. The clinical presentation and therapy of diseases related to anti-neutrophil cytoplasmic antibodies (ANCA). Autoimmun Rev 2016;15(10):978–82.
32. Bischof A, Manigold T, Barro C, et al. Serum neurofilament light chain: a biomarker of neuronal injury in vasculitic neuropathy. Ann Rheum Dis 2017. https://doi.org/10.1136/annrheumdis-2017-212045.
33. Sakai K, Komai K, Yanase D, et al. Plasma VEGF as a marker for the diagnosis and treatment of vasculitic neuropathy. J Neurol Neurosurg Psychiatry 2005;76(2):296.
34. Vrancken AFJE, Gathier CS, Cats EA, et al. The additional yield of combined nerve/muscle biopsy in vasculitic neuropathy. Eur J Neurol 2011;18(1):49–58.

35. Tracy JA, Engelstad JK, Dyck PJB. Microvasculitis in diabetic lumbosacral radiculoplexus neuropathy. J Clin Neuromuscul Dis 2009;11(1):44–8.
36. Nukada H, Dyck PJ. Microsphere embolization of nerve capillaries and fiber degeneration. Am J Pathol 1984;115(2):275–87. Available at: http://www.pubmedcentral. nih.gov/articlerender.fcgi?artid=1900501&tool=pmcentrez&rendertype=abstract. Accessed March 20, 2013.
37. Nukada H, Dyck PJ, Karnes JL. Spatial distribution of capillaries in rat nerves: correlation to ischemic damage. Exp Neurol 1985;87(2):369–76. Available at: http://www.ncbi.nlm.nih.gov/pubmed/3967721. Accessed April 7, 2013.
38. Benstead TJ, Dyck PJ, Sangalang V. Inner perineurial cell vulnerability in ischemia. Brain Res 1989;489(1):177–81. Available at: http://www.ncbi.nlm. nih.gov/pubmed/2743147. Accessed April 7, 2013.
39. Collins MP, Periquet-Collins I, Sahenk Z, et al. Direct immunofluorescence in vasculitic neuropathy: specificity of vascular immune deposits. Muscle Nerve 2010;42(1):62–9.
40. Karadag O, Jayne DJ. Polyarteritis nodosa revisited: a review of historical approaches, subphenotypes and a research agenda. Clin Exp Rheumatol 2018; 36. Suppl 111(2):135–42. Available at: http://www.ncbi.nlm.nih.gov/pubmed/ 29465365.
41. Pagnoux C, Seror R, Henegar C, et al. Clinical features and outcomes in 348 patients with polyarteritis nodosa: a systematic retrospective study of patients diagnosed between 1963 and 2005 and entered into the French Vasculitis Study Group Database. Arthritis Rheum 2010;62(2):616–26.
42. de Menthon M, Mahr A. Treating polyarteritis nodosa: current state of the art. Clin Exp Rheumatol 2011;29(1 Suppl 64):S110–6. Available at: http://www. ncbi.nlm.nih.gov/pubmed/21586205.
43. Wu W, Chaer RA. Nonarteriosclerotic vascular disease. Surg Clin North Am 2013;93(4):833–75, viii.
44. Chasset F, Francès C. Cutaneous manifestations of medium- and large-vessel vasculitis. Clin Rev Allergy Immunol 2017;53(3):452–68.
45. Forbess L, Bannykh S. Polyarteritis nodosa. Rheum Dis Clin North Am 2015; 41(1):33–46, vii.
46. Stone JH. Polyarteritis nodosa. JAMA 2002;288(13):1632–9. Available at: http:// www.ncbi.nlm.nih.gov/pubmed/12350194. Accessed April 7, 2013.
47. Guillevin L. Infections in vasculitis. Best Pract Res Clin Rheumatol 2013;27(1): 19–31.
48. Wiik AS. Autoantibodies in ANCA-associated vasculitis. Rheum Dis Clin North Am 2010;36(3):479–89.
49. Ntatsaki E, Watts RA, Scott DGI. Epidemiology of ANCA-associated vasculitis. Rheum Dis Clin North Am 2010;36(3):447–61.
50. Mahr AD. Epidemiological features of Wegener's granulomatosis and microscopic polyangiitis: two diseases or one "anti-neutrophil cytoplasm antibodies-associated vasculitis" entity? APMIS Suppl 2009;117(127):41–7.
51. Mohammad AJ, Jacobsson LTH, Westman KWA, et al. Incidence and survival rates in Wegener's granulomatosis, microscopic polyangiitis, Churg-Strauss syndrome and polyarteritis nodosa. Rheumatology (Oxford) 2009;48(12): 1560–5.
52. Guillevin L, Durand-Gasselin B, Cevallos R, et al. Microscopic polyangiitis: clinical and laboratory findings in eighty-five patients. Arthritis Rheum 1999;42(3): 421–30.

53. Cattaneo L, Chierici E, Pavone L, et al. Peripheral neuropathy in Wegener's granulomatosis, Churg-Strauss syndrome and microscopic polyangiitis. J Neurol Neurosurg Psychiatry 2007;78(10):1119–23.

54. Lauque D, Cadranel J, Lazor R, et al. Microscopic polyangiitis with alveolar hemorrhage. A study of 29 cases and review of the literature. Groupe d'Etudes et de Recherche sur les Maladies "Orphelines" Pulmonaires (GERM"O"P). Medicine (Baltimore) 2000;79(4):222–33. Available at: http://www.ncbi.nlm.nih.gov/pubmed/10941351.

55. Collins CE, Quismorio FP. Pulmonary involvement in microscopic polyangiitis. Curr Opin Pulm Med 2005;11(5):447–51. Available at: http://www.ncbi.nlm.nih.gov/pubmed/16093820.

56. Chung SA, Seo P. Microscopic polyangiitis. Rheum Dis Clin North Am 2010; 36(3):545–58.

57. Wilke L, Prince-Fiocco M, Fiocco GP. Microscopic polyangiitis: a large single-center series. J Clin Rheumatol 2014;20(4):179–82.

58. Savage CO, Winearls CG, Evans DJ, et al. Microscopic polyarteritis: presentation, pathology and prognosis. Q J Med 1985;56(220):467–83. Available at: http://www.ncbi.nlm.nih.gov/pubmed/4048389.

59. Lhote F, Cohen P, Guillevin L. Polyarteritis nodosa, microscopic polyangiitis and Churg-Strauss syndrome. Lupus 1998;7(4):238–58.

60. Kluger N, Pagnoux C, Guillevin L, et al, French Vasculitis Study Group. Comparison of cutaneous manifestations in systemic polyarteritis nodosa and microscopic polyangiitis. Br J Dermatol 2008;159(3):615–20.

61. Eriksson P, Segelmark M, Hallböök O. Frequency, diagnosis, treatment, and outcome of gastrointestinal disease in granulomatosis with polyangiitis and microscopic polyangiitis. J Rheumatol 2018;45(4):529–37.

62. de Lind van Wijngaarden RAF, van Rijn L, Hagen EC, et al. Hypotheses on the etiology of antineutrophil cytoplasmic autoantibody associated vasculitis: the cause is hidden, but the result is known. Clin J Am Soc Nephrol 2008;3(1): 237–52.

63. Marzano AV, Raimondo MG, Berti E, et al. Cutaneous manifestations of ANCA-associated small vessels vasculitis. Clin Rev Allergy Immunol 2017;53(3): 428–38.

64. Keogh KA, Specks U. Churg-Strauss syndrome: clinical presentation, antineutrophil cytoplasmic antibodies, and leukotriene receptor antagonists. Am J Med 2003;115(4):284–90. Available at: http://www.ncbi.nlm.nih.gov/pubmed/12967693. Accessed August 23, 2013.

65. Sinico RA, Di Toma L, Maggiore U, et al. Prevalence and clinical significance of antineutrophil cytoplasmic antibodies in Churg-Strauss syndrome. Arthritis Rheum 2005;52(9):2926–35.

66. Masi AT, Hunder GG, Lie JT, et al. The American College of Rheumatology 1990 criteria for the classification of Churg-Strauss syndrome (allergic granulomatosis and angiitis). Arthritis Rheum 1990;33(8):1094–100. Available at: http://www.ncbi.nlm.nih.gov/pubmed/2202307. Accessed April 7, 2013.

67. Sablé-Fourtassou R, Cohen P, Mahr A, et al. Antineutrophil cytoplasmic antibodies and the Churg-Strauss syndrome. Ann Intern Med 2005;143(9):632–8. Available at: http://www.ncbi.nlm.nih.gov/pubmed/16263885.

68. Lanham JG, Elkon KB, Pusey CD, et al. Systemic vasculitis with asthma and eosinophilia: a clinical approach to the Churg-Strauss syndrome. Medicine (Baltimore) 1984;63(2):65–81. Available at: http://www.ncbi.nlm.nih.gov/pubmed/6366453. Accessed August 23, 2013.

69. Wu EY, Hernandez ML, Jennette JC, et al. Eosinophilic granulomatosis with polyangiitis: clinical pathology conference and review. J Allergy Clin Immunol Pract 2018;6(5):1496–504.

70. Collins MP, Periquet MI. Isolated vasculitis of the peripheral nervous system. Clin Exp Rheumatol 2008;26(3 Suppl 49):S118–30. Available at: http://www.ncbi.nlm.nih.gov/pubmed/18799069. Accessed April 30, 2013.

71. Vinit J, Muller G, Bielefeld P, et al. Churg-Strauss syndrome: retrospective study in Burgundian population in France in past 10 years. Rheumatol Int 2011;31(5):587–93.

72. Moosig F, Bremer JP, Hellmich B, et al. A vasculitis centre based management strategy leads to improved outcome in eosinophilic granulomatosis and polyangiitis (Churg-Strauss, EGPA): monocentric experiences in 150 patients. Ann Rheum Dis 2012;1–7. https://doi.org/10.1136/annrheumdis-2012-201531.

73. Scott DG, Watts RA. Systemic vasculitis: epidemiology, classification and environmental factors. Ann Rheum Dis 2000;59(3):161–3. Available at: http://www.ncbi.nlm.nih.gov/pubmed/10700420.

74. Comarmond C, Cacoub P. Granulomatosis with polyangiitis (Wegener): clinical aspects and treatment. Autoimmun Rev 2014;13(11):1121–5.

75. Tarabishy AB, Schulte M, Papaliodis GN, et al. Wegener's granulomatosis: clinical manifestations, differential diagnosis, and management of ocular and systemic disease. Surv Ophthalmol 2010;55(5):429–44.

76. Seo P, Stone JH. The antineutrophil cytoplasmic antibody-associated vasculitides. Am J Med 2004;117(1):39–50.

77. Gómez-Puerta JA, Hernández-Rodríguez J, López-Soto A, et al. Antineutrophil cytoplasmic antibody-associated vasculitides and respiratory disease. Chest 2009;136(4):1101–11.

78. Pagnoux C, Mahr A, Cohen P, et al. Presentation and outcome of gastrointestinal involvement in systemic necrotizing vasculitides: analysis of 62 patients with polyarteritis nodosa, microscopic polyangiitis, Wegener granulomatosis, Churg-Strauss syndrome, or rheumatoid arthritis-associated. Medicine (Baltimore) 2005;84(2):115–28. Available at: http://www.ncbi.nlm.nih.gov/pubmed/15758841.

79. Holle JU, Laudien M, Gross WL. Clinical manifestations and treatment of Wegener's granulomatosis. Rheum Dis Clin North Am 2010;36(3):507–26. https://doi.org/10.1016/j.rdc.2010.05.008.

80. Collins MP, Periquet MI. Prevalence of vasculitic neuropathy in Wegener granulomatosis. Arch Neurol 2002;59(8):1333–4 [author reply: 1334]. Available at: http://www.ncbi.nlm.nih.gov/pubmed/12164733. Accessed May 4, 2013.

81. Gwathmey KG, Burns TM, Collins MP, et al. Vasculitic neuropathies. Lancet Neurol 2014;13(1):67–82.

82. Zhang W, Zhou G, Shi Q, et al. Clinical analysis of nervous system involvement in ANCA-associated systemic vasculitides. Clin Exp Rheumatol 2009;27(1 Suppl 52):S65–9. Available at: http://www.ncbi.nlm.nih.gov/pubmed/19646349. Accessed April 7, 2013.

83. Suppiah R, Hadden RDM, Batra R, et al. Peripheral neuropathy in ANCA-associated vasculitis: outcomes from the European Vasculitis Study Group trials. Rheumatology (Oxford) 2011;50(12):2214–22.

84. Hoffman GS, Kerr GS, Leavitt RY, et al. Wegener granulomatosis: an analysis of 158 patients. Ann Intern Med 1992;116(6):488–98. Available at: http://www.ncbi.nlm.nih.gov/pubmed/1739240. Accessed August 23, 2013.

85. Holle JU, Gross WL, Latza U, et al. Improved outcome in 445 patients with We-gener's granulomatosis in a German vasculitis center over four decades. Arthritis Rheum 2011;63(1):257–66.

86. Makol A, Crowson CS, Wetter DA, et al. Vasculitis associated with rheumatoid arthritis: a case-control study. Rheumatology (Oxford) 2014;53(5):890–9.

87. Kishore S, Maher L, Majithia V. Rheumatoid vasculitis: a diminishing yet devas-tating menace. Curr Rheumatol Rep 2017;19(7):39.

88. Scott DG, Bacon PA, Tribe CR. Systemic rheumatoid vasculitis: a clinical and laboratory study of 50 cases. Medicine (Baltimore) 1981;60(4):288–97. Available at: http://journals.lww.com/md-journal/Abstract/1981/07000/Systemic_Rheumatoid_Vasculitis__A_Clinical_and.4.aspx. Accessed April 8, 2013.

89. Watts RA, Scott DGI. Vasculitis and inflammatory arthritis. Best Pract Res Clin Rheumatol 2016;30(5):916–31.

90. Grant IA, Hunder GG, Homburger HA, et al. Peripheral neuropathy associated with sicca complex. Neurology 1997;48(4):855–62. Available at: http://www.ncbi.nlm.nih.gov/pubmed/9109867. Accessed November 5, 2014.

91. Mori K, Iijima M, Koike H, et al. The wide spectrum of clinical manifestations in Sjögren's syndrome-associated neuropathy. Brain 2005;128(Pt 11):2518–34.

92. Delalande S, de Seze J, Fauchais A-L, et al. Neurologic manifestations in pri-mary Sjögren syndrome: a study of 82 patients. Medicine (Baltimore) 2004; 83(5):280–91. Available at: http://www.ncbi.nlm.nih.gov/pubmed/15342972. Ac-cessed November 5, 2014.

93. Birnbaum J. Peripheral nervous system manifestations of Sjögren syndrome: clinical patterns, diagnostic paradigms, etiopathogenesis, and therapeutic stra-tegies. Neurologist 2010;16(5):287–97.

94. Quartuccio L, Baldini C, Priori R, et al. Cryoglobulinemia in Sjögren syndrome: a disease subset that links higher systemic disease activity, autoimmunity, and local B cell proliferation in mucosa-associated lymphoid tissue. J Rheumatol 2017;44(8):1179–83.

95. Baimpa E, Dahabreh IJ, Voulgarelis M, et al. Hematologic manifestations and predictors of lymphoma development in primary Sjögren syndrome: clinical and pathophysiologic aspects. Medicine (Baltimore) 2009;88(5):284–93.

96. Lenglet T, Haroche J, Schnuriger A, et al. Mononeuropathy multiplex associated with acute parvovirus B19 infection: characteristics, treatment and outcome. J Neurol 2011;258(7):1321–6.

97. Pagnoux C, Cohen P, Guillevin L. Vasculitides secondary to infections. Clin Exp Rheumatol 2006;2(Suppl 41):S71–81.

98. Lidar M, Lipschitz N, Langevitz P, et al. The infectious etiology of vasculitis. Autoimmunity 2009;42(5):432–8. Available at: http://www.ncbi.nlm.nih.gov/pubmed/19811260. Accessed August 26, 2013.

99. Cacoub P, Terrier B. Hepatitis B-related autoimmune manifestations. Rheum Dis Clin North Am 2009;35(1):125–37.

100. Ramos-Casals M, Muñoz S, Medina F, et al. Systemic autoimmune diseases in patients with hepatitis C virus infection: characterization of 1020 cases (The HIS-PAMEC Registry). J Rheumatol 2009;36(7):1442–8.

101. Saadoun D, Terrier B, Semoun O, et al. Hepatitis C virus-associated polyarteritis nodosa. Arthritis Care Res (Hoboken) 2011;63(3):427–35.

102. Khella SL, Souayah N. Hepatitis C: a review of its neurologic complications. Neurologist 2002;8(2):101–6. Available at: http://www.ncbi.nlm.nih.gov/pubmed/12803695. Accessed April 8, 2013.

103. Gemignani F, Brindani F, Alfieri S, et al. Clinical spectrum of cryoglobulinaemic neuropathy. J Neurol Neurosurg Psychiatry 2005;76(10):1410–4.

104. de Freitas MRG. Infectious neuropathy. Curr Opin Neurol 2007;20(5):548–52.

105. Gherardi R, Belec L, Mhiri C, et al. The spectrum of vasculitis in human immunodeficiency virus-infected patients. A clinicopathologic evaluation. Arthritis Rheum 1993;36(8):1164–74. Available at: http://www.ncbi.nlm.nih.gov/pubmed/8343192.

106. Patel N, Patel N, Khan T, et al. HIV infection and clinical spectrum of associated vasculitides. Curr Rheumatol Rep 2011;13(6):506–12.

107. Merkel PA. Drug-induced vasculitis. Rheum Dis Clin North Am 2001;27(4):849–62. Available at: http://www.ncbi.nlm.nih.gov/pubmed/11723768.

108. Grau RG. Drug-induced vasculitis: new insights and a changing lineup of suspects. Curr Rheumatol Rep 2015;17(12):71.

109. Sokumbi O, Wetter DA, Makol A, et al. Vasculitis associated with tumor necrosis factor-α inhibitors. Mayo Clin Proc 2012;87(8):739–45.

110. Subesinghe S, van Leuven S, Yalakki L, et al. Cocaine and ANCA associated vasculitis-like syndromes—a case series. Autoimmun Rev 2018;17(1):73–7.

111. Friedman DR, Wolfsthal SD. Cocaine-induced pseudovasculitis. Mayo Clin Proc 2005;80(5):671–3.

112. Kang MK, Gupta RK, Srinivasan J. Peripheral vasculitic neuropathy associated with minocycline use. J Clin Neuromuscul Dis 2018;19(3):138–41.

113. Baratta JM, Dyck PJB, Brand P, et al. Vasculitic neuropathy following exposure to minocycline. Neurol Neuroimmunol Neuroinflamm 2016;3(1):e180.

114. Thaisetthawatkul P, Sundell R, Robertson CE, et al. Vasculitic neuropathy associated with minocycline use. J Clin Neuromuscul Dis 2011;12(4):231–4.

115. Daxini A, Cronin K, Sreih AG. Vasculitis associated with immune checkpoint inhibitors-a systematic review. Clin Rheumatol 2018. https://doi.org/10.1007/s10067-018-4177-0.

116. Kao JC, Liao B, Markovic SN, et al. Neurological complications associated with anti-programmed death 1 (PD-1) antibodies. JAMA Neurol 2017;74(10):1216–22.

117. Aya F, Ruiz-Esquide V, Viladot M, et al. Vasculitic neuropathy induced by pembrolizumab. Ann Oncol 2017;28(2):433–4.

118. Choi HS, Kim DH, Yang SN, et al. A case of paraneoplastic vasculitic neuropathy associated with gastric cancer. Clin Neurol Neurosurg 2013;115(2):218–21.

119. Kannan MA, Challa S, Kandadai RM, et al. Series of paraneoplastic vasculitic neuropathy: a rare, potentially treatable neuropathy. Neurol India 2015;63(1):30–4.

120. Oh SJ. Paraneoplastic vasculitis of the peripheral nervous system. Neurol Clin 1997;15(4):849–63. Available at: http://www.ncbi.nlm.nih.gov/pubmed/9367968. Accessed April 8, 2013.

121. Correia C da C, Teixeira HM, Melo RV de. Vasculitic neuropathy presenting as Churg-Strauss paraneoplastic syndrome: a rare association. Arq Neuropsiquiatr 2011;69(6):994–5. Available at: http://www.ncbi.nlm.nih.gov/pubmed/22297897.

122. Ashok Muley S, Brown K, Parry GJ. Paraneoplastic vasculitic neuropathy related to carcinoid tumor. J Neurol 2008;255(7):1085–7.

123. Ansari J, Nagabhushan N, Syed R, et al. Small cell lung cancer associated with anti-Hu paraneoplastic sensory neuropathy and peripheral nerve microvasculitis: case report and literature review. Clin Oncol (R Coll Radiol) 2004;16(1):71–6.

Available at: http://www.ncbi.nlm.nih.gov/pubmed/14768759. Accessed August 4, 2013.

124. Takahashi M, Koike H, Ikeda S, et al. Distinct pathogenesis in nonsystemic vasculitic neuropathy and microscopic polyangiitis. Neurol Neuroimmunol Neuroinflamm 2017;4(6):e407.

125. Bennett DLH, Groves M, Blake J, et al. The use of nerve and muscle biopsy in the diagnosis of vasculitis: a 5 year retrospective study. J Neurol Neurosurg Psychiatry 2008;79(12):1376–81.

126. Collins MP, Periquet MI, Mendell JR, et al. Nonsystemic vasculitic neuropathy: insights from a clinical cohort. Neurology 2003;61(5):623–30. Available at: http://www.ncbi.nlm.nih.gov/pubmed/12963752.

127. Davies L, Spies JM, Pollard JD, et al. Vasculitis confined to peripheral nerves. Brain 1996;119(Pt 5):1441–8. Available at: http://www.ncbi.nlm.nih.gov/pubmed/8931569.

128. Dyck PJ, Benstead TJ, Conn DL, et al. Nonsystemic vasculitic neuropathy. Brain 1987;110(Pt 4):843–53. Available at: http://www.ncbi.nlm.nih.gov/pubmed/3651797. Accessed April 7, 2013.

129. Agadi JB, Raghav G, Mahadevan A, et al. Usefulness of superficial peroneal nerve/peroneus brevis muscle biopsy in the diagnosis of vasculitic neuropathy. J Clin Neurosci 2012;19(10):1392–6.

130. Stork ACJ, van der Meulen MFG, van der Pol W-L, et al. Wartenberg's migrant sensory neuritis: a prospective follow-up study. J Neurol 2010;257(8):1344–8.

131. Laterre C, Ghilain S, Tassin S, et al. Wartenberg's disseminated sensory neuropathy. Rev Neurol (Paris) 1988;144(5):358–64 [in French]. Available at: http://www.ncbi.nlm.nih.gov/pubmed/2843980.

132. Simmad VI, Juel VC, Phillips LH. Clinical and electrophysiological findings in the migrant sensory "neuritis" of Wartenberg. J Clin Neuromuscul Dis 1999;1(1):6–10. Available at: http://www.ncbi.nlm.nih.gov/pubmed/19078541.

133. Hamano T, Kaji R, Oka N, et al. Migrant sensory neuritis–electrophysiological and pathological study. Rinsho Shinkeigaku 1992;32(10):1112–6 [in Japanese]. Available at: http://www.ncbi.nlm.nih.gov/pubmed/1297555.

134. Rattananan W, Thaisetthawatkul P, Dyck PJB. Postsurgical inflammatory neuropathy: a report of five cases. J Neurol Sci 2014;337(1–2):137–40.

135. Staff NP, Engelstad J, Klein CJ, et al. Post-surgical inflammatory neuropathy. Brain 2010;133(10):2866–80.

136. Dyck PJ, Norell JE. Microvasculitis and ischemia in diabetic lumbosacral radiculoplexus neuropathy. Neurology 1999;53(9):2113–21. Available at: http://www.ncbi.nlm.nih.gov/pubmed/10599791. Accessed May 27, 2013.

137. Dyck PJ, Norell JE, Dyck PJ. Non-diabetic lumbosacral radiculoplexus neuropathy: natural history, outcome and comparison with the diabetic variety. Brain 2001;124(Pt 6):1197–207. Available at: http://www.ncbi.nlm.nih.gov/pubmed/11353735.

138. Massie R, Mauermann ML, Staff NP, et al. Diabetic cervical radiculoplexus neuropathy: a distinct syndrome expanding the spectrum of diabetic radiculoplexus neuropathies. Brain 2012;135(Pt 10):3074–88.

139. Garces-Sanchez M, Laughlin RS, Dyck PJB, et al. Painless diabetic motor neuropathy: a variant of diabetic lumbosacral radiculoplexus neuropathy? Ann Neurol 2011;69(6):1043–54.

140. Ferrante MA. The distribution of neuralgic amyotrophy lesions is overwhelmingly extraplexal. Muscle Nerve 2018;58(3):325–6.

141. Dyck PJ, Engelstad J, Norell J. Microvasculitis in non-diabetic lumbosacral radiculoplexus neuropathy (LSRPN): similarity to the diabetic variety (DLSRPN). J Neuropathol Exp Neurol 2000;59(6):525–38. Available at: http://www.ncbi. nlm.nih.gov/pubmed/10850865. Accessed May 2, 2013.

142. Watts RA, Scott DG, Pusey CD, et al. Vasculitis-aims of therapy. An overview. Rheumatology (Oxford) 2000;39(3):229–32. Available at: http://www.ncbi.nlm. nih.gov/pubmed/10788527.

143. Pagnoux C, Guillevin L. Peripheral neuropathy in systemic vasculitides. Curr Opin Rheumatol 2005;17(1):41–8. Available at: http://www.ncbi.nlm.nih.gov/ pubmed/15604903.

144. Gorson KC. Vasculitic neuropathies: an update. Neurologist 2007;13(1):12–9.

145. Lapraik C, Watts R, Bacon P, et al. BSR and BHPR guidelines for the management of adults with ANCA associated vasculitis. Rheumatology (Oxford) 2007; 46(10):1615–6.

146. Mukhtyar C, Guillevin L, Cid MC, et al. EULAR recommendations for the management of primary small and medium vessel vasculitis. Ann Rheum Dis 2009;68(3):310–7.

147. Smith RM, Jones RB, Jayne DRW. Progress in treatment of ANCA-associated vasculitis. Arthritis Res Ther 2012;14(2):210.

148. Yates M, Watts RA, Bajema IM, et al. EULAR/ERA-EDTA recommendations for the management of ANCA-associated vasculitis. Ann Rheum Dis 2016;75(9): 1583–94.

149. Ntatsaki E, Carruthers D, Chakravarty K, et al. BSR and BHPR guideline for the management of adults with ANCA-associated vasculitis. Rheumatology (Oxford) 2014;53(12):2306–9.

150. Harigai M, Nagasaka K, Amano K, et al. 2017 Clinical practice guidelines of the Japan Research Committee of the Ministry of Health, Labour, and Welfare for Intractable Vasculitis for the management of ANCA-associated vasculitis. Mod Rheumatol 2018;1–11. https://doi.org/10.1080/14397595.2018.1500437.

151. Naddaf E, Dyck PJB. Vasculitic neuropathies. Curr Treat Options Neurol 2015; 17(10):374.

152. Gorson KC. Therapy for vasculitic neuropathies. Curr Treat Options Neurol 2006; 8(2):105–17. Available at: http://www.ncbi.nlm.nih.gov/pubmed/16464407. Accessed May 5, 2013.

153. Pepper RJ, McAdoo SP, Moran SM, et al. A novel glucocorticoid-free maintenance regimen for anti-neutrophil cytoplasm antibody-associated vasculitis. Rheumatology (Oxford) 2018. https://doi.org/10.1093/rheumatology/key288.

154. Jones RB, Tervaert JWC, Hauser T, et al. Rituximab versus cyclophosphamide in ANCA-associated renal vasculitis. N Engl J Med 2010;363(3):211–20.

155. Stone JH, Merkel PA, Spiera R, et al. Rituximab versus cyclophosphamide for ANCA-associated vasculitis. N Engl J Med 2010;363(3):221–32.

156. Guillevin L, Pagnoux C, Seror R, et al. The Five-Factor Score revisited: assessment of prognoses of systemic necrotizing vasculitides based on the French Vasculitis Study Group (FVSG) cohort. Medicine (Baltimore) 2011;90(1):19–27.

157. Puéchal X. Targeted immunotherapy strategies in ANCA-associated vasculitis. Joint Bone Spine 2018. https://doi.org/10.1016/j.jbspin.2018.09.002.

158. Ribi C, Cohen P, Pagnoux C, et al. Treatment of polyarteritis nodosa and microscopic polyangiitis without poor-prognosis factors: a prospective randomized study of one hundred twenty-four patients. Arthritis Rheum 2010;62(4):1186–97.

159. Walters G. Role of therapeutic plasmapheresis in ANCA-associated vasculitis. Pediatr Nephrol 2016;31(2):217–25.

160. Mahr A, Chaigne-Delalande S, De Menthon M. Therapeutic plasma exchange in systemic vasculitis: an update on indications and results. Curr Opin Rheumatol 2012;24(3):261–6.

161. Levy Y, Uziel Y, Zandman G, et al. Response of vasculitic peripheral neuropathy to intravenous immunoglobulin. Ann N Y Acad Sci 2005;1051:779–86.

162. Tsurikisawa N, Taniguchi M, Saito H, et al. Treatment of Churg-Strauss syndrome with high-dose intravenous immunoglobulin. Ann Allergy Asthma Immunol 2004; 92(1):80–7.

163. Martinez V, Cohen P, Pagnoux C, et al. Intravenous immunoglobulins for relapses of systemic vasculitides associated with antineutrophil cytoplasmic autoantibodies: results of a multicenter, prospective, open-label study of twenty-two patients. Arthritis Rheum 2008;58(1):308–17.

164. Jayne DR, Chapel H, Adu D, et al. Intravenous immunoglobulin for ANCA-associated systemic vasculitis with persistent disease activity. QJM 2000; 93(7):433–9.

165. Matsuo S, Hayashi K, Morimoto E, et al. The successful treatment of refractory polyarteritis nodosa using infliximab. Intern Med 2017;56(11):1435–8.

166. Teixeira V, Oliveira-Ramos F, Costa M. Severe and refractory polyarteritis nodosa associated with CECR1 mutation and dramatic response to infliximab in adulthood. J Clin Rheumatol 2018. https://doi.org/10.1097/RHU.0000000000000839.

167. Wechsler ME, Akuthota P, Jayne D, et al. Mepolizumab or placebo for eosinophilic granulomatosis with polyangiitis. N Engl J Med 2017;376(20):1921–32.

168. Dyck PJ, Norell JE. Methylprednisolone may improve lumbosacral radiculoplexus neuropathy. Can J Neurol Sci 2001;28(3):224–7. Available at: http://www.ncbi.nlm.nih.gov/pubmed/11513340. Accessed April 9, 2013.

169. Tamburin S, Zanette G. Intravenous immunoglobulin for the treatment of diabetic lumbosacral radiculoplexus neuropathy. Pain Med 2009;10(8):1476–80.

170. Kilfoyle D, Kelkar P, Parry GJ. Pulsed methylprednisolone is a safe and effective treatment for diabetic amyotrophy. J Clin Neuromuscul Dis 2003;4(4):168–70. Available at: http://www.ncbi.nlm.nih.gov/pubmed/19078710.

171. Dyck PJB, O'Brien P, Bosch P, et al. The multi-center double-blind controlled trial of IV methylprednisolone in diabetic lumbosacral radiculoplexus neuropathy [abstract]. Neurology 2006;66(5 supp):A191.

172. Chan YC, Lo YL, Chan ES. Immunotherapy for diabetic amyotrophy. Cochrane Database Syst Rev 2017;(7):CD006521.

173. Maritati F, Alberici F, Oliva E, et al. Methotrexate versus cyclophosphamide for remission maintenance in ANCA-associated vasculitis: a randomised trial. PLoS One 2017;12(10):e0185880.

174. Puéchal X, Pagnoux C, Baron G, et al. Adding azathioprine to remission-induction glucocorticoids for eosinophilic granulomatosis with polyangiitis (churg-strauss), microscopic polyangiitis, or polyarteritis nodosa without poor prognosis factors: a randomized, controlled trial. Arthritis Rheumatol 2017; 69(11):2175–86.

175. Pagnoux C, Guillevin L, French Vasculitis Study Group. MAINRITSAN investigators. Rituximab or azathioprine maintenance in ANCA-associated vasculitis. N Engl J Med 2015;372(4):386–7.

176. Pawlotsky J-M. NS5A inhibitors in the treatment of hepatitis C. J Hepatol 2013; 59(2):375–82. https://doi.org/10.1016/j.jhep.2013.03.030.

177. Ahmed M. Era of direct acting anti-viral agents for the treatment of hepatitis C. World J Hepatol 2018;10(10):670–84.

178. Roccatello D, Sciascia S, Rossi D, et al. The challenge of treating hepatitis C virus-associated cryoglobulinemic vasculitis in the era of anti-CD20 monoclonal antibodies and direct antiviral agents. Oncotarget 2017;8(25):41764–77.

179. Ramos-Casals M, Stone JH, Cid MC, et al. The cryoglobulinaemias. Lancet 2012;379(9813):348–60.

180. Collins MP. The vasculitic neuropathies: an update. Curr Opin Neurol 2012; 25(5):573–85.

181. Saadoun D, Resche Rigon M, Sene D, et al. Rituximab plus Peg-interferon-alpha/ribavirin compared with Peg-interferon-alpha/ribavirin in hepatitis C-related mixed cryoglobulinemia. Blood 2010;116(3):326–34 [quiz: 504–5].

182. Dammacco F, Tucci FA, Lauletta G, et al. Pegylated interferon-alpha, ribavirin, and rituximab combined therapy of hepatitis C virus-related mixed cryoglobulinemia: a long-term study. Blood 2010;116(3):343–53.

183. Cacoub P, Si Ahmed SN, Ferfar Y, et al. Long-term efficacy of interferon-free antiviral treatment regimens in patients with hepatitis C virus-associated cryoglobulinemia vasculitis. Clin Gastroenterol Hepatol 2018. https://doi.org/10.1016/j.cgh.2018.05.021.

184. Marson P, Monti G, Montani F, et al. Apheresis treatment of cryoglobulinemic vasculitis: a multicentre cohort study of 159 patients. Transfus Apher Sci 2018. https://doi.org/10.1016/j.transci.2018.06.005.

185. Kallenberg CGM, Tadema H. Vasculitis and infections: contribution to the issue of autoimmunity reviews devoted to "autoimmunity and infection". Autoimmun Rev 2008;8(1):29–32.

186. Lam KC, Lai CL, Trepo C, et al. Deleterious effect of prednisolone in HBsAg-positive chronic active hepatitis. N Engl J Med 1981;304(7):380–6.

187. Guillevin L, Mahr A, Callard P, et al. Hepatitis B virus-associated polyarteritis nodosa. Medicine (Baltimore) 2005;84(5):313–22.

188. Guillevin L, Lhote F, Gayraud M, et al. Prognostic factors in polyarteritis nodosa and Churg-Strauss syndrome. A prospective study in 342 patients. Medicine (Baltimore) 1996;75(1):17–28. Available at: http://www.ncbi.nlm.nih.gov/pubmed/8569467.

Giant Cell Arteritis

David S. Younger, MD, MPH, MS[a,b,*]

KEYWORDS

- Primary • Secondary • Vasculitis • Autoimmune • Nervous system

KEY POINTS

- Giant cell arteritis (GCA) or large-vessel GCA is a chronic, idiopathic, granulomatous vasculitis.
- Vascular complications are generally due to delay in diagnosis and initiation of effective treatment.
- Advancements have been made in MRI and MR angiography, computed tomography angiography, 18fluoro-deoxyglucose/PET and color duplex ultrasonography.
- Corticosteroids are the mainstay of therapy in GCA and tocilizumab is an alternative agent.

INTRODUCTION

In 1890, Hutchinson[1] described painful inflamed temporal arteries that prevented a man from wearing his hat. Giant cell arteritis (GCA) was characterized as a distinct entity by Horton and colleagues in 1932.[2] It is the most common primary systemic vasculitis of the Western world in people older than 50. The 2012 Revised Chapel Hill Consensus Conference nomenclature[3] categorizes GCA as a large-vessel vasculitis, prompting use of the equivalent term, large-vessel GCA. This article reviews the epidemiologic, clinicopathologic features, diagnosis, and treatment of GCA.

EPIDEMIOLOGY

The lifetime risk of developing GCA is estimated at 1% for women and 0.5% for men.[4] The disease rarely occurs in individuals younger than 50 years and peaks in the eighth decade of life. It more commonly affects Scandinavian individuals and North Americans of Scandinavian decent than Southern Europeans and rarely occurs in Black

Disclosure Statement: The author has nothing to disclose.
[a] Department of Neurology, Division of Neuro-Epidemiology, New York University School of Medicine, New York, NY 10016, USA; [b] School of Public Health, City University of New York, New York, NY, USA
* 333 East 34th Street, Suite 1J, New York, NY 10016.
E-mail address: youngd01@nyu.edu
Website: http://www.davidsyounger.com

Neurol Clin 37 (2019) 335–344
https://doi.org/10.1016/j.ncl.2019.01.008
0733-8619/19/© 2019 Elsevier Inc. All rights reserved.

and Asian individuals. There is a genetic predisposition to the disease and an association with the HLA-DRB1*04 allele.[5]

PATHOLOGY

The classic histologic changes of GCA include arterial wall inflammation, internal elastic lamina fragmentation, and intimal thickening (**Fig. 1**). Although GCA derives its name from the presence of multinucleated giant cells, the latter are seen in only approximately one-half of positive temporal artery biopsies (TABs), in association with a granulomatous inflammatory infiltrate composed of CD4+ T-cells and macrophages located at the intima-media junction near fragments of the internal elastic lamina. Other TAB specimens manifest lympho-mononuclear–predominant panarteritis with occasional neutrophils and eosinophils without giant cells. In a minority of cases, inflammation may be seen in periadventitial vessels or the vasa vasorum. There is considerable variation in histopathology between patients and within a given TAB tissue sample. Arteritic involvement of a given artery may be focal and segmental, leading to skip lesions. There may be healed arteritis suggested by intimal thickening, fragmented elastic lamina, and scarred media, although these may in part be age-related changes. Arterial wall thickening can lead to partial or complete occlusion of the lumen and ischemic complications, such as anterior ischemic optic neuropathy (AION). A subset of patients had small-vessel vasculitis surrounding noninflamed temporal artery segments in TAB tissue specimens.[6] Arteritis of the temporal artery is not entirely specific for GCA, and can be encountered with polyarteritis nodosa, antineutrophil cytoplasm antibody–associated vasculitis, malignancy, and atypical polymyalgia rheumatica (PMR).

IMMUNOPATHOGENESIS

Inappropriate activation, maturation, and retention of antigen-presenting adventitial dendritic cells are early steps in the pathogenesis of GCA. These cells sample the surrounding environment for viral and bacterial pathogens through the action of toll-like receptors (TLRs) wherein particular TLR profiles appear to be vessel specific,[7] which may explain why some blood vessels are more prone to be targeted by GCA than others. Mouse models[8] show activated vessel wall–embedded dendritic cells that release chemokines that recruit CD4+ T-cells and macrophages. The pattern of

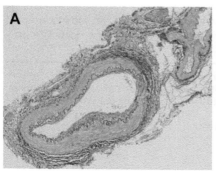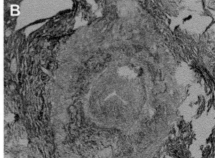

Fig. 1. TABs. (*A*) Normal. (*B*) Typical GCA showing inflammation of the arterial wall, fragmentation of the internal elastic lamina, intimal thickening, and luminal occlusion.

arterial inflammation corresponds to TLR4 stimulation that induces panarteritis, and TLR5 that stimulates perivasculitis.[9]

CLINICAL FEATURES

The onset of GCA tends to be insidious over weeks to months, and abrupt in up to 20% of patients, with a spectrum of initial disease manifestations attributable to the localized effects of vascular and systemic inflammation, including new-onset headache, scalp tenderness, jaw claudication, fever, fatigue, malaise, anorexia, weight loss polymyalgia, and visual loss. The artificial separation of cranial and extracranial features is misleading, as postmortem studies show that the intracranial arteries are largely spared.[10] Although headache is a prominent feature, it is not universal. The headache is classically constant, sudden in onset, and located in the temporal region where it is severe enough to disturb sleep. It can vary greatly in intensity and location. It may become progressively worse, or wax and wane, temporarily subsiding in the absence of treatment. A key feature is that it typically differs from any other previously experienced headache, and for this reason, the patient may deny headache, instead calling the symptom head pain. The headache may be associated with scalp tenderness, especially on hair brushing/combing or wearing glasses. The slightest pressure on resting the head on a pillow may be intolerable. The pain may be generalized, spare the scalp altogether, or affect the eye, ear, face, jaw, or neck. Tenderness, prominence, and decreased temporal artery pulsation (**Fig. 2**) increase the likelihood of GCA, although a third of TAB-proven GCA cases have normal temporal arteries on clinical examination.

An estimated 15% of patients with GCA experience ophthalmologic complications, notably ischemic optic neuropathy (AION) due to arteritic involvement of the short posterior ciliary arteries supplying the optic nerve head, with the remainder composed mainly of retinal blindness due to central retinal artery involvement.[11,12] Visual loss is painless, partial or complete, and unilateral or bilateral; and once established it is

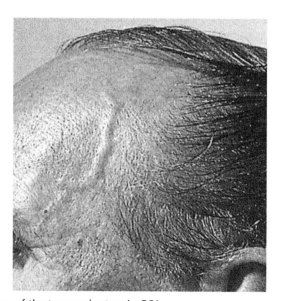

Fig. 2. Prominence of the temporal artery in GCA.

irreversible. It may be preceded by fleeting visual blurring with exercise, amaurosis fugax, or diplopia, but commonly occurs without warning and may be the presenting symptom. Ophthalmoplegia is usually due to a partial or complete oculomotor or abducens nerve palsy, and is a recognized complication of ischemia affecting the extraocular muscles, cranial nerves, or brainstem.

Other ischemic complications of GCA include transient ischemic attack and stroke, which may occur due to thrombosis, microembolism, or a combination of intimal hyperplasia and distal thrombosis. Although the vertebral arteries are inflamed in the large majority of patients at postmortem examination, clinically significant vertebrobasilar insufficiency is uncommon.

Large-Vessel Involvement

Aortic inflammation can be observed in surgical biopsies or at postmortem examination in GCA; however, the true frequency is difficult to ascertain. Computed tomography angiography (CTA) and helical aortic computed tomodensitometry discern aortic involvement in 45% to 65% of patients with GCA, with the thoracic aorta most often affected. The relationship between aortitis and subsequent aortic aneurysm remains unclear. In a cross-sectional study using CT, 12 (22.2%) of 54 patients with GCA developed aortic aneurysms after 4.0 to 10.5 years[13] with relative risks ranging from 3.0 to 17.3. Distal stenotic lesions of the subclavian, axillary, and brachial arteries occur in 3% to 15% of patients. Lower extremity arteries are infrequently affected; however, the identification of claudication and vascular bruits is important to ascertain before initiation of empiric corticosteroids (CS) because such findings, which add weight to the formal diagnosis of GCA, may resolve with effective treatment. The management of peripheral arterial involvement rarely requires surgical intervention.

DIAGNOSIS
Classification Criteria

The American College of Rheumatology (ACR) 1990 criteria for the classification of GCA[14] requires the presence of 3 or more of the following: age older than 50 years, new-onset localized headache, temporal artery tenderness or decreased pulsation, erythrocyte sedimentation rate (ESR) >50 mm/h, and abnormal TAB, yielding a sensitivity of 93.5% and specificity of 91.2% to discern GCA from other vasculitides. Jaw claudication in association with diplopia or decreased vision, or scalp tenderness and new headache are predictive of GCA (**Table 1**). The ACR Classification criteria have been mistakenly used for diagnosis, where they function poorly and (without TAB) are very insensitive.

Laboratory Studies

Blood studies
Acute-phase markers of inflammation are often significantly elevated, and a normocytic normochromic anemia and thrombocytosis may be present, as may elevation of liver transaminase levels with a reduced albumin level. The presence of rheumatoid factor, antinuclear and other autoantibodies are not present in greater frequency than in the general population. Although the ESR has historically been the acute-phase measure of choice in the diagnosis of GCA, up to a quarter of patients may have a normal value and elevation of the C-reactive protein (CRP) is a better predictor of obtaining a diagnostic TAB. The combination of an elevated CRP and positive TAB render the highest sensitivity and specificity for the diagnosis of GCA.

Table 1		
Positive predictive value of clinical features of GCA		
Clinical Features Associated With a Positive TAB	**PPV, %**	**Percentage of Patients, %**
New headache	46	49
Scalp tenderness	61	18
Jaw claudication	78	17
Double vision	65	10
Jaw claudication + Scalp tenderness + New headache	90	6
Jaw claudication + Double vision or decreased vision	100	0.7

Abbreviations: GCA, giant cell arteritis; PPV, positive predictive value; TAB, temporal artery biopsy.
   Adapted from Younge BR, Cook BE, Bartley GB, et al. Initiation of glucocorticoid therapy: before or after temporal artery biopsy? Mayo Clin Proc 2004;79:486; with permission.

Temporal artery biopsy

TAB has been the gold standard test representing definitive pathologic diagnosis. Performed correctly, TAB carries a low procedural risk of significant complications and a positive result removes later doubts about diagnosis, particularly if treatment causes complications, or if the patient fails to respond promptly to therapy, whereas a negative biopsy is important in averting the long-term risk of empiric corticosteroid therapy.[15] The true sensitivity of unilateral TAB was 87% using Bayesian analysis with a variation in sensitivity of 24% to 94% in clinical cohorts.[16] The likelihood of a false-negative TAB may be influenced by the length of the specimen, the duration of prior glucocorticoid therapy, pathologic sectioning techniques, and the presence of predominantly noncranial disease. Retrospective reviews suggest a postfixation biopsy length of 1 to 2 cm is adequate. Whether bilateral biopsies should be performed depends on the rate of discordance, which in a pooled analysis of 4 studies looking at 439 synchronous bilateral biopsies was 5.9%.[17] The side selected for TAB should be the one, if present, with lateralizing symptoms or signs.

Temporal artery ultrasound

Temporal artery ultrasound studies, which are cost-effective, noninvasive, and lack significant complications, take approximately 5 minutes to perform, and render an image of the inflamed temporal artery characterized by edematous wall swelling. The latter conforms to a dark hypoechoic circumferential halo sign that represents continuous or segmental wall thickening (**Fig. 3**). Stenosis and occlusion common in elderly patients due to atherosclerosis, neither of which are specific or sensitive for GCA, also may be noted.

Three meta-analyses[18–21] demonstrated the usefulness of the halo sign in the diagnosis of GCA with a sensitivity of 68% and specificity of 91%, and 100% specificity for s bilateral halo sign.

Other imaging studies

Conventional angiography has little if any role unless a surgical intervention is contemplated. Ultrasound of the thoracic aorta is generally inadequate but it may provide useful information in proximal upper limb arteries to increases the diagnostic yield of GCA. Both MRI, MR angiography (MRA), and contrast-enhanced CTA provide useful images of mural and luminal changes suggestive of large-vessel vasculitis in GCA that include circumferential wall swelling, smoothly tapered luminal narrowing of aortic branches, and aortic aneurysm formation. Moreover, MRI and MRA are favored over CTA by

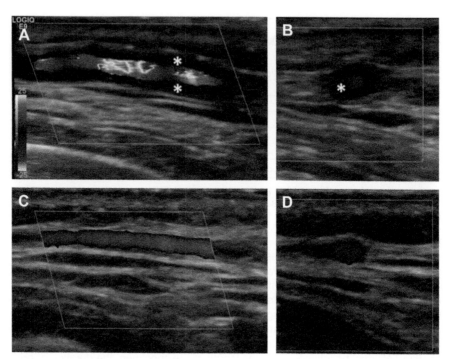

Fig. 3. TAUS. The hypoechoic "halo" sign (*asterisks*) on (*A*) longitudinal and (*B*) transverse section. (*C*) and (*D*) Normal artery.

most experts. Bright mural enhancement of the temporal artery on contrast-enhanced high-resolution MRI had comparable sensitivity and specificity to temporal artery ultrasound (TAUS) in the diagnosis of GCA in one retrospective single-center analysis, the latter of which decreased in sensitivity over the first few days of corticosteroid treatment (85% after 0–1 days, 64% after 2–4 days, 56% after >4 days).[12,22]

Whole-body [18]Fluorodeoxyglucose (FDG)-PET increases the overall diagnostic accuracy of large-vessel involvement in GCA from 54% to 70%.[23] One meta-analysis[24] found that the absence of FDG uptake conferred a negative predictive value of 88% of GCA, whereas thoracic vascular uptake was highly suggestive of GCA. However, there have not been properly designed trials to assess the sensitivity and specificity of ^{18}F-FDG PET in GCA, nor does it reliably distinguish between atherosclerosis and vasculitis.[25] The radiographic features of large-vessel involvement so noted in CTA and PET imaging decrease rapidly after the initiation of CS treatment; features of large-vessel vasculitis including concentric wall thickening were significantly more frequent in treatment-naïve patients compared with patients treated with CS for 1 to 3 days (77% vs 29%, $P = .005$).[26] The diagnostic accuracy of PET in detecting large-vessel involvement was significantly higher in patients not receiving immunosuppressive therapy (93.3% vs 64.5%).[23]

PROGNOSIS

Clinical studies have not validated the relation of existent classification criteria for GCA to clinical and laboratory measures to prognosticate relapse likelihood and outcome. It seems reasonable to consider a return to higher-dose treatment to improve prognosis in patients experiencing a returning headache, PMR-like symptoms, jaw claudication, and visual symptoms. Since the advent of CS for GCA, the long-term outcome and survival rates have been similar to age-matched population including those with large-vessel complications,[26] although before CS, the estimated mortality was 12.5%.[27]

TREATMENT AND OUTCOME

Most experts recommend early initiation of high-dose CS therapy. The case can be made for early intervention with empiric treatment in patients with visual loss because untreated, the other eye is at heightened similar risk in up to one-third of cases for the ensuing 3 weeks, moreover partial visual improvement in vision is more likely if treatment commences within the first day of visual loss. A similar approach is advocated in those with features of impending visual loss, such as amaurosis fugax, diplopia, and jaw claudication. However, if the likelihood of GCA is low to moderate, withholding treatment and awaiting TAB that later returns negative would avoid unnecessary treatment.

Although there are no randomized controlled trials (RCTs) of the use of CS in GCA, most experts agree with daily morning treatment of prednisone at dosages of 40 mg to 60 mg until symptoms and laboratory abnormalities resolve. Alternate daily CS is not as effective as a daily regimen, alone or in association with adjuvant methotrexate for GCA. In fact, the symptomatic response that follows CS treatment is so striking and rapid in GCA, that it is a diagnostic criterion of the disease. Patients with PMR experience improvement in symptoms related to systemic inflammation over 2 to 3 days, whereas symptoms related to impaired blood flow, such as jaw claudication and visual disturbance, generally take longer to respond and resolve. Although sustained visual loss may be permanent and unresponsive to therapy, the risk of further progression is low. Although prednisone in the dose range of 10 mg to 40 mg per day was effective in several cohorts,[28,29] the results were not considered conclusive because of small sample sizes and apparent selection bias. Pulsed intravenous methylprednisolone was advocated in patients with GCA and visual disturbances[30,31]; however, one observational study[32] and another RCT[33] failed to demonstrate improved efficacy in preventing visual loss compared with high-dose oral therapy. Moreover, intravenous pulsed methylprednisolone, which demonstrated no significant long-term CS-sparing effects in the treatment of simple forms of GCA, was reserved for complicated forms of GCA. One small RCT[34] that administered 3 consecutive days of 1 g intravenous pulsed methylprednisolone induction, followed by oral CS found higher rates of remission, fewer relapses, and more rapid tapering compared with patients treated with oral high-dose CS. The CS dose can be gradually tapered in the first month after the resolution of reversible clinical symptoms and the levels of acute-phase reactants falls by 50%. Treatment should be continued for at least 2 years, with most patients weaned off of medication by 4 to 5 years. A minority of them may need continued low-dose CS.

A multicenter RCT[35] concluded that tocilizumab, received weekly or every other week, combined with a 26-week prednisone taper, was superior to either 26-week or 52-week prednisone tapering plus placebo with regard to sustained CS-free remission in patients with GCA. Longer follow-up is necessary to determine the durability of remission and safety of tocilizumab. Sustained remission at week 52 occurred in 56% of the patients treated with tocilizumab weekly and in 53% of those treated with tocilizumab every other week, as compared with 14% of those in the placebo group who underwent the 26-week prednisone taper and 18% of those in the placebo group who underwent the 52-week prednisone taper ($P<.001$ for the comparisons of either active treatment with placebo). The cumulative median prednisone dose over the 52-week period was 1862 mg in each tocilizumab group, as compared with 3296 mg in the placebo group that underwent the 26-week taper ($P<.001$ for both comparisons) and 3818 mg in the placebo group that underwent the 52-week taper ($P<.001$ for both comparisons). Serious adverse events occurred in 15% of the patients in the group that received tocilizumab weekly, 14% of those in the group that received tocilizumab every other week, 22% of those in the placebo group that underwent the 26-week taper, and 25% of those in the placebo group that underwent the 52-week taper.

SUMMARY

GCA is a common, serious, and treatable vasculitis that affects older adults. Rapid access and management care pathways ensure the early referral of untreated suspected patients for readily available TAB especially warranted in those with low to moderate probability of disease, and appropriate primary and secondary care to prevent excess morbidity and mortality associated with empiric and often unwarranted high-dose CS therapy. Published guidelines for GCA diagnosis and management need to be rigorously examined to assess the impact of CRP, TAUS signs, large-vessel imaging, and TAB in any given patient, especially those who warrant empiric high-dose CS due to impending visual loss. Moreover, guidelines need to reflect a unified definition of clinical relapse. Studies assessing the link among clinical symptoms, inflammatory markers, imaging techniques, and mimicking conditions will be very valuable. Finally, long-term vascular complications are increasingly recognized in GCA, and this is blurring the margin between atherosclerosis and vasculitis, which may improve our understanding of both these conditions (65). Biological agents, including tocilizumab, are emerging as effective and safe CS-sparing therapy in treating GCA.

REFERENCES

1. Hutchinson J. Diseases of the arteries: on a peculiar form of thrombotic arteritis of the aged which is sometimes productive of gangrene. Arch Surg 1890;1:323–9.
2. Horton BT, Magath TB, Brown GE. An undescribed form of arteritis of temporal vessels. Mayo Clin Proc 1932;7:700–1.
3. Jennette JC, Falk RJ, Bacon PA, et al. 2012 revised International Chapel Hill Consensus Conference nomenclature of vasculitides. Arthritis Rheum 2013;65: 1–11.
4. Crowson CS, Matteson EL, Myasoedova E, et al. The lifetime risk of adult-onset rheumatoid arthritis and other inflammatory autoimmune rheumatic diseases. Arthritis Rheum 2011;63:633–9.
5. Weyand CM, Hicok KC, Hunder GG, et al. The HLA-DRB1 locus as a genetic component in giant cell arteritis: mapping of a disease-linked sequence motif to the antigen binding site of the HLA-DR molecule. J Clin Invest 1992;90: 2355–61.
6. Cooke WT, Cloake PCP, Govan ADT, et al. Temporal arteritis: a generalized vascular disease. Q J Med 1946;15:47–75.
7. Salvarani C, Cantini F, Hunder GG. Polymyalgia rheumatica and giant-cell arteritis. Lancet 2008;372:234–45.
8. Garcia-Martinez A, Hernandez-Rodriguez J, Arguis P, et al. Development of aortic aneurysm/dilatation during the follow up of patients with giant cell arteritis: a cross-sectional screening of fifty-four prospectively followed patients. Arthritis Care Res 2008;59:422–30.

9. Agard C, Barrier J, Dupas B, et al. Aortic involvement in recent-onset giant cell (temporal) arteritis: a case–control prospective study using helical aortic computed tomodensitometric scan. Arthritis Care Res 2008;59:670–6.

10. Brack A, Martinez-Taboada V, Stanson A, et al. Disease pattern in cranial and large-vessel giant cell arteritis. Arthritis Rheum 1999;42:311–7.

11. Parikh M, Miller NR, Lee AD, et al. Prevalence of a normal C-reactive protein with an elevated erythrocyte sedimentation rate in biopsy-proven giant cell arteritis. Ophthalmology 2006;113:1842–5.

12. Salvarani C, Hunder GG. Giant cell arteritis with low erythrocyte sedimentation rate: frequency of occurrence in a population-based study. Arthritis Care Res 2001;45:140–5.

13. Pipitone N, Salvarani C. Improving therapeutic options for patients with giant cell arteritis. Curr Opin Rheumatol 2008;20:17–22.

14. Murchison AP, Bilyk JR, Eagle RC, et al. Shrinkage revisited: how long is long enough? Ophthalmic Plast Reconstr Surg 2012;28:261–3.

15. Schmidt WA. Imaging in vasculitis. Best Pract Res Clin Rheumatol 2013;27:107–18.

16. Clifford A, Burrell S, Hanly JG. Positron emission tomography/computed tomography for the diagnosis and assessment of giant cell arteritis: when to consider it and why. J Rheumatol 2012;39:1909–11.

17. Hauenstein C, Reinhard M, Geiger J, et al. Effects of early corticosteroid treatment on magnetic resonance imaging and ultrasonography findings in giant cell arteritis. Rheumatology 2012;51:1999–2003.

18. Hayreh SS, Zimmerman B. Management of giant cell arteritis: our 27-year clinical study: new light on old controversies. Ophthalmologica 2003;217:239–59.

19. Spiera RF, Spiera H. Therapy for giant cell arteritis: can we do better? Arthritis Rheum 2006;54:3071–4.

20. Agard C, Espitia O, Neel A. Prognosis of giant cell arteritis. Presse Med 2012;41:966–74 [in French].

21. Bury D, Joseph J, Dawson T. Does preoperative steroid treatment affect the histology in giant cell (cranial) arteritis? J Clin Pathol 2012;65:1138–40.

22. Hall S, Persellin S, Lie JT, et al. The therapeutic impact of temporal artery biopsy. Lancet 1983;2:1217.

23. Murchison AP, Gilbert ME, Jurij R, et al. Validity of the American College of Rheumatology criteria for the diagnosis of giant cell arteritis. Am J Ophthalmol 2012;154:722–9.

24. Hunder GG, Sheps SG, Allen GL, et al. Daily and alternate-day corticosteroid regimens in treatment of giant cell arteritis: comparison in a prospective study. Ann Intern Med 1975;82:613–8.

25. Proven A, Gabriel SE, Orces C, et al. Glucocorticoid therapy in giant cell arteritis: duration and adverse outcomes. Arthritis Rheum 2003;49:703–8.

26. Nordborg E, Nordborg C. Giant cell arteritis: strategies in diagnosis and treatment. Curr Opin Rheumatol 2004;16:25–30.

27. Kyle V, Hazleman BL. Treatment of polymyalgia rheumatica and giant cell arteritis. II. Relation between steroid dosing and steroid associated side effects. Ann Rheum Dis 1989;48:662–6.

28. Unizony SH, Dasgupta B, Fisheleva E, et al. Design of the tocilizumab in giant cell arteritis trial. Int J Rheumatol 2013;2013:912562.

29. Nesher G, Berkun Y, Mates M, et al. Risk factors for cranial ischemic complications in giant cell arteritis. Medicine 2004;83:114–22.

30. Mukhtyar C, Guillevin L, Cid MC, et al. EULAR recommendations for the management of large vessel vasculitis. Ann Rheum Dis 2009;68:318–23.
31. Dasgupta B, Borg FA, Hassan N, et al. BSR and BHPR guidelines for the management of giant cell arteritis. Rheumatology 2010;49:1594–7.
32. Narvaez J, Nolla-Sole JM, Clavaguera MT, et al. Longterm therapy in polymyalgia rheumatica: effect of coexistent temporal arteritis. J Rheumatol 1999;26:1945–52.
33. Narvaez J, Bernard B, Gomez-Vaquero C, et al. Impact of antiplatelet therapy in the development of severe ischaemic complications and in the outcome of patients with giant cell arteritis. Clin Exp Rheumatol 2008;26(Suppl 49):S57–62.
34. Berger CT, Wolbers M, Meyer P, et al. High incidence of severe ischaemic complications in patients with giant cell arteritis irrespective of platelet count and size, and platelet inhibition. Rheumatology 2009;48:258–61.
35. Stone JH, Tuckwell K, Dimonaco S, et al. Trial of tocilizumab in giant-cell arteritis. N Engl J Med 2017;377:317–28.

Polyarteritis Nodosa Neurologic Manifestations

Hubert de Boysson, MD[a], Loïc Guillevin, MD[b],*

KEYWORDS

- Polyarteritis nodosa • Peripheral neuropathy • Vasculitis • ANCA • Stroke
- Hepatitis B virus

KEY POINTS

- Peripheral neuropathy is often the most frequent and earliest symptom of polyarteritis no-dosa (PAN).
- Peripheral neuropathy does not affect survival but can be responsible for severe functional sequelae.
- Central nervous system (CNS) involvement is rare in PAN but outcome of CNS manifestations can be lethal.
- Treatment varies according to cause (eg, hepatitis B virus [HBV] positivity or not, deficit of adenosine deaminase-2 [DADA2]) and severity: corticosteroids and sometimes immuno-suppressants in the absence of HBV infection; corticosteroids, then antiviral treatment and plasma exchanges in cases of HBV-PAN; antitumor necrosis factor in DADA2 patients.

Polyarteritis nodosa (PAN), first described by Küssmaul and Maier,[1] is a necrotizing vasculitis mainly manifested by weight loss; fever; asthenia; peripheral neuropathy; renal, musculoskeletal, and/or gastrointestinal (GI) tract involvement; cutaneous lesions; hypertension; and/or cardiac failure. Peripheral neuropathy is often the most frequent and earliest symptom of PAN. Central nervous system (CNS) manifestations are less frequent.[2,3]

In light of its potential causes, primary and secondary forms of PAN can also be distinguished. Notably, PAN can be the consequence of hepatitis B virus (HBV) infection (HBV-PAN).[4] This cause was frequent in the 1980s but is becoming extremely rare since the implementation of the anti-HBV vaccination and enhanced blood transfusion

Disclosure statement: None.
[a] Department of Internal Medicine, Centre Hospitalier Universitaire de Caen, Caen, France;
[b] Vasculitides and Scleroderma, Department of Internal Medicine, Referral Center for Rare Autoimmune and Systemic Diseases, Hôpital Cochin, Université Paris Descartes, 27, rue Fg Saint-Jacques, Paris 75679 Cedex 14, France
* Corresponding author.
E-mail address: loic.guillevin@aphp.fr

Neurol Clin 37 (2019) 345–357
https://doi.org/10.1016/j.ncl.2019.01.007
0733-8619/19/© 2019 Elsevier Inc. All rights reserved.

safety and hygiene procedures. This article reviews the clinical PAN manifestations, focusing on the peripheral nervous system (PNS) and CNS symptoms.

DEFINITIONS, CLASSIFICATION, AND DIAGNOSIS

Vasculitides are mainly defined based on their histologic features. However, more recently, pathogenic mechanisms and the presence or absence of immunologic markers have also been considered.[5] PAN is a necrotizing vasculitis in which histologic characteristics include fibrinoid necrosis of the artery media, perivascular inflammatory infiltrates, and vessel thrombosis following intima infiltration. Lesions progress to fibrotic scar replacement, causing tissue ischemia and damage.

Vasculitic lesions are segmentally distributed, with a predilection for arterial bifurcations. Early inflammatory infiltrates contain lymphocytes, plasmocytes, histiocytes, and some neutrophils. Fibrinoid necrosis of the artery media leads to thrombosis development. Segmental necrosis of medium-sized vessels may also give rise to microaneurysms.[6] Because PAN activity consists of successive flares, different histologic stages may be seen in the same tissue sample. Arterial lesions are ubiquitous and can be present in all medium-sized arteries. Some unusual localizations have been described; for example, fibrinoid necrosis in a temporal artery mimicking the clinical symptoms of giant cell arteritis.[7] Granulomatous inflammation in biopsied tissue excludes PAN; it is mainly characteristic of granulomatosis with polyangiitis or eosinophilic granulomatosis with polyangiitis (EGPA). The latter 2 vasculitides affect small-sized vessels, whereas medium-size vessels are the predominant sites of PAN.

The 1990 American College of Rheumatology classification criteria are no longer useful for PAN because they do not separate PAN and microscopic polyangiitis (MPA), a small-sized vessel antineutrophil cytoplasm antibody (ANCA)-associated vasculitis.[8] The 1994 and 2012 Chapel Hill Consensus Conference Nomenclature versions[9,10] provide a precise definition of PAN (**Box 1**).

Specific guidelines have also been elaborated by the Peripheral Nerve Society to diagnose and classify vasculitides affecting peripheral nerves.[11]

Diagnosis of vasculitis theoretically requires histologic proof. However, because tissues from sites easy to biopsy may show only nonspecific inflammation or may be normal, the diagnosis can be based on a combination of clinical, immunologic, and radiological findings. ANCA-negativity and angiography-detected stenoses or microaneurysms are useful for diagnosis. Immunofluorescence-linked and/or enzyme-linked immunosorbent assay (ELISA)-detected ANCA should be considered an exclusionary criterion for PAN diagnosis. The angiograms of approximately two-thirds of PAN patients investigated visualize celiomesenteric and renal angiographic findings;

Box 1
Definition of polyarteritis nodosa adopted by the 2012 International Chapel Hill Consensus Conference on the Nomenclature of Vasculitides

Medium-sized vessel vasculitides: vasculitis predominantly affecting medium-sized arteries, defined as the main visceral arteries and their branches. However, any size artery may be affected. Inflammatory aneurysms and stenoses are common.

PAN: necrotizing arteritis of medium-sized or small-sized arteries, without glomerulonephritis or vasculitis in arterioles, capillaries, or venules, and not associated with ANCA.

Adapted from Jennette JC, Falk RJ, Bacon PA, et al. 2012 revised International Chapel Hill Consensus Conference Nomenclature of Vasculitides. Arthritis Rheum 2013;65:1–11; with permission.

for example, multiple 1 to 5-mm diameter microaneurysms or irregular stenoses.[12] Although highly suggestive, those findings are not absolutely specific. Visceral artery aneurysms are also found in thrombotic thrombocytopenic purpura, mycotic infections, fibromuscular dysplasia, atrial myxoma, malignant hypertension, and rare patients with small-sized vessel vasculitides.[13] Henegar and colleagues[5] established diagnostic criteria for PAN comprising positive and negative items which, when combined, are relevant for diagnosis (**Table 1**).

PAN may develop in a setting of infection, mainly HBV and rarely human immunodeficiency virus (HIV) or other viruses.[14] When hepatitis C virus (HCV) is found, it is more frequently an HBV coinfection than a specific cause of PAN. In the late 1980s, HBV was responsible for one-third of the PAN cases.[4] HBV-PAN is no longer observed in developed countries. The last rare cases the authors observed were the consequence of a probable reactivation of a dormant nonreplicating HBV.

A cat eye syndrome critical region protein-1 (*CECR1*) mutation, responsible for a deficit of adenosine deaminase-2 (DADA2) was recently described in children. DADA2 usually becomes manifest in childhood, with 24% of reported patients consulting before 1 year of age, and 77% before the age of 10 years.[15] It is the first molecularly described monogenic vasculitis syndrome. Patients carrying this mutation have PAN symptoms, with strokes occurring more frequently than in other PAN forms.[15–18] Systemic symptoms are comparable to those of PAN but DADA2 is more severe.[15] Patients can be siblings, sometimes twins. This new form of PAN demonstrates that PAN causes are probably multifactorial.

Table 1	
Polyarteritis nodosa diagnostic or exclusionary criteria	
PAN Criteria	**Comment**
Diagnostic	
Poor condition and/or weight loss	Present for several weeks or months, with loss of appetite
Myalgias and/or arthralgias	Proximal or distal muscle pain without deficit, inflammatory arthralgias with or without arthritis
Testicular tenderness	With or without concomitant orchitis; no infectious cause found
Mononeuritis multiplex	Recent, not attributable to metabolic or toxic cause
Hypertension	Recent-onset arterial hypertension not related to an organic cause other than a vasculitic process
Renal insufficiency	Recent-onset renal insufficiency or acute impairment of renal function
Replicating HBV	Should occur <24 mo before vasculitis onset; replication proven by viral DNA and hepatitis B e antigen positivity
Exclusionary	
Glomerulonephritis	Suggested by hematuria and proteinuria, without renal insufficiency; histologically proven
Alveolar hemorrhage	Hemoptysis with alveolar pneumonia or positive bronchoalveolar lavage Golde test
Asthma	Severe and recent asthma onset with hypereosinophilia or history of asthma with recent worsening
ANCA+	Identified by immunofluorescence and confirmed by ELISA
Cryoglobulinemia	Mixed type II or III cryoglobulinemia

EPIDEMIOLOGY

No recent data on PAN prevalence and incidence are available. In a study on biopsy-proven forms, the annual PAN incidence and prevalence were, respectively, 0.7 and 6.3 per 100,000 habitants.[19] Estimates of the annual PAN-type systemic vasculitis incidence in the general population range from 4.6 per 1,000,000 in England to 9.0 per 1,000,000 in Olmsted County, MN, to 77 per 1,000,000 in a hepatitis B hyperendemic Alaskan Eskimo.[20,21] PAN affects men and women with a male predominance, all racial groups, at every age, usually starting between 40 and 60 years but can develop in children and patients older than 65 years old.[4] Based on follow-up of a vasculitis cohort, PAN is now extremely rare, even though its recrudescence has been seen in the 2 past 2 years; however, there is no precise data on its frequency, which might have been biased by the referral center's specialty and tertiary nature. HBV-PAN has almost completely disappeared in the French population. In France, vaccination is strongly encouraged for teenagers and populations at risk. Blood transfusion is safe, with specific polymerase chain reaction detection of viruses (HBV, HCV, and HIV) and the hospital hygiene measures implemented nationwide, including systematic single use of materiel.

EXTRANEUROLOGICAL MANIFESTATIONS

Two-thirds of PAN patients are in poor general condition, with anorexia and weight loss occurring early during the course of the disease, and perhaps being the sole manifestations. Patients may be febrile. They usually complain of myalgias and arthralgias, most often affecting the major joints: knees, ankles, elbows, and wrists. Pain can be localized to nerve territories.

Renal Manifestations

Vascular nephropathy can lead to renal insufficiency of variable intensity, which, in turn, can cause severe or malignant arterial hypertension as a complication.[22]

Acute renal failure can be an early manifestation or occur at the time of a flare. Some patients may require renal dialysis early or at some later time, when renal insufficiency progresses as a consequence of chronic worsening of renal ischemia. However, the outcome of renal insufficiency is not predictable and improvement may occur.

Angiograms of patients with renal involvement show renal infarcts, multiple stenoses, and/or microaneurysms of digestive and renal artery branches. Renal infarcts are responsible for renal insufficiency.

Orchitis

Noninfectious orchitis, attesting to testicular artery involvement, is rarely the first sign of PAN but it is characteristic. With rapid initiation of corticosteroids, orchitis may regress.[6,12]

Skin Manifestations

Vascular purpura is frequent in PAN. Because the skin contains medium-sized vessels, nodules can form in the dermis and hypodermis, and predominately on the legs. They appear and disappear within a few days. Livedo racemosa or reticularis can be observed. Postinflammatory ischemic leg ulcers can develop and are recognized by their topography. They must be differentiated from cholesterol crystal emboli in patients with atherosclerosis.[6,12]

Peripheral Vascular Manifestations

Distal digital gangrene can result from arterial obstruction. Angiography can demonstrate the presence of stenoses and/or microaneurysms. Raynaud phenomenon, when present, can remain isolated or be complicated by necrosis.[6,12]

Gastrointestinal Involvement

GI tract involvement is among the most severe PAN manifestations,[23] especially in HBV-PAN.[24] Abdominal pain occurs in one-quarter to one-third of the patients and can be the first symptom. Most patients have ischemia of the small intestine but rarely the colon or stomach. Small intestine perforation and GI bleeding are the most severe signs.[24]

Chronic pancreatitis with pseudocysts[25] has a particularly poor prognosis. Vasculitis of the appendix or gallbladder can be the first symptom. The prognoses of those manifestations depend on whether either is the first overt vasculitis sign or a complication of previously diagnosed and treated PAN.

Cardiac Manifestations

Cardiac involvement results from vasculitis of the coronary arteries and/or their branches, or severe or malignant hypertension. Despite coronary artery vasculitis, angina is rare and coronary angiography is usually normal. Stenoses of the main coronary arteries were found during autopsies in less than half of the PAN patients.[26] Arteriolar involvement and myocardial necrotic foci can be seen.

Left heart failure, the most common cardiac involvement manifestation, occurs early during the course of PAN. Supraventricular rhythm disturbances occur more often than ventricular rhythm disturbances. Pericardium involvement by the vasculitic process is rare. One-third of PAN patients have arterial hypertension but rarely have malignant hypertension.

Hepatitis B Virus–Polyarteritis Nodosa

When HBV is involved, PAN usually appears during the year following infection. Hepatitis is usually present before PAN onset. The authors previously observed that some patients developed PAN several years after contamination and hypothesized that those cases were caused by mutant HBVs. Clinical manifestations are basically the same as those commonly seen in non–HBV-PAN.[4] Seroconversion usually leads to recovery. Vascular nephropathy can be responsible for sequelae but recovery is possible, even in renal insufficient patients, with little residual impairment of renal function.

Abdominal manifestations and vascular nephropathy are common.

NEUROLOGIC MANIFESTATIONS
Peripheral Nervous System Involvement

Half to three-quarters of PAN patients experience peripheral neuropathy.[27,28] PNS involvement typically results from focal or multifocal, axonal, ischemic neuropathy caused by arteriolar occlusion of the vasa nervorum, usually of epineurial arteries.[2,3] For 36.4% (8/22) to 55.6% (15/27) of patients with systemic necrotizing vasculitides,[29,30] signs of PNS involvement are the initial symptoms. Patients commonly complain of pain or inexplicable sensory symptoms in the days preceding palsy onset. At that time, the physical examination is normal. PAN onset is usually acute but may be more progressive, particularly in the elderly. Sensory signs are responsible for hypoesthesias or hyperesthesias, dysesthesias, or frank pain as the prominent and earliest features. Usually, motor deficits start later but are also of sudden onset, sometimes preceding the sensory loss.

The first manifestations often affect the lower limbs, with 1 particular nerve initially involved. Later, other nerves become affected. This pattern is referred to as mononeuritis multiplex. In its late stage, so many nerves can be involved that mononeuritis multiplex can be mistaken for a symmetric process. In those cases, only careful history-taking will be able to identify the patchy asymmetric pattern of early involvement. Less frequently, distal symmetric sensorimotor polyneuropathy and pure sensory neuropathy may occur. The nerves most frequently affected (in decreasing order), respectively unilaterally and bilaterally, are: the sciatic nerve or its peroneal branch, 62.5% to 84% of the patients and one-third but asynchronously; the tibial nerve, 27.5% to 41% and 5%; the ulnar nerve, 25.5% to 56% and 8%; the median nerve, 21.5% and 3%; the radial nerve 8% to 29% and 2%; the femoral nerve, 2% unilaterally; and the proximal sciatic nerve or sciatic root unilaterally in another 2%.[24,31,32] A Guillain-Barré syndrome–like clinical picture has been described, as have radicular syndromes and plexopathies.[33] Exceptionally, some patients with DADA2 have polyneuropathy or mononeuritis multiplex.[15]

Some patients with histologically proven peripheral nerve vasculitis seem to have PNS-limited PAN.[34] This form has been referred to as nonsystemic vasculitis[35] and is called single-organ vasculitis in the 2012 Chapel Hill Nomenclature.[10] This form of PAN is called PAN but, except for the neurologic signs, the disease is not systemic. Hence, it is unclear whether it is the same disease or 2 entities. Notably, the single-organ form relapses frequently, without systemic inflammation.

In PAN limited to the skin, PNS involvement has also been described. The authors think that it too should be considered a different entity, even though it is referred to as PAN. However, that "an isolated vasculitis is a limited expression of a systemic vasculitis does not imply that the vasculitis will or will not subsequently evolve into systemic disease."[10] Indeed, Said[32] showed that 37% of the patients with initially isolated peripheral nerve vasculitis subsequently developed systemic vasculitis manifestations and that 24% of them experienced neuropathy relapses. Although some sporadic cases reported had poor outcomes,[34] most nonsystemic vasculitides, clearly restricted to peripheral nerves, respond favorably to treatment (mainly corticosteroids and immunosuppressants)[35,36]; however, improvement may occur very slowly and sometimes only partially. Severe pain and sensory symptoms can sometimes persist for years, or even indefinitely, after the first clinical symptoms and, evidently, negatively impact the patient's quality of life.

Because cerebrospinal fluid (CSF) findings are usually normal, lumbar puncture is not done routinely. For the rare patients with such analyses, CSF had moderately increased protein concentrations and rare cellular contents. However, CSF analysis is indicated for patients with plexopathies, clinical manifestations mimicking Guillain-Barré syndrome, or to look for a differential diagnosis.

With treatment, mononeuritis multiplex progressively regresses and patients can recover without sequelae. Cranial nerve palsies, most often involving the oculomotor (III), trochlear (IV), abducent (VI), facial (VII), and acoustic VIII nerves, affects less than 2% of PAN patients. Bladder neuropathy is rarely observed.[37]

Central Nervous System Involvement

PAN affects the CNS in 2% to 10% of subjects.[6,38] Previously, 20% to 40% of the subjects had CNS involvement but headaches had been included among CNS symptoms and some subjects with MPA had probably been included in the series.[2,28]

CNS involvement usually arises late during the course of the vasculitis; pertinently, a CNS event renders a PAN link questionable. Some investigators suggested that hypertension-associated microangiopathy and a prothrombotic state are more frequent components of a CNS event than a vasculitic process.[39] Parenchymal biopsy would demonstrate vasculitis but is rarely obtained, given its invasive nature. Only a few cases of biopsy-proven PAN-related CNS vasculitis have been reported.[40] Most often, clinical and radiological findings and extraneurological signs of disease activity lead the clinician to suspect PAN-related CNS involvement.

Clinical manifestations

Neurologic symptoms of PAN-related CNS involvement are highly variable and depend on the territory affected. Their onset can be acute (eg, stroke or seizures) or more chronic and insidious, such as headaches or encephalopathic symptoms (cognitive and vigilance disorders or psychiatric manifestations). Although headaches are common, not all patients have them.[3]

Motor deficits are common and often explained by small to large brain infarctions. Other potential neurologic deficits include speech disorders, sensory deficits, or cerebellar ataxia. Although cranial nerve involvement is possible, it has rarely been reported. Encephalopathic manifestations include confusion, cognitive disorders, psychiatric manifestations (mainly depression), and vigilance disorders (ranging from psychomotor retardation to coma). Seizures are also common.

Frequent visual loss can result from anterior optic neuropathy or posterior (retrobulbar) optic neuropathy.[3,41,42]

In addition to a neurologic work-up, other extraneurological symptoms should be actively sought because they are frequently present.

Computed tomography scan and MRI

Despite its poor sensitivity and specificity, CT scan is often the first imaging examination. MRI is essential for all patients and, when available, should include the following sequences: T1, T2, T2*, fluid-attenuated inversion recovery (FLAIR), diffusion-weighted imaging (DWI) or apparent diffusion coefficient mapping, and gadolinium-enhanced T1. Vascular sequences should be also obtained.

Different lesion patterns can be discerned within a single imaging procedure. Ischemic lesions, isolated or disseminated, are common. Subacute and chronic ischemic lesions are also seen, often associated with acute lesions. Cortical and subcortical regions are frequently involved.[38] Multiple ischemic lesions are suggestive of a vasculitic process but can also be seen in atherosclerosis, infections, or other vasculopathies. Disseminated lesions of different ages are also suggestive of vasculitis. Multiple patterns of acute ischemic lesions can be seen in gray and white matter (subcortical, peripheral, superficial, or deep lesions).

Subcortical and white matter FLAIR hyperintense lesions are frequently seen but are nonspecific because they are also found in other inflammatory and noninflammatory conditions. FLAIR lesions in the cortex or posterior areas are rare and more evocative of vasculitis. Gadolinium injection is required in the diagnostic workup of CNS vasculitis and gadolinium-enhanced lesions are suggestive of an inflammatory process. Meningeal tissues, as well as the parenchyma, can be gadolinium-enhanced. Pachymeningitis is only exceptionally reported in PAN[43] and is more often found in granulomatous diseases or primary CNS vasculitis. In the authors' experience, pachymeningitis in PAN was not observed.

Hemorrhagic lesions can be observed within acute ischemic lesions, indicating hemorrhagic transformation. However, spontaneous parenchymal or subarachnoid hemorrhages, possibly attributable to microaneurysm rupture, have been described.[44–46] Some hemorrhagic lesions might also be caused by hypertensive microangiopathy.[2,39]

The presence of different MRI abnormalities is frequent and suggestive of vasculitis when multiple ischemic lesions are seen concomitantly with small hemorrhages, FLAIR lesions, and gadolinium enhancements. Conversely, PAN-related CNS vasculitis is highly improbable in a patient whose MRI is normal.

Cerebral Angiography

For patients with imagery-documented ischemic CNS lesions or those suspected of having specific PAN-related CNS vasculitis, angiography is required. Although aneurysm formations are frequent in extraneurological medium-sized vessels, they are more rarely reported in brain vessels.[38,46,47] Magnetic resonance angiography (MRA), brain CT angiography, or digital subtraction angiography are the 3 main procedures used. The latter technique has the best spatial resolution, enabling analysis of vessels greater than or equal to 500 μm but it is an invasive procedure. Although MRA's ability to explore vessels greater than 700 μm is limited, the development of 3T MRA has increased the procedure's spatial resolution.

In addition to microaneurysms, which occur more frequently in PAN, multiple arterial segmental and focal stenoses (>80% of lumen narrowings) and occlusions are other typical vasculitis findings.[38,46,47] Importantly, those stenoses can also be found in other conditions (eg, atherosclerosis or reversible cerebral vasoconstriction syndrome). However, in the last 2 entities, lesions are often diffuse and involve more vessels than vasculitis.

Deficit of Adenosine deaminase-2

In 2 2014 reports, patients with DADA2 and early-onset PAN with lacunar strokes, livedoid rash, and intermittent fevers were described.[16,17] Since then, fewer than 200 patients have been reported. Skin (mainly livedo) and CNS are commonly involved.[15,18] Observed in more than 50% of those patients, CNS events were predominantly multiple acute or chronic ischemic lacunar infarcts located in the deep-brain nuclei and/or the brain stem, sparing the subcortical white matter. Hemorrhagic events seemed to be a part of the clinical spectrum, even though they occurred more frequently in patients taking aspirin or warfarin.[15] Other rare manifestations included spastic diplegia or paraplegia, peripheral polyneuropathy (with perineuritis), ataxia, neurosensory hearing loss, mononeuritis multiplex, labyrinthitis, encephalopathy, and cerebral atrophy.[15]

In addition to neurologic and skin manifestations, peripheral vascular symptoms, renal and intestinal involvements, and hepatic and splenic involvements leading to portal hypertension have been described. Finally, cytopenias, including some bone-marrow failures and hypogammaglobulinemia, can be present.[15–17,48,49]

TREATMENT

Although codified, PAN treatment is essentially based on therapeutics already prescribed for other vasculitides. The newest targeted monoclonal antibodies have been tried anecdotally for PAN patients but were not effective, in sharp contrast to their proven efficacy against ANCA-associated vasculitides. Therefore, PAN treatment remains based on corticosteroids and immunosuppressants for non–HBV-PAN, and antiviral agents combined with plasma exchanges (PEs) for HBV-PAN.

Treatment Stratification According to Polyarteritis Nodosa Form and/or Its Subgroups

To help clinicians choose the most effective therapy and avoid overtreating patients, the authors revisited the 1996 Five-Factor Score (FFS) in 2011.[50] The revised FFS, whose items were associated with higher mortality (renal insufficiency [creatininemia >150 μmol/L]; cardiomyopathy; GI manifestations; age greater than 65 years old; and absence of ear, nose, and throat involvement), has significant prognostic value. When FFS at diagnosis was 0, 1, or greater than or equal to 2, respective 5-year mortality reached 9%, 21%, or 40%. The 1996 FFS version included CNS involvement[51] but it was no longer a poor-prognosis factor in the revised FFS, mainly because of the small number of PAN patients with CNS manifestations in a vasculitis patient cohort.[50]

Corticosteroids Alone

Corticosteroids alone can effectively treat PAN without poor-prognosis factors; that is, FFS equals 0,[52] obtaining survival rates similar to those of patients whose induction regimen combined corticosteroids and cyclophosphamide. When PAN fails to respond to corticosteroids alone, adjunction of an immunosuppressant (cyclophosphamide or azathioprine) should be beneficial. A recent study on subjects with PAN, EGPA, or MPA[53] confirmed that adding azathioprine to corticosteroids for subjects with FFS equals 0 was not more effective than steroids alone and was unable to prevent relapses.

The benefit of adding an immunosuppressant to the induction regimen of patients with CNS involvement has not been proven. However, given that severe clinical manifestations of CNS involvement frequently coexist with other systemic involvements, corticosteroids are rarely prescribed alone.

Corticosteroids and Cyclophosphamide

Combining an immunosuppressant with induction corticosteroids has transformed the prognosis of severe non–HBV-PAN. When cyclophosphamide is indicated for PAN patients, 1 to 3 intravenous pulses should be preferred to oral intake because systemic administration achieves a more rapid clinical response. In combination with corticosteroids, 6 intravenous cyclophosphamide pulses usually suffice to induce remission. An azathioprine or methotrexate maintenance-therapy regimen is then prescribed for 12 to 18 months.

Treatment of Hepatitis B Virus and Other Virus-Related Polyarteritis Nodosa

Virus-associated vasculitides require specific therapeutics. In the context of chronic HBV infections, the PAN can be successfully treated with corticosteroids and immunosuppressants, obtaining short-term outcomes comparable to those obtained with PEs and antiviral agents.[4] However, in the virus-infection setting, immunosuppressants can be deleterious, enhancing virus replication, and, over the long term, perpetuating chronic HBV infection and facilitating progression toward cirrhosis, which may subsequently evolve to hepatocellular carcinoma.

Because antiviral drug efficacies against chronic hepatitis and PEs for PAN have been demonstrated, the authors devised an etiologic therapeutic regimen for HBV-PAN. Initial corticosteroids, to rapidly control the most severe life-threatening PAN manifestations common during the first weeks of overt vasculitis, were stopped abruptly to enhance immunologic clearance of HBV-infected hepatocytes and favor hepatitis B e (HBe) antigen to anti–HBe-antibody seroconversion; then, PEs were added to control the course of PAN.

An induction regimen combining an antiviral (eg, vidarabine; interferon alpha-2b; or, more recently, lamivudine, entecavir) and PEs to treat HBV-PAN was able to achieve excellent overall therapeutic outcomes in several weeks. That antiviral-PE strategy amplified the seroconversion rate from 14.7% with conventional treatment to 49.4%.[4]

Plasma Exchanges

At present, no trial-documented proof supports the systematic prescription of PEs at the time of non–HBV-PAN diagnosis, even for patients with poor prognosis factors.[52,54]

In contrast, for HBV-PAN, because corticosteroids and immunosuppressants cannot be recommended, PEs are essential to clear immune complexes and immediately control serious disease symptoms, while buying time for the antiviral's effect to take hold.

Specific Considerations on Peripheral Neuropathy

A long-term analyses of subjects included in prospective studies confirmed the initial results in terms of survival and relapse rates, and showed that subjects with peripheral neuropathy at PAN onset more frequently required an immunosuppressant combined with corticosteroids to manage their relapses than those without that symptom initially.[55,56] That observation over the long term leads the authors to hypothesize that induction with corticosteroids and an immunosuppressant, independent of disease severity, could prevent late relapses. However, that hypothesis should be tested in a prospective trial.

Adenosine Deaminase-2

The first DADA2 patients with severe symptoms received corticosteroids and immunosuppressants, which yielded various outcomes, including several flares at corticosteroid tapering.[15] To date, treatment of DADA2 symptoms mainly relies on antitumor necrosis factor agents, which limits stroke recurrences. Rituximab has been used to treat DADA2-associated cytopenias and hypogammaglobulinemia can be managed with gammaglobulin substitution.[15] Bone-marrow failure and severe immune deficiency might require hematopoietic stem cell transplantation.[48,49] Because plasma ADA2 levels can be measured, infusions of fresh-frozen plasma were considered to replace insufficient ADA2. However, the ADA2 half-life and the large plasma volumes required to be effective render this approach impractical.[15]

REFERENCES

1. Küssmaul A, Maier R. Ueber eine bischer nicht beschriebene eigenthumliche Arterienerkrankung (Periarteritis nodosa), die mit Morbus Brightii und rapid fortschreitender allgemeiner Muskellhamung einhergeht. Dtsch Arch Klin Med 1866;1:484–518.
2. Ford RG, Siekert RG. Central nervous system manifestations of periarteritis nodosa. Neurology 1965;15:114–22.
3. Minagar A, Fowler M, Harris MK, et al. Neurologic presentations of systemic vasculitides. Neurol Clin 2010;28:171–84.
4. Guillevin L, Mahr A, Callard P, et al. Hepatitis B virus-associated polyarteritis nodosa: clinical characteristics, outcome, and impact of treatment in 115 patients. Medicine (Baltimore) 2005;84:313–22.

5. Henegar C, Pagnoux C, Puéchal X, et al. A paradigm of diagnostic criteria for polyarteritis nodosa: analysis of a series of 949 patients with vasculitides. Arthritis Rheum 2008;58:1528–38.

6. Hernandez-Rodriguez J, Alba MA, Prieto-Gonzalez S, et al. Diagnosis and classification of polyarteritis nodosa. J Autoimmun 2014;48-49:84–9.

7. Nesher G, Oren S, Lijovetzky G, et al. Vasculitis of the temporal arteries in the young. Semin Arthritis Rheum 2009;39:96–107.

8. Lightfoot RW Jr, Michel BA, Bloch DA, et al. The American College of Rheumatology 1990 criteria for the classification of polyarteritis nodosa. Arthritis Rheum 1990;33:1088–93.

9. Jennette JC, Falk RJ, Andrassy K, et al. Nomenclature of systemic vasculitides. Proposal of an international consensus conference. Arthritis Rheum 1994;37:187–92.

10. Jennette JC, Falk RJ, Bacon PA, et al. 2012 revised International Chapel Hill Consensus Conference Nomenclature of Vasculitides. Arthritis Rheum 2013;65:1–11.

11. Collins MP, Dyck PJ, Gronseth GS, et al. Peripheral Nerve Society guidelines on the classification, diagnosis, investigation, and immunosuppressive therapy of non-systemic vasculitic neuropathy: executive summary. J Peripher Nerv Syst 2010;15:176–84.

12. Guillevin L, Lhote F. Polyarteritis nodosa and microscopic polyangiitis. Clin Exp Immunol 1995;101(Suppl 1):22–3.

13. van Rijn MJ, Ten Raa S, Hendriks JM, et al. Visceral aneurysms: old paradigms, new insights? Best Pract Res Clin Gastroenterol 2017;31:97–104.

14. Gisselbrecht M, Cohen P, Lortholary O, et al. HIV-related vasculitis: clinical presentation and therapeutic approach on six patients. AIDS 1997;11:121–3.

15. Meyts I, Aksentijevich I. Deficiency of adenosine deaminase 2 (DADA2): updates on the phenotype, genetics, pathogenesis, and treatment. J Clin Immunol 2018; 38:569–78.

16. Navon Elkan P, Pierce SB, Segel R, et al. Mutant adenosine deaminase 2 in a polyarteritis nodosa vasculopathy. N Engl J Med 2014;370:921–31.

17. Zhou Q, Yang D, Ombrello AK, et al. Early-onset stroke and vasculopathy associated with mutations in ADA2. N Engl J Med 2014;370:911–20.

18. Barron K, Ombrello A, Stone D, et al. Ho. The expanding clinical spectrum of patients with deficiency of adenosine deaminase 2 (DADA2). Arthritis Rheumatol 2018;70 [abstract: 1911].

19. Scott DG, Bacon PA, Elliott PJ, et al. Systemic vasculitis in a district general hospital 1972–1980: clinical and laboratory features, classification and prognosis of 80 cases. Q J Med 1982;51:292–311.

20. McMahon BJ, Bender TR, Templin DW, et al. Vasculitis in Eskimos living in an area hyperendemic for hepatitis B. JAMA 1980;244:2180–2.

21. Watts RA, Gonzalez-Gay MA, Lane SE, et al. Geoepidemiology of systemic vasculitis: comparison of the incidence in two regions of Europe. Ann Rheum Dis 2001;60:170–2.

22. Cohen L, Guillevin L, Meyrier A, et al. L'hypertension arterielle maligne de la periarterite noueuse. Incidence, particularites clinicobiologiques et pronostic a partir d'une serie de 165 cas. Arch Mal Coeur Vaiss 1986;79:773–8.

23. Pagnoux C, Seror R, Henegar C, et al. Clinical features and outcomes in 348 patients with polyarteritis nodosa: a systematic retrospective study of patients diagnosed between 1963 and 2005 and entered into the French Vasculitis Study Group Database. Arthritis Rheum 2010;62:616–26.

24. Pagnoux C, Mahr A, Cohen P, et al. Presentation and outcome of gastrointestinal involvement in systemic necrotizing vasculitides: analysis of 62 patients with polyarteritis nodosa, microscopic polyangiitis, Wegener granulomatosis, Churg–Strauss syndrome, or rheumatoid arthritis-associated vasculitis. Medicine (Baltimore) 2005;84:115–28.

25. Suresh E, Beadles W, Welsby P, et al. Acute pancreatitis with pseudocyst formation in a patient with polyarteritis nodosa. J Rheumatol 2005;32:386–8.

26. Holsinger DR, Osmundson PJ, Edwards JE. The heart in periarteritis nodosa. Circulation 1962;25:610–8.

27. Frohnert PP, Sheps SG. Long-term follow-up study of periarteritis nodosa. Am J Med 1967;43:8–14.

28. Moore PM, Fauci AS. Neurologic manifestations of systemic vasculitis. A retrospective and prospective study of the clinicopathologic features and responses to therapy in 25 patients. Am J Med 1981;71:517–24.

29. Bouche P, Leger JM, Travers MA, et al. Peripheral neuropathy in systemic vasculitis: clinical and electrophysiologic study of 22 patients. Neurology 1986;36: 1598–602.

30. Castaigne P, Brunet P, Hauw JJ, et al. Système nerveux périphérique et périartérite noueuse. Revue de 27 observations. Rev Neurol (Paris) 1984;140:343–52.

31. Pagnoux C, Guillevin L. Peripheral neuropathy in systemic vasculitides. Curr Opin Rheumatol 2005;17:41–8.

32. Said G. Necrotizing peripheral nerve vasculitis. Neurol Clin 1997;15:835–48.

33. Suggs SP, Thomas TD, Joy JL, et al. Vasculitic neuropathy mimicking Guillain-Barré syndrome. Arthritis Rheum 1992;35:975–8.

34. Abgrall S, Mouthon L, Cohen P, et al. Localized neurological necrotizing vasculitides. Three cases with isolated mononeuritis multiplex. J Rheumatol 2001;28: 631–3.

35. Griffin JW. Vasculitic neuropathies. Rheum Dis Clin North Am 2001;27:751–60.

36. Dyck PJ, Benstead TJ, Conn DL, et al. Nonsystemic vasculitic neuropathy. Brain 1987;110(Pt 4):843–53.

37. Lortholary O, Molinie V, Jaccard A, et al. Bladder neuropathy and gastric paralysis in polyarteritis nodosa associated with hepatitis B virus. Scand J Rheumatol 1990;19:442–3.

38. Provenzale JM, Allen NB. Neuroradiologic findings in polyarteritis nodosa. AJNR Am J Neuroradiol 1996;17:1119–26.

39. Reichart MD, Bogousslavsky J, Janzer RC. Early lacunar strokes complicating polyarteritis nodosa: thrombotic microangiopathy. Neurology 2000;54:883–9.

40. Kasantikul V, Suwanwela N, Pongsabutr S. Magnetic resonance images of brain stem infarct in periarteritis nodosa. Surg Neurol 1991;36:133–6.

41. Hsu CT, Kerrison JB, Miller NR, et al. Choroidal infarction, anterior ischemic optic neuropathy, and central retinal artery occlusion from polyarteritis nodosa. Retina 2001;21:348–51.

42. Kostina-O'Neil Y, Jirawuthiworavong GV, Podell DN, et al. Choroidal and optic nerve infarction in hepatitis C-associated polyarteritis nodosa. J Neuroophthalmol 2007;27:184–8.

43. Song JS, Lim MK, Park BH, et al. Acute pachymeningitis mimicking subdural hematoma in a patient with polyarteritis nodosa. Rheumatol Int 2005;25:637–40.

44. Dutra LA, de Souza AW, Grinberg-Dias G, et al. Central nervous system vasculitis in adults: an update. Autoimmun Rev 2017;16:123–31.

45. Oomura M, Yamawaki T, Naritomi H, et al. Polyarteritis nodosa in association with subarachnoid hemorrhage. Intern Med 2006;45:655–8.

46. Takahashi JC, Sakai N, Iihara K, et al. Subarachnoid hemorrhage from a ruptured anterior cerebral artery aneurysm caused by polyarteritis nodosa. Case report. J Neurosurg 2002;96:132–4.
47. Alhalabi M, Moore PM. Serial angiography in isolated angiitis of the central nervous system. Neurology 1994;44:1221–6.
48. Hashem H, Kelly SJ, Ganson NJ, et al. Deficiency of adenosine deaminase 2 (DADA2), an inherited cause of polyarteritis nodosa and a mimic of other systemic rheumatologic disorders. Curr Rheumatol Rep 2017;19:70.
49. Springer JM, Gierer SA, Jiang H, et al. Deficiency of adenosine deaminase 2 in adult siblings: many years of a misdiagnosed disease with severe consequences. Front Immunol 2018;9:1361.1–4.
50. Guillevin L, Pagnoux C, Seror R, et al. The Five-Factor Score revisited: assessment of prognoses of systemic necrotizing vasculitides based on the French Vasculitis Study Group (FVSG) cohort. Medicine (Baltimore) 2011;90:19–27.
51. Guillevin L, Lhote F, Gayraud M, et al. Prognostic factors in polyarteritis nodosa and Churg–Strauss syndrome. A prospective study in 342 patients. Medicine (Baltimore) 1996;75:17–28.
52. Ribi C, Cohen P, Pagnoux C, et al. Treatment of polyarteritis nodosa and microscopic polyangiitis without poor-prognosis factors: a prospective randomized study of one hundred twenty-four patients. Arthritis Rheum 2010;62:1186–97.
53. Puéchal X, Pagnoux C, Baron G, et al. Adding azathioprine to remission-induction glucocorticoids for eosinophilic granulomatosis with polyangiitis (Churg–Strauss), microscopic polyangiitis, or polyarteritis nodosa without poor prognosis factors: a randomized, controlled trial. Arthritis Rheumatol 2017;69:2175–86.
54. Guillevin L, Lhote F, Cohen P, et al. Corticosteroids plus pulse cyclophosphamide and plasma exchanges versus corticosteroids plus pulse cyclophosphamide alone in the treatment of polyarteritis nodosa and Churg–Strauss syndrome patients with factors predicting poor prognosis. A prospective, randomized trial in sixty-two patients. Arthritis Rheum 1995;38:1638–45.
55. Samson M, Puéchal X, Devilliers H, et al. Long-term follow-up of a randomized trial on 118 patients with polyarteritis nodosa or microscopic polyangiitis without poor-prognosis factors. Autoimmun Rev 2014;13:197–205.
56. Samson M, Puéchal X, Devilliers H, et al. Mononeuritis multiplex predicts the need for immunosuppressive or immunomodulatory drugs for EGPA, PAN and MPA patients without poor-prognosis factors. Autoimmun Rev 2014;13:945–53.

Autoimmune Encephalitides

David S. Younger, MD, MPH, MS[a,b,*]

KEYWORDS

- Autoimmune • Encephalitides • Hashimoto encephalopathy
- Central nervous system vasculitis

KEY POINTS

- Autoimmune encephalitis is a severe inflammatory disorder of the brain with diverse causes and a complex differential diagnosis including central nervous system vasculitis, and autoimmune encephalitis associated with serum and intrathecal antibodies to intracellular and surface neuronal antigens against constituents of the limbic system neuropil.
- This association has led to a reconsideration of several neuropsychiatric and neurocognitive disorders as having shared mechanisms of origin.
- The successful use of serum and intrathecal antibodies to diagnose affected patients, and their subsequent improvement with effective treatment, has resulted in few biopsy and postmortem examinations.
- In those available, there can be variable infiltrating inflammatory T cells with cytotoxic granules in close apposition to neurons, analogous to microscopic vasculitis.
- One particular type of autoimmune encephalitis is associated with Hashimoto thyroiditis and uniquely associated with true central nervous system vasculitis.

INTRODUCTION

According to Dalmau,[1] myasthenia gravis and Lambert-Eaton myasthenic syndrome are 2 prototypical B-cell peripheral nervous system disorders with targeted antibodies to acetylcholine receptors and voltage-gated calcium channels resulting from disturbed B-cell immunity. In the central nervous system (CNS), paraneoplastic disorders were analogously associated with onconeural antibodies, cross-reactive with tumor nuclear and cytoplasmic neuronal antigens, and mediated by cytotoxic T-cells. In solving the mystery of the large group of undiagnosed neuropsychiatric disorders leading to autoimmune encephalitis (AE) and limbic

Disclosure: The author has nothing to disclose.
[a] Department of Neurology, Division of Neuro-Epidemiology, New York University School of Medicine, New York, NY 10016, USA; [b] School of Public Health, City University of New York, New York, NY, USA
* 333 East 34th Street, 1J, New York, NY 10016.
E-mail address: youngd01@nyu.edu
Website: http://www.davidsyounger.com

encephalitis (LE), investigators returned to the laboratory to study patterns of newly recognized autoantibodies that recognized surface antigen (SAg) and intracellular antigen (IAg) of the brain neuropil.[2,3] The successful use of serum and intrathecal antibodies to diagnose affected patients, and their subsequent improvement with effective treatment, resulted in few CNS tissue biopsy and postmortem examinations. However, in those available, the associated histopathology appeared to result from infiltrating inflammatory T-cells, with cytotoxic granules in close apposition to neurons, analogous but distinct from microscopic vasculitis. With the ease of screening the serum and cerebrospinal fluid (CSF) from a panel of pathogenic autoantibodies, and obtaining detailed morphologic and metabolic images of the brain specific for the disorders, AE is included in the differential diagnosis of adult primary angiitis of the CNS (PACNS) and childhood PACNS (cPACNS).[4–7] This article reviews the historical background, epidemiology, clinical presentation, laboratory evaluation, histopathology, diagnosis, and management of autoimmune encephalitides relevant to CNS vasculitis, in particular Hashimoto encephalopathy (HE).

BACKGROUND

Corsellis and colleagues[8] coined LE, noting a relation to bronchial cancer in 3 patients in the sixth to eighth decades of life. All 3 cases had subacute temporal lobe seizures, neuropsychiatric disturbances, and memory disturbances for 2 years before death. Postmortem examination revealed inflammatory lesions in limbic gray-matter sections of the brain, notably in medial temporal lobe structures, including the hippocampal gyrus. Case 2 had an undifferentiated nonmetastatic lung carcinoma removed 6 months after onset of neurologic symptoms, whereas 2 others had unsuspected cancer at postmortem examination. Case 1 had a bronchial carcinoma restricted to a mediastinal lymph node without a primary lesion, whereas case 3 had an unsuspected oat cell carcinoma infiltrating the main bronchi of both lungs and adjacent mediastinal nodes. Attention turned away from LE and toward neurologic autoimmune paraneoplastic syndromes with the discovery of several neuronal target antigens including Hu (ANNA-1), responsible for paraneoplastic encephalomyelitis[9] in association with small cell lung cancer (SCLC); Ri (ANNA-2) responsible for paraneoplastic cerebellar degeneration[10] and motor neuronopathy[11] in association with breast cancer; and PCA-1 responsible for paraneoplastic cerebellar degeneration[12] in association with gynecologic tumors. Other autoantibodies included anti-MA1 and MA2 and testicular cancer, and the collapsin response mediator protein-5 (CRMP5/Cv2) in association with thymoma.[13,14] Each with an intracellular target antigen, the resultant histopathology of these antibodies consisted of infiltrative cytotoxic (CD8+) T-cell destruction of neurons, with variable immunoglobulin G (IgG) and complement deposits in the CNS, with fewer helper (CD4+) T-cells, and generally absent B-cells. The role of infiltrating CD8+ T-cells in cell death was suggested by its close apposition to neurons.[15]

Bien and colleagues[16] revisited noncancerous cases of LE in its relation to temporal lobe epilepsy, whereas the interface of strictly paraneoplastic and autoimmune mechanisms was highlighted by recognition of patients with stiff person syndrome (SPS) in association with glutamic acid decarboxylase (GAD) antibodies; and neurologic syndromes associated with voltage-gated potassium channel (VGKC)–complex antibodies. Nonparaneoplastic CNS autoimmunity was investigated in a patient with SPS, epilepsy, and type-1 diabetes (T1D), and increased titers of oligoclonal CSF

IgG,[17] in whom serum and CSF produced identical intense staining of all gray-matter regions. GAD65 was an important autoantigen in T1D, being highly expressed in the cytoplasm of pancreatic β cells. However, only patients with very high titers of GAD were associated with LE; they typically presented with recent-onset temporal lobe epilepsy (TLE) and intrathecal secretion defining a form of nonparaneoplastic LE. Other patients within the SPS spectrum harbored antibodies against other proteins of the GABAergic synapse associated with lymphoma, and malignant tumors of the breast, colon, lung, and thymus.[18]

The clinical phenotypes associated with autoantibodies to VGKC complex ranging from peripheral nerve hyperexcitability (PNH) to Morvan syndrome (MoS) and LE and autoimmune epilepsy[19,20] were described in 2 patients with reversible LE.[21] By 2010, Graus and colleagues[22] had classified neuronal antibodies associated with syndromes resulting from CNS neuronal dysfunction into 2 groups according to the location of the target antigen. One group of well-characterized autoantibodies recognized onconeuronal IAg antigens, including Ri, Yo, Hu, Ma2, CRMP5/Cv2, and GAD, that were useful in the designation of a specific paraneoplastic neurologic disorder. Bien and colleagues[23] described qualitative and quantitative immunopathologic features of biopsy or postmortem brain tissue in 17 cases of AE associated with IAg (Hu, Ma2, GAD) or SAg (VGKC-C and N-methyl-D-aspartate receptor [NMDAR]). Their studies noted higher CD8+/CD3+ ratio and more frequent appositions of granzyme-B (GrB) (+) cytotoxic T-cells to neurons, with associated cell loss in the IAg-onconeural group compared with those in the SAg group. The exceptions were GAD cases that showed less intense inflammation and low CD8/CD3 ratios compared with the IAg-onconeural cases. A role for T-cell–mediated neuronal cytotoxicity was found in LE associated with IAg-directed autoantibodies, whereas a complement-mediated humoral immune mechanism was suggested in VDKC-complex encephalitis. There was apparent absence of both mechanisms in NMDA receptor encephalitis.

Bauer and Bien[24] suggested that neurodegeneration in brains of patients with antibodies against IAg was not simply induced by antibody reactivity with the target antigen but rather by the inflammatory T-cells. To be pathogenic, the imputed antibody had to first transit the blood-brain barrier (BBB) and the cell membrane of the target cell to a location where it could bind the pathogenic IAg. Depending on protein conformation and folding, the antigenic site might be readily accessible before inactivation and ensuing irreparable cell damage. A major concern in managing these disorders has not only been prompt treatment of the tumor but commencement of effective immunotherapy targeting mainly cytotoxic T-cells.[25] Vasculitis is not a recognized mechanism of injury in intraneuronal antibodies, either in life or at postmortem examination. The exception is the dubious association of extralimbic AE in association with increased serum GAD antibody levels suggested by Najjar and colleagues. A 31-year-old man had new onset of tonic-clonic seizures in association with an enhancing right anterior frontal lobe lesion on brain MRI and irregularity of the distal frontal right middle cerebral artery branches on cerebral angiography. Brain biopsy showed perivascular and intramural inflammation associated with microglia and histiocytic nodules. Serum GAD antibodies tested 6 months after treatment with oral corticosteroids and high-dose intravenous immunoglobulin (IVIg) therapy were increased 20-fold.

The past decade has witnessed the emergence of serum autoantibodies against SAg and synaptic-enriched regions leading to LE that spares the cytoplasm and nuclei of neurons.[26–29] Supportive of LE or AE, these new antibodies share the property of strong immunolabeling of areas of dense dendritic network and synaptic-enriched regions in the neuropil of hippocampus. The clinical phenotype associated with novel neuropil antibodies includes dominant behavioral and psychiatric symptoms and seizures but with inconstant features of cognition and memory, and brain MRI and 2-deoxy-2-[fluorine-18] fluoro-D-glucose (^{18}F-FDG) PET abnormalities that defined a neuronal tropism for structures associated with the medial temporal lobe.

In retrospect, a role for autoimmune dysfunction in neuropsychiatric illness had been sought since the 1930s, when autoantibodies were first reported in a schizophrenia patient.[30] Since then, there have been reports of specific autoimmune responses to self-antigens in psychosis, affective disorders, and other neurobehavioral and neurocognitive disturbances[31–33] endogenous to the limbic system of the temporal lobe, which includes hippocampal connections to other brain regions. The hippocampus is a highly plastic, stress-sensitive region that plays a central role in mood disorders and the consolidation and transformation of discrete short-term memories and long-term cortical storage.[34] In particular, normal regulation of mood depends on the integrity of brain circuits, including the orbitofrontal-amygdala network, which supports emotions and moods, whereas the hippocampal-cingulate system supports the encoding of memory using all major neurotransmitters, including glutamate, γ-aminobutyric acid, acetylcholine, noradrenalin, and serotonin. Maintenance of the delicate balance of intact cell signaling and neurotransmitter balance seems to be most important in optimal hippocampal functioning. Animal models of major depressive disorder support a role for antidepressant medications as neuroprotective agents because of their effect on the induction of neuronal sprouting, whereas neurogenesis seems to be linked to the enhanced expression of brain-derived nerve growth factor associated with developmental stresses such as early-life maternal separation.[35] Long-term treatment with antidepressant medications is thought to act on monoamine systems neurotransmitter systems that increase cyclic adenosine monophosphate (cAMP)–dependent phosphorylation, and the upregulation of cAMP response element–binding protein (CREB) messenger RNA levels, dysfunction of which has also been implicated in MDD.[36] MRI fused with ^{18}F-FDG-PET and volumetric analysis have been used to study hippocampal morphology and metabolism revealing reduced hippocampal volume,[37] all of which seem to predict vulnerability to neuropsychiatric disturbances[38]. The mechanisms by which genetic vulnerability, early disturbed CNS neurodevelopment, infection, trauma, and neuroinflammation confer a vulnerability to mood disorders and neurocognitive disturbances are not well understood.

AUTOIMMUNE LIMBIC ENCEPHALITIDES

Three autoantibodies found in children and adults with LE target intracellular GAD65, and surface antigens of the NMDAR and VGKC complex. Classically, the associated symptoms, which evolve over days to weeks, include short-term memory loss, sleep disturbances, seizures, irritability, depression, hallucinations, and personality change.

Anti–Glutamic Acid Decarboxylase 65 Encephalitis

Autoimmunity targeting the 65-kDa isoform of GAD65 encompass diverse autoimmune disorders such as T1D and rare neurologic disorders including LE, TLE, cerebellar ataxia, and large and small fiber peripheral and autonomic neuropathy.[39] A review of adult-onset SPS showed a prevalence estimate of 1 in 1.25 million[40] with a predominance of women, and average age of onset of 40 years. The frequency of high titers of anti-GAD antibodies defined a radioimmunoassay (RIA) value greater than 1000 IU/mL in TLE of unknown origin is 21%[41] of cases, with the highest titers related to TLE. Affected patients are typically women with T1D, early-onset epilepsy, and concomitant hypothyroidism, psoriatic arthritis, and Celiac disease, a third of whom reported onset of LE as the predominant feature, with supportive findings of amygdala and hippocampus signal intensities on brain MRI, and medial temporal hypometabolism on FDG brain PET. The levels of anti-GAD ranged from 1207 to 87,510 IU/mL, with absent oligoclonal bands (OCBs), and a ratio of serum/CSF GAD antibody levels greater than 1 suggesting intrathecal synthesis. Malter and colleagues[42] estimated the prevalence of GAD antibodies in LE to be 17%, noting a subgroup of patients with TLE who had very high titers equivalent to those with SPS, medial temporal inflammation on MRI, and concomitant LE. In the TLE cohort, GAD antibody encephalitis proved to be as common as VGKC-complex antibodies but differed in younger age, female sex, presentation of first seizure, CSF OCBs, and intrathecal autoantibody synthesis. Patients with high levels of GAD antibodies, and classic or other neurologic syndromes not typically associated with GAD antibodies were at higher risk for an underlying cancer.

Gagnon and Savard[43] reviewed the clinical experience of 58 cases of GAD65-antibody LE beginning with the first reported case[44] and inclusively through 2016, in 7 observational studies, 3 case series, and 21 published case reports, providing a useful summary of the literature of anti-GAD65–associated LE. Diabetes alone, generally T1D, was noted in 50% of cases, in association with thyroiditis, diabetes, celiac disease, psoriasis, and common variable immune deficiency respectively in 73%, 18%, 9%, and 9%. Cancer was noted in 6 (10%) cases, including 4 SCLC and 2 malignant thymomas, generally in men of mean age 61 years (range, 38–70 years). The commonest presenting clinical features were seizures in 56 (97%) cases, most commonly refractory status epilepticus; cognitive impairment in 38 (59%), mainly affecting memory, language, executive function, and attention; psychiatric symptoms in 16 (28%) cases, most commonly depression, behavior, perception, and anxiety. The most common seizure presentation was refractory status epilepticus.

Low titers of anti-GAD65 antibodies, generally less than 20 nmol/L, occur in T1D and in the general population, whereas cases of anti-GAD65–associated neurologic disorders, including LE, are seen in the hundreds of nanomoles per liter. GAD65 is located predominantly in nerve terminals anchored to the cytoplasm-facing side of synaptic vesicles where it thought to synthesize GABA for neurotransmission supplementary to basal levels. The classification of high titers of anti-GAD65 autoantibodies has been problematic in being grouped with onconeural autoantibodies.

The dominant clinical phenotype of seizures, neurocognitive disturbances, and neuropsychiatric disturbances in most patients with anti-GAD autoantibody–associated LE is explained by the frequent involvement of the medial temporal lobes; an inflammatory CSF with intrathecal secretion of the anti-GAD65 autoantibody, and OCBs. Bien and colleagues[45] described a 24-year-old woman with frequent temporal lobe seizures, nonparaneoplastic LE, and a serum anti-GAD65 antibody titer of 1:32,000, in whom T_2/fluid-attenuated inversion recovery (FLAIR) MRI evolved over a period of 8 months, showing right hippocampal swelling and signal increase to sclerosis and atrophy on MRI commensurate with clinical progression. Among 58 literature patients,[43] 45 out of 58 (78%) patient MRIs were abnormal, with specific involvement of the temporal lobes in 34 (59%), and multifocal abnormalities in 9 (16%); 7 patient MRIs were normal. The results of electroencephalography (EEG), available in 35 cases, showed epileptiform discharges in 27 (77%) and focal temporal involvement in 19 (70%). Lumbar CSF was studied in 41 cases, showed pleocytosis in 11 (27%) with white blood cell (WBC) counts ranging from 7 to 114 cells/μL, and present OCBs in one-half of cases. There were significantly increased titers of anti-GAD65 antibodies in both serum and CSF in 35 patients, and in either serum (in 18) or CSF alone in 3.

Bien and colleagues[23,45] summarized the histopathologic features of selective resection of the sclerotic hippocampus in a patient, which included neuronal loss and astrogliosis and a strong accumulation of inflammatory cells in the resected hippocampus. There was marked invasion of the hippocampus by lymphocytes, which were mainly CD8+ T-cells with the cytotoxic effector molecule GrB, in addition to CD20+ B-cells and CD138+ plasma cells. The pattern of pyramidal cell loss was severe in sectors CA4 and CA3, with selective sparing of CA1 and CA2. Surviving neurons were positive for major histocompatibility complex class I, fulfilling the prerequisite for attack by CD8+ T-cells. The investigators[23] quantitated the number of parenchymal T-, B-, and plasma cells; macrophages; and glial cells in 3 cases of anti-GAD65 autoantibody LE, which included a previously reported case,[40] differentiating them from the IAg-onconeural cases (Ma2 in 3 cases; Hu in 4 cases); SAg types associated with VGKC complex (4 cases) and NMDA receptor (3 cases); and Rasmussen encephalitis (22 cases) and neurodegeneration controls (25 cases). The percentage of CD8 T cells in the IAg-GAD cases was intermediate (54%) between the IAg-onconeural and SAg cases. The CD8+/CD3+ ratio of the SAg cases was significantly different from the Rasmussen encephalitis controls. Apposition of multiple GrB+ lymphocytes to single neurons was consistent with a specific cytotoxic T-cell attack in case GAD/3. Bien and colleagues[23] noted diffuse cytoplasmic IgG detected by anti–human IgG in both neurons and astrocytes in all cases similar to that of controls, which they attributed to leakiness of damaged neuronal membranes. Staining of C9neo indicating complement activation was negative in the IAg-GAD cases.

The diagnosis of anti-GAD LE should be considered in patients with a clinical syndrome of temporal lobe seizures, cognitive and psychiatric disturbances, and brain MRI abnormalities on T_2FLAIR MRI implicating the medial temporal lobes; CSF pleocytosis, present OCB; and an EEG revealing temporal lobe epileptic or slow-wave activity in association with high levels of anti-GAD65 autoantibodies on RIA. In the case series summarized by Gagnon and Savard,[43] full recovery was noted in 8% of patients who were treated with corticosteroids alone, with IVIg, or in combination with plasma exchange (PE), as well as another who received no immunosuppressant therapy and recovered. Death occurred in 8% of patients, several of whom had an associated cancer. Sustained improvement was noted 43% of cases with follow-up of 8 years.

There are unsubstantiated cases of biopsy-proven seronegative encephalitis reported by Najjar and colleagues[46,47] in association with isolated neuropsychiatric disorders with a questionable relationship to prototypical AE.

Anti–N-Methyl-D-aspartate Receptor Encephalitis

Dalmau and Bataller[48] identified a new CNS antigen as NR1/NR2B12 heteromers of the NMDAR with predominantly neuropsychiatric symptoms from a cohort of 526 cases of noninfectious LE with antibodies against CNS proteins. The anti-NMDA antibody seems to play a critical role in synaptic plasticity and memory. Although anti-NMDA receptor encephalitis is not by definition associated with cancer, 59% of patients had a tumor, most commonly benign-appearing cystic mature or immature teratoma tumors of the ovary. All showed serum or CSF antibodies to the NMDAR. A year later, the same investigators[26] described a case series of 100 patients with antibodies against NR1-NR2 heteromers of the NMDAR as measured by enzyme-linked immunosorbent assay (ELISA), 91 of whom were women, all with psychiatric symptoms or memory complaints. Seizures were seen in 76 patients; 88 were unresponsive or had altered consciousness, 86 had dyskinesias, 69 had autonomic instability, and 66 showed hypoventilation. Three-quarters presented initially to a psychiatric service.

Given its characteristic disease course, it is assumed that a relevant proportion of patients previously diagnosed with encephalitis of unknown origin have anti-NMDAR encephalitis,[49] representing about 1% of all young patients' admissions to intensive care units (ICUs). A French study[50] noted a frequency of anti-NMDAR encephalitis of 2% in febrile encephalitis, which may be an underestimate because it excluded children. A multicenter, population-based, prospective study showed that anti-NMDAR encephalitis accounted for 4% of case of encephalitis in the United Kingdom, making it the most common cause of AE after acute demyelinating encephalomyelitis (ADEM) in children.[51]

Clinically, anti-NMDAR encephalitis commences with nonspecific prodromal symptoms of headache, fever, nausea, or viral-infection–like illness,[52] but over days to weeks, seizures and neurocognitive and neurobehavioral complaints emerge, including memory loss and frank neuropsychiatric manifestations of insomnia, mania, anxiety, depression, and paranoia.[53,54] There can be movement disorders with orolingual-facial dyskinesia, autonomic manifestations, central hypoventilation, tachycardia, and bradycardia. The eventual outcome is favorable in up to three-quarters of all patients, who recover and have mild deficits with immunotherapy, whereas one-quarter have severe persistent deficits or die. Relapses in 25% to 30% of cases[55] are partly attributed to lack of treatment, whereas 12% of treated cases relapsed in the first 2 years in one long-term outcome cohort analysis.[56]

Most patients with anti-NMDAR encephalitis have intrathecal synthesis of antibodies and numerous CD 138+ antibody–secreting plasma cells in perivascular, interstitial, and Virchow-Robin spaces with complement-fixing IgG and IgG3 sub-types, as well as B- and T-cells in perivascular regions. Complement-mediated mechanisms in anti-NMDA receptor encephalitis studied in cultured rat hippocampal neurons tested for complement fixation[57] show complement binding in vitro, although not in the brains of affected patients.

Testing for NMDAR antibodies is recommended in patients who manifest encephalitic signs, psychiatric symptoms, seizures, and CSF inflammation, after exclusion of viral and bacterial causes of infection regardless of neuroradiologic investigation because the disorder may be associated with normal MRI findings in up to 50% of cases. The remaining one-half include nonspecific changes and abnormal T_2/FLAIR MRI hyperintensities in the mesial temporal lobe, cerebral or cerebellar cortex, basal ganglia, or brainstem. FDG brain PET shows hypermetabolism or hypometabolism in the affected regions.[58] Up to 25% of patients have electrographic seizures. CSF analysis can show moderate lymphocytic pleocytosis, increased protein content, increased IgG index, and CSF-specific OCBs, which are typically negative at first testing, but can become positive later with disease progression in up to one-half of cases.

The histopathologic aspects of NMDAR encephalitis were studied in 14 cases, including 9 at postmortem examination and 5 in brain biopsy tissue. Dalmau and colleagues[59] described 12 women with prominent psychiatric symptoms, amnesia, seizures, dyskinesia, autonomic dysfunction, and altered consciousness. All had serum/CSF antibodies that immunolabeled the neuropil of hippocampus/forebrain, in particular the cell surface of hippocampal neurons, and reacted with NR2B, and to a lesser extent NR2A, subunits of the NMDA receptor. NR2B binds glutamate and forms heteromers (NR1/NR2B or NR1/NR2A/NR2B) that are preferentially expressed in the adult hippocampus/forebrain. Expression of functional heteromers, and no single subunits, was required for antibody binding. The CSF and serum of all

12 patients showed a distinctive pattern of reactivity with the neuropil of rat hippocampus, and the immunolabeling predominantly occurred with the cell membrane of neurons and was intense in the molecular layer of the hippocampus. Three patients, aged 14, 24, and 35 years (cases 2, 6, 10) died, including 1 (case 10) previously reported,[60] 3 to 6 months after symptom presentation. MRI showed T_2/FLAIR hyperintensities in the medial temporal lobes (case 2), hyperintensity of the parietal sulci and enhancement of overlying meninges (case 6), and a third (case 10) showed normal findings. CSF in all 3 showed pleocytosis varying from 115 (case 10) to 219 WBCs (case 6) with minimally increased or normal protein content, and positive OCBs. Immunofluorescence microscopy experiments showed colocalization of antigens reacting with patient antisera and antibodies against NR2B, and colocalization of these antibodies in patients' tumor samples and in brain. Postmortem examination showed extensive gliosis, rare T-cell infiltrates, and neuronal degeneration predominantly involving, but not restricted to, the hippocampus in all 3. Microglial nodules and neuronophagia were rarely seen. In all cases, these findings predominated in the hippocampus, where there was intense IgG immunostaining.

The main epitope targeted by the antibodies is the extracellular N-terminal domain of the NR1 subunit. Patients' antibodies decrease the numbers of cell-surface NMDAR and clusters in postsynaptic dendrites, an effect that is reversed by antibody removal. Tüzün and colleagues[61] extended the immunopathologic analysis of cases 6 and 10 reported previously by Dalmau and colleagues,[59] noting that lymphocytic infiltrates were uncommon, being rarely noted in the perivascular and leptomeningeal regions, and scarcely distributed in brain parenchyma. CD20+ B-cells and CD79a plasma cells were identified in the perivascular space, including 1% cytotoxic T-cells and absence of GrB+, Fas, and Fas ligand–positive cells. IgG, including deposits, was noted in all areas of the CNS but most intensely in the hippocampus. Using HEK293 cells expressing NR1/NR2B, the NMDAR IgG were mainly IgG_1 but included IgG_2 and IgG_3 types.

Camdessanché and colleagues[62] reported the postmortem findings of a brain biopsy specimen from an 18-year-old woman with NMDAR encephalitis who presented with subacute mood changes and facial jerks. Brain MRI showed foci of T_2 hyperintensities in the right frontal lobe, and CSF showed 21 WBCs and OCBs. The frontal lobe showed perivascular cuffing of CD20+ B-cells and a few CD138+ plasma cells, with few CD3+ T-cells or CD68+ macrophages scattered throughout gray and white matter and in perivascular spaces. Retrospective screening for anti-NMDAR antibodies was performed on a CSF sample that was positive at a dilution of 1:10, both in the neuropil of the rat hippocampus and in transfected HEK293 cells.

Martinez-Hernandez and colleagues[57] described 2 male patients, aged 7 and 59 years, and 3 female patients aged 5, 24, and 35 years, the last 2 with ovarian teratomas and anti-NMDAR encephalitis, who presented with subacute short-term memory deficits, psychiatric disturbances, seizures, movement disorders, and dysautonomia ranging from 22 days to 4 months. CSF showed increased protein levels ranging from 94 to 219 mg/dL with OCBs, and brain MRI showed increased FLAIR signal in medial temporal lobes (case 1), parietal cortex (case 2), and left temporal cortex (case 3), in the insula and anterior temporal lobes with atrophy in another (case 5). Brain MRI was normal in case 4. Treatment with combined immunotherapy in 1 patient who underwent a brain biopsy was effective, whereas the others died. One patient who died underwent earlier brain biopsy, and the remaining 3 patients were studied at postmortem examination. Patients' antibodies were able to fix complement on cultures of rat hippocampal neuron but this was not detected in any of the brain regions of

3 patients, or in biopsies of 2 patients, all with anti-NMDAR encephalitis. The main histologic findings were an abundance of infiltrating CD138+ plasma cells and plasmablasts in perivascular regions cuffing blood vessels, Virchow-Robin spaces, and lining the meningeal-brain surface in proximity to the CSF.

Bien and colleagues[23] examined brain biopsy tissue from 2 women and 1 man, aged 17 to 22 years with NMDAR encephalitis, all 3 with encephalopathy lasting 2 months to 12 months, none with an associated tumor. Two were treated with immunotherapy before frontal (2 patients) or temporal lobe cortical biopsy. Serial MRI in 1 patient did not show hippocampal atrophy. Histopathology of the tissue specimens showed low density of T cells, in the range of neurodegeneration controls. The ratio of perivascular CD8+/CD3+ was slightly increased, and there were cytotoxic granules in some parenchymal T cells, but no apposition of CD8++ T-cells to single neurons. Diffuse cytoplasmic IgG was evident in both neurons and astrocytes and C9neo deposition was present in the cytoplasm and on the surface of hippocampal CA4, dentate, and cortical neurons. The neocortex of NMDAR antibody–positive patients showed almost no inflammation, and no clear signs of neuronal loss. Even though NMDA receptor antibodies seemed to be involved in the clinical disease process, there was no evidence to suggest a classic mechanism of cytotoxic T-cell or humoral immune-mediated neuronal cell death. The possibility that a more active inflammatory infiltrate or antibody deposition could be found at an earlier disease stage in both the hippocampus and cortex could not be excluded, although it was striking that MRI evidence of inflammation in the hippocampus was rare.

Collectively, the histopathologic findings were consistent with a selective and reversible decrease in NMDAR surface density and synaptic localization that correlated with patients' antibody titers. The mechanism of this decrease was selective antibody-mediated capping and internalization of surface NMDARs, which was supported by the experimental finding of Hughes and colleagues[63] who studied Fab fragments prepared from patients' antibodies that did not decrease surface receptor density. Subsequent cross-linking with anti-Fab antibodies recapitulated the decrease caused by intact patient NMDA receptor antibodies. These cellular mechanisms seem to be the cause of the specific titer-dependent and reversible loss of NMDARs. The loss of the subtype of glutamate receptors that eliminates NMDAR–mediated synaptic function may underlie the learning, memory, and other behavioral deficits observed in affected patients.

Suggested criteria for the definite diagnosis of anti-NMDAR LE[3] include the presence of IgG anti-GluN1 antibodies in a suspected patient with subacute onset of psychiatric behavior or cognitive disturbances, seizures, movement disorder, and autonomic dysfunction; abnormal EEG that shows focal or diffuse slowing or epileptic activity; and CSF pleocytosis or OCBs. Prompt diagnosis of anti-NMDAR encephalitis leads to improvement typically after removal and treatment of an offending cancer, or in the absence thereof. The demonstration of copious infiltrates of antibody-secreting cells in the CNS of affected patients provides an explanation for the intrathecal synthesis of antibodies, and implications for treatment used to arrest and reverse the disorder using IVIg, corticosteroids, cyclophosphamide, or rituximab.

It is now assumed that a relevant proportion of patients previously diagnosed with encephalitis of unknown origin would have anti-NMDAR encephalitis,[49] representing about 1% of all young patients' admissions to ICU. A French study[50] noted a frequency of anti-NMDAR encephalitis of 2% in febrile encephalitis, which could be an underestimate because of the exclusion of children. A multicenter population-based prospective study showed that anti-NDMAR encephalitis accounted for 4%

of case of encephalitis in the United Kingdom, making it the most common cause of AE after ADEM in children.[51]

Anti–Voltage-gated Potassium Channel Complex Encephalitis

About the same time that MoS was described, anti–VGKC complex antibodies were determined using RIA in patients with noninfectious AE.[19] Although the disorder was generally termed LE, the term limbic encephalopathy was also used because more patients were found to be seropositive without evidence of classic features of hyperintense signal in the medial temporal lobes on brain MRI, and CSF inflammation.[19] Autoantibodies against the VGKC complex detected by RIA in the sera of patients with AE did not bind directly to VGKC-complex channel proteins proper, but instead to synaptic and axonal neuronal proteins that coprecipitated with detergent-solubilized VGKC.[64,65]

Attention has focused on identifying the principal autoantigens in the VGKC complex and expanding the spectrum of corresponding phenotypes. Initial reports[66,67] suggested that patients' antibodies were bound to the VGKCs Kv1.1 and Kv1.2. Subsequent studies showed that leucine-rich glioma-inactivated protein 1 (LGI1), and contactin-associated protein–like 2 (CASPR2) were the main autoantigens[64,65] and associated with transiently expressed axonal glycoprotein (TAG1), postsynaptic density protein-*Drosophila* disc large tumor suppressor-zonula occludens-1 protein (PDZ), and the ankyrin-spectrin protein in both the PNS and CNS. Antibodies against contactin-2 usually occur in association with those targeting LGI1 or Caspr2 and were identified in other disorders, raising doubts about their importance. There is a diversity and overlap of neurologic phenotypes associated with VGKC complex IgG in the serum and CSF, and distinct immunoglobulin-subtype specificity. The commonest presentation of VGKC-complex autoantibodies is LE in the CNS, and neuromyotonia or MoS in the periphery.

In the United Kingdom, where the incidence of encephalitis is estimated at 5.23 cases per 100,000 population per year based on admissions to the National Health Service between 2005 and 2009, Granerod and colleagues[68] estimated the incidence of encephalitis as 4.32 cases/100,000/y. A capture-recapture model estimated the incidence of encephalitis to be 8.66 cases/100,000/y. Two percent of patients (n = 216) had more than 1 encephalitis admission during the study period, and the incidence did not change (4.20 cases/100,000/y) when subsequent admissions of these patients were excluded from the analysis. By using data restricted to the primary diagnostic field, the overall mean incidence was 2.75 cases/100,000/y (95% confidence interval, 2.39–3.10 cases/100,000/y). The results of multivariable analyses showed that, compared with 2005 to 2006, incidences in all subsequent years were slightly higher but with little evidence of a trend (P = .19). The incidence rate was highest among patients less than 1 year of age and in those greater than 65 years of age. A retrospective study that reviewed antibodies to VGKC, LGI1, and CASPR2 in 46 children with severe acute encephalitis identified only 1 affected child (2.2%) among 46 children.[69]

Among 64 patients with VGKC-complex encephalitis,[70] the clinical features included neuropsychiatric features, disorientation, confusion, or amnesia in 100% of patients; tonic-clonic seizures in 92%; delusions in 21%; hallucinations in 17%; agitation in 6%; pain in 4.7%; and peripheral neuropathy in 1.6% of cases. Neurocognitive complaints, psychiatric symptoms, and seizures typical evolve over days to weeks, occasionally acutely, but more often insidiously over months before coming to medical attention. Flanagan and colleagues[71] studied the finding of an apparent dementia in 72 affected patients. Responsiveness to immunosuppressant and immunomodulatory therapy was predicted by seropositivity for neuronal VGKC-complex antibody more than calcium channel or neuronal acetylcholine receptor (P = .01). Up to 40% of patients may also manifest frontal lobe and frank psychiatric features. Parthasarathi and colleagues[72] described a 58-year-old man with panic attacks and psychogenic non-epileptic seizures who later developed delusions and hallucinations followed by confusion. He was found to have VGKC-complex antibodies and was treated with immunomodulatory therapy leading to near-complete recovery. Bettcher and colleagues[73] delineated cognitive strengths and weaknesses among 12 patients with VGKC-complex encephalitis, noting mild to moderate impairment in memory and executive functions, with variable impairments in language and sparing of visuospatial skills that correlated with MRI findings of T_2/FLAIR hyperintensities in medial temporal lobe (10 out of 10) and basal ganglia (2 out of 10). Serial cognitive examination revealed heterogeneity in cognitive function.

Seizures occur in 90% of cases and are most commonly focal, with infrequent generalization, manifesting typical medial temporal lobe signature with hand and orofacial automatisms. Three seizure semiologies, ictal bradycardia, piloerection, and fasciobrachial dystonic seizures (FBDS), show a strong association to LE associated with LGI1 antibodies. FBDSs consist of brief frequent episodes of abnormal unilateral and bilateral movements of the arms, sometimes the ipsilateral muscles of the face, and more rarely the leg. Video EEG shows an epileptic origin of these myocloniclike movements; however, regular EEG with scalp electrodes often misses an interictal focus. If FBDSs are recognized early, and serum LGI1 antibodies are detected, immunotherapy prevents progression to frank LE, which in one study arose after a median delay of 36 days. Kalachikov and colleagues[74] described autosomal dominant lateral temporal epilepsy (ADLTE) characterized by partial seizures and preceding auditory signs in the LGI1/*epitempin* gene expressed on chromosome 10q24. Mutations in this gene introduce premature stop codons and prevent production of full-length protein from the affected allele. Although LGI1 haploinsufficiency causes ADLTE, the underlying molecular mechanism that results in abnormal brain excitability has instead been attributed to dysregulation of synaptic α-amino-3-hydroxy-5-methyl-4-isoxazolepropionic acid receptors (AMPARs) in hippocampal neurons in the epileptic LGI1 knockout mouse.[75] Fukata and colleagues[76] proposed that extracellularly secreted LGI1 linking 2 epilepsy-related brain receptors, a disintegrin and metalloproteinase domain 22 (ADAM22) and ADAM23, organize a transsynaptic protein complex that includes presynaptic potassium channels and postsynaptic AMPA receptor scaffolds. The lack of LGI1 disrupts this synaptic protein connection and selectively reduces AMPA receptor–mediated synaptic transmission in the hippocampus.

Younger[77] described new-onset FBDS and memory disturbances in association with distal large and painful small fiber peripheral neuropathy and dysautonomia without systemic malignancy in a patient with extrathecal VGKC-complex antibody production. Epidermal nerve fiber studies confirmed small fiber neuropathy in association with abnormal autonomic laboratory testing.

Neuropathic pain as a manifestation of VGKC-complex autoimmunity was noted in 316 (4%) of 1992 patients evaluated neurologically at a tertiary referral center[78] and was typically subacute in onset, nociceptive, regional, or diffuse. In cases suspected of peripheral neuropathy with mild subjective loss of temperature and pain attributed to small fiber dysfunction, electrodiagnostic studies show variable minor reduction of sural sensory nerve action potential amplitudes with motor hyperexcitability. The VGKC-complex antibody titers were often low (0.02–0.1 nM) and antibodies to GLI1 or CASPR2 were present in 28% overall, with the latter most common (7%).

Autonomic involvement was noted in 29% of the cohort studied by Klein and colleagues,[78] and in 3 (60%) of the patients described by Lahoria and colleagues.[79] Hypothermia was described in association with VGKC-complex antibody–associated LE in 4 patients,[22] 1 of whom had concomitant neuropathic pain, and, in the absence thereof, the others were conjectured to have otherwise disturbed hypothalamic thermoregulatory mechanisms as the cause for dysautonomia.

LGI1 is a secreted synaptic protein that associates with and regulates Kv1.1 and Kv1.2, as well as AMPA. Caspr2 is a transmembrane axonal protein of the neurexin IV superfamily that localizes to the juxtaparanode of myelinated axons, and its extracellular domain interacts with contactin-2, where it connects with the cytoskeleton via protein 4.1B. Caspr2, contactin-2, and protein 4.1B are all necessary to concentrate Kv1.1 and Kv1.2 channels in the juxtaparanode. Lai and colleagues[64] studied proteins associated with Kv1.1 and Kv1.2, noting that VGKCs themselves were the autoantibody targets, explaining the diversity of symptoms among patients with these antibodies. LGI1 is primarily a CNS protein, and LGI1 antibodies are associated with LE, seizures, and hyponatremia. LGI1 antibodies cause reversible CNS synaptic dysfunction by several mechanisms. The antibodies may prevent binding of LGI1 to the receptors that it regulates, or they might act on the LGI1-ADAM protein complex. Alternatively, LGI1 antibodies could disrupt currents mediated by Kv1.1 and Kv1.2, and/or impair AMPAR function, either indirectly by blocking LGI1-mediated regulation of these proteins or directly by disrupting the entire protein complex. The identification of LGI1 as a major target of so-called VGKC antibodies clarifies several aspects of the associated disorder.

Caspr2 antibodies are associated with AE, PNH, and MoS. Peripheral nervous system manifestations may precede or follow those of the CNS by up to several years. Some affected patients have an associated thymic tumor, but most do not. Mutations in the human gene encoding Caspr2 (*CNTNAP2*) are associated with autism, epilepsy, Tourette syndrome, cortical dysplasia, obsessive-compulsive disorder, Pitt-Hopkins syndrome, and other mental disabilities. Mice with a *caspr2* deletion show analogous behavioral defects and symptoms.[80] Note that common variants of the *CNTNAP2* gene in healthy individuals are associated with abnormal language processing and are a risk factor for autism.[81] Caspr2 antibodies act by disrupting axonal potassium currents. Factors such as differences in time to establishment of intrathecal antibody synthesis or in the structure of tight, septatelike junctions of myelinating cells around the axons may explain this variability. The VGKC-complex antibody levels broadly differ between the different syndromes, with highest levels in LE and FBDS, moderate levels in MoS, and lowest levels (often <400 pM) in PNH.

The high proportion of VGKC-complex IgG-seropositive patients whose serum samples lack LGI1 IgG and CASPR2 IgG specificities suggests that other VGKC-complex molecular targets remain to be discovered. Only about 4% to 5.5% of unselected cases were seropositive by RIA with confirmatory retesting using 125I-α-dendrotoxin alone (radioligand for Kv1.1, Kv1.2, and Kv1.6 channels),[77,78] making the test unreliable as a screen for LE without further subtyping for LGI1 and CASPR2-IgG. So selected, 26% to 28% of seropositive VGKC sera revealed reactivity with LGI1 and/or CASPR2-IgG, with a significant association between LGI1-IgG positivity and cognitive impairment and seizures ($P<.05$), and CASPR2-IgG positivity and peripheral motor excitability ($P = .004$); however, neither autoantibody was pathognomonic for a specific neurologic presentation. There has been concern for screening of unselected sera for VGKC-complex antibodies by RIA. It can be argued that VGKC-complex RIA antibody test should be used as initial screening to select positive samples that could then be confirmed by LGI1 or CASPR2-IgG antibody subtyping;

however, the latter may also be positive in selected VGKC-complex antibody-negative sera by RIA. Paterson and colleagues[82] noted positive VGKC-complex antibody values (>400 pM; >0.4 nM) that were likely to be relevant in LE and related syndromes, as well as low-positive values (<400 pM; 0.1–0.4 nM) in 32 out of 44 cases considered to be nonautoimmune, 4 (13%) cases of which were found to have a definite or probable paraneoplastic neurologic disorder, neuromyotonia, or MoS. Ances and colleagues[29] noted that the RIA used in the clinical analysis of VGKC-complex antibodies identified a limited number of subunits (Kv1.1, Kv1.2, and Kv1.6) but that it was reasonable to speculate that antibodies to other subunits, K (+) channel families, and VGKC ion channels might also associate with LE.

Neuroimaging studies in VGKC-complex antibody-associated LE show highly variable results. Both mesial temporal lobe hypometabolism on FDG brain PET and hypermetabolism have been described.[83–85] In a patient with VGKC-complex LE[84] who did not definitively show structure abnormalities on serial brain MRI over time despite ongoing temporal lobe seizures captured on video-EEG, FDG brain PET fused with gadolinium-enhanced MRI later showed bitemporal hypometabolism. Baumgartner and colleagues[85] identified 9 out of 18 (50%) patients positive for nonparaneoplastic antibodies against neuronal surface antigens (VGKC or NMDA-R), 2 of whom displayed mesiotemporal hypermetabolism on FDG brain PET, with 4 others who were rated normal, and 3 who displayed hypermetabolism outside the mesiotemporal region. The fraction of abnormal scans using MRI was lower (10 out of 16; 62.3%) than for FDG brain PET (14 out of 18; 77.7%).

CSF results were equally variable in VGKC-complex autoimmunity. Jarius and colleagues[86] performed 29 lumbar punctures in 17 patients with VGKC-complex LE, noting normal findings in up to 53% of CSF specimens. There were no significant differences between the CSF findings and the titers of serum VGKC-complex autoantibodies. Slight pleocytosis, mainly consisting of lymphocytes and monocytes, and increased total protein concentrations were present in 41% and 47%, respectively. A disturbance of the integrity of the BBB was found in 6 (35%) patients based on an abnormal CSF/serum humoral immune response. Absence of CSF-specific OCB, considered a marker of autochthonous antibody synthesis within the CNS in all patients,[87] suggested an extrathecal origin of VGKC-complex autoantibodies. Vincent and colleagues[19] reported the CSF findings in 10 patients, all with VGKC-complex antibody-associated LE, noting mild lymphocytosis and mild or moderately increased protein content in one-half. OCBs were noted in 1 patient, whereas 6 other OCBs were identical to serum. VGKC-complex antibody assays on matched serum and CSF showed antibodies levels of the latter present in 4 patients that varied between less than 1% and 10% of the serum, and less than 10% in 1 patient with the lowest serum value. These findings were consistent with extrathecal synthesis of VGKC-complex antibodies.

Irani and Vincent[70] estimated features of peripheral neuropathy in 1.6% of VGKC-complex antibody-positive LE cases. Lahoria and colleagues[79] described 5 patients with painful polyneuropathy, all positive for VGKC-complex autoantibodies (range, 0.08–1.18 nM), 2 of whom had antigens positive for CASPR2 and LGI1-IgG, both at low VGKC-complex antibody titers (respectively 0.08 and 0.16 nM/L). Electrodiagnostic studies showed length-dependent sensorimotor polyneuropathy that was concordant with abnormal indices of axonal degeneration or demyelination in 4 nerves, and the latter with quantitative analysis of semithin sections in 2. All 5 showed absence of inflammatory cell infiltration. By comparison, the symptoms of small fiber neuropathy, which arise from dysfunction in nociception, temperature, and autonomic modalities, are most adequately assessed by epidermal nerve fiber density in a 3-mm punch biopsy of skin from the lateral calf and thigh, and a combination of cardiovagal, sudomotor, and adrenergic function tests in comparison with controls.

Eight patients with VGKC-complex LE were studied histopathologically, including stereotactic brain biopsy in 3,[19,23] at epilepsy surgery in 1 case,[23] and at postmortem examination in 4 patients.[23,82–84] Vincent and colleagues[19] described a 56-year-old man with 7-month history of confusion and memory impairment who developed partial focal seizures, anxiety, and delusions. CSF showed mild pleocytosis and brain MRI showed unilateral left medial temporal lobe signal change with focal slow activity on EEG. The serum VGKC antibody titer was 2224 pM (normal, 0–100 pM; >400 pM highly increased). Histopathology of a stereotactic biopsy of the left amygdala showed positive staining for perivascular and parenchymal CD45+ lymphocyte infiltrates, astrogliosis, and CD68+ microglial activation. He was received a course of intravenous dexamethasone with a slight beneficial response but persistent memory deficits. Follow-up brain MRI showed evolution of bilateral hippocampus atrophy and signal changes.

Dunstan and Winer[87] reported a 78-year-old man with a 2-week history of confusion, cognitive impairment, and hyponatremia. Brain MRI showed increased signal in the right medial temporal lobe with subcortical white matter changes. CSF was normal. Assay for VGKC antibodies was 1637 pM by RIA. He received anticonvulsants but deteriorated because of sepsis and died. Postmortem examination showed no evidence of a malignancy. The brain showed severe neuronal loss with multiple reactive astrocytes, macrophages, and scattered T cells in the right amygdala nucleus and adjacent hippocampus.

Park and colleagues[88] described a 65-year-old woman with a 3-month history of amnesia, disorientation, memory loss, and partial complex seizures. Brain MRI was normal and CSF showed 17 WBCs. EEG showed mild diffuse slowing. She later developed hyponatremia, and serum VGKC-complex antibodies were 1.73 nmol/L (normal, <0.02 nmol/L) by RIA. Whole-body FDG-PET showed mediastinal adenopathy. She was treated with intravenous corticosteroids for 5 weeks without improvement and later died. General autopsy limited to the chest showed no malignancy. Postmortem examination of the brain showed mild focal perivascular T-cell lymphocyte cuffing and infiltrates of overlying meninges and parenchyma of the cingulate gyrus, hippocampus, amygdala and midbrain.

Khan and colleagues[89] reported a 56-year old man with a 4-month history of confusion, disorientation, and seizures. A serum VGKC antibody titer was 3327 pM by RIA and there was hyponatremia. Brain MRI showed left hippocampal atrophy on T_2/FLAIR images. General postmortem examination showed no malignancy. Examination of the brain showed pathologic changes in both hippocampi and right amygdala regions comprising pyramidal neuronal cell loss in the CA4 region, marked activation of CD68+ microglia, and reactive GFAP+ astrocytosis extending to the subiculum, less so near the joining of the parahippocampal gyrus. There were perivascular infiltrates of CD20+ B-cells and a few CD4+ T-cells, especially in the right hippocampus.

Bien and colleagues[23] summarized the histopathologic findings in the brain of 4 cases, 3 men and 1 woman, aged 33 to 68 years, with LE (3 patients) and multifocal encephalitis (1 patient), ranging from 5 to 9 months. Serum VGKC antibody titers were 167, 288, 958, and 2224 pM respectively. Serial MRI showed an evolution from hippocampal swelling with T_2/FLAIR signal increase to frank hippocampal atrophy and increased signal intensities. Histopathologic examinations, including quantitative immunocytochemical studies, showed variably intense inflammation and overall lower CD8/CD3 ratios, although there were GrB+ T-cells present in the lesions without opposition to neurons or release of FrB, therefore T-cell cytotoxicity was not a major contributor. Immunoglobulin and complement deposition on neurons was a prominent finding, and terminal deoxynucleotidyl transferase dUTP nick and labeling (TUNEL) reaction in the same area showed acute neuron cell death, suggesting antibody and complement-mediated neuronal cell damage in these patients. The investigators[23] noted that IgG4 rather than IgG1 antibodies dominated in the sera of patients with VGKC-complex LE.

Suspected patients with new onset and rapid progression of memory deficits, seizures, or psychiatric symptoms suggesting involvement of the limbic system, bilateral medial temporal lobe abnormalities on T2/FLAIR MRI, and CSF pleocytosis combined with TLE or slow-wave activity on EEG should be screened for VGKC-complex antibodies, with detection of LGI1 and CSFPR2 by RIA. The diagnosis of VGKC-complex LE can be established in suspected cases when serologic studies are combined with clinical, neuroradiologic, and CSF inflammatory parameters and a reasonable exclusion of alternative diagnoses. If so, immunomodulatory and immunosuppressive therapy should begin. Less than one-half of affected patients fail to improve with first-line therapy using IVIg, PE, or corticosteroids, needing to advance to second-line agents, including cyclophosphamide and rituximab.

Bataller and colleagues[90] noted that treatment responsiveness of LE was especially favorable among patients with antibodies to the VGKC complex, with overall improvement in two-thirds or more of patients. However, a favorable response to therapy was not limited to patients with VGKC-complex antibodies but extended to novel-cell-membrane antigens expressed in the hippocampus. The salutary effect of immunotherapy in the management of seizures in VGKC-complex antibody-associated LE is well supported by the autoimmune basis of FBDS.[91]

HASHIMOTO THYROIDITIS AND ENCEPHALOPATHY

For nearly half a decade, investigators have pursued the association of Hashimoto thyroiditis (HT) and a reversible encephalopathy with clinicopathologic resemblance to CNS vasculitis. In 1966, the British neurologist Brain and colleagues[92] described HE in a 40-year-old man with 12 ictal and strokelike episodes of confusion and agitation 1 year after onset of treated hypothyroidism. The cerebral disorder remitted completely after 19 months commensurate with a decline in high serum thyroid-antibody levels. Treatment with prednisone and an anticoagulant for 3 months was ineffective. His neurologic symptoms remitted while he was taking only levothyroxine. The investigators concluded that the likeliest explanation for this protracted and stuttering brain disorder was localized cerebral edema caused by antibody-mediated autoimmunity. Jellinek and Ball[93] extended the results of Brain and colleagues,[92] describing the original patient, who, at age 62 years, died 12 years later of an unrelated cause. Postmortem examination showed virtually no remaining thyroid tissue and atheromatous cerebrovascular changes with splenic atrophy. The investigators postulated that underlying autoimmunity was the cause of HT, HE, and splenic atrophy. A half decade later, Rowland and colleagues[94] characterized the clinicopathologic aspects of HE, beginning with the patient described by Brain and colleagues[92] and ending in 2002, adding a case of their own. The diagnosis of HE, as described by Rowland and colleagues,[94] which rested on the presence of HT (**Fig. 1**) with measurably high titers of thyroid peroxidase (TPO) or antithyroglobulin (Tg) antibodies, clinical encephalopathy, and absence of CSF evidence of bacterial or viral infection, has served as the standard for future case selection.

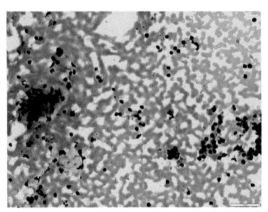

Fig. 1. HT. Fine-needle aspiration in a goiter in a background of lymphocytic thyroiditis. There is a thin background of purple colloid in between gray staining red blood cells amid follicular cells and dark blue staining nucleated lymphocytes recognized by crush or stringing effects (Diff-Quik, original magnification ×200).

Clinical Presentation

In the series of Rowland and colleagues,[94] the mean age at onset of symptoms of HE was 44 years (range, 9–78 years). In addition to encephalopathy as required, strokelike signs presented in 23 (27%) cases, seizure in 56 (66%), myoclonus in 32 (38%), and visual hallucination or paranoid delusion in 31 (36%). The course was relapsing and remitting in 51 (60%) cases.

Laboratory Findings

In the series of Rowland and colleagues,[94] both Tg and microsomal or TPO antibodies were found together in 60 (71%) cases, with 1 antibody of the 2 normal in 20 (24%) cases. There was no relationship between the neurologic symptoms and signs and the type or serum concentration of antithyroid antibodies. Altogether, 30 (35%) cases were subclinically hypothyroid, 19 (22%) were euthyroid, and 17 (20%) were overtly hypothyroid. Fourteen (16%) cases had an increased erythrocyte sedimentation rate or antinuclear antibodies, and 3 had a concomitant connective tissue disease. An increased CSF protein level was noted in 66 (78%) patients, with abnormal findings in neuroimaging in 40 out of 82 (49%) or EEG in 80 out of 82 (98%) patients. A goiter was detected in 24 out of 39 (62%) patients. ^{18}F-FDG-PET of the brain fused with MRI may show signal abnormality in the hippocampus with hypometabolism in the mesial temporal lobes. Nuclear medicine cerebral perfusion with single-photon emission computed tomography may disclose regions of hypoperfusion that overlap with areas of hypometabolism, suggesting concomitant disruption of the BBB.

Immunopathogenic Mechanisms

Unlike the close relationship between antithyroid antibodies and HT, in HE neither high titers of antithyroid antibodies nor the presence of subclinical or overt hypothyroidism seems to account for the observed encephalopathy.[94] The neurologic findings in euthyroid patients are similar to those in patients with subclinical or overt hypothyroidism.

Ochi and colleagues[95] provided a link between HT autoimmunity and the CNS using human brain proteome map and two-dimensional electrophoresis to screen brain proteins reactive to serum antithyroid antibodies. The investigators[95] identified α-enolase, a candidate marker for HE-related disorder, encoded on 1p36.23. Kishitani and colleagues[96] extended the findings of Ochi and colleagues,[95] noting anti–NH2 terminal of α-enolase antibodies in sera of 24% of patients with HE and limbic abnormalities on MRI showing abnormal signal in unilateral or bilateral medial temporal lobes, and diffuse slow-wave activity with epileptogenic discharges. These findings suggested that LE associated with anti–NH$_2$ terminal of α-enolase antibodies may be an etiopathogenic factor of HE in some cases. Graus and colleagues[3] proposed HE as a recognizable autoimmune encephalopathy after exclusion of other syndromes associated with well-defined autoantibodies. It is still unclear whether antithyroid antibodies represent an immune epiphenomenon in a subset of patients with encephalopathy or are associated with pathogenic mechanisms of the disorder.

According to Rowland and colleagues,[94] one subgroup of patients with HE present with strokelike episodes. Inoue and colleagues[97] described a patient with progressive parkinsonism and normal cognitive and intellectual performance. Slow background activity on EEG was the only sign of encephalopathy, which normalized after treatment with corticosteroids. Younger[98] described a patient with hemiparkinsonism in a strokelike onset. ^{18}F-FDG-PET metabolic imaging showed severe hypometabolism within the posterior aspect of the left putamen, suggesting focal vascular injury, with superimposed left temporal and left parietal hypometabolism and mild volume loss relative to the rest of the brain (**Fig. 2**).

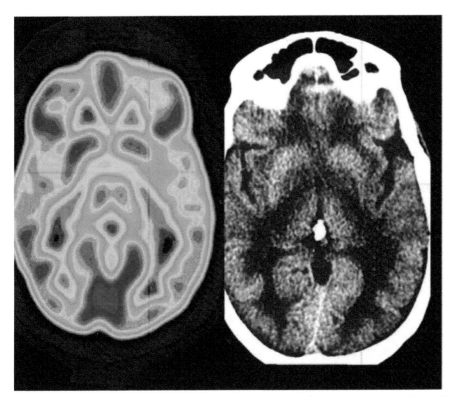

Fig. 2. HE. PET imaging from the vertex to foramen magnum following injection of 10-mCi ^{18}F-FDG (*left*) shows severely reduced metabolic activity in the posterior half of the left putamen, with correlative morphologic changes (*right*) with fusion to gadolinium-enhanced MRI.

A vasculitic pathogenesis seems to be equally likely in some cases of HE based on the tendency for increased autoimmunity in HT. In addition, the available histopathology in HE supports an inflammatory vasculopathy, so noted in 1 postmortem case that showed lymphocytic infiltration of brainstem veins,[99] and in brain biopsy tissue from another case categorized as isolated angiitis caused by lymphocytic infiltration of the walls of arterioles and veins.[100] Brain biopsy tissue of a second living patient showed perivascular cuffs of lymphocytic cells.[94] It is noteworthy that patients with HE and circulating α-enolase antibodies are at risk for heightened autoimmune activity and a tendency for systemic and invasive autoimmune disorders, including systemic vasculitis.[101,102]

Treatment

The significance of corticosteroid sensitivity in HE is widely accepted as a criterion for the diagnosis. However, as Rowland and colleagues[94] suggested, it would be unwise to define any condition by response to any particular therapy, especially if not replacing a specific deficit or directing it at a particular target. Patients with HE improve in association with, but not necessarily because of, corticosteroid therapy. Moreover, those that respond to corticosteroids have no distinguishing clinical characteristics nor receive treatment in other fashions for a meaningful comparison.

SUMMARY

There has been a rapid expansion in knowledge of AE neurologic and neuropsychiatric disorders. Three well-described disorders targeting antigens on the surface or in the cells of the temporal lobe neuropil manifest limbic and extralimbic dysfunction. Patients with HT may develop a rare autoimmune encephalopathy. Recognition of these cases has shifted clinical paradigms and led to new insights into the mechanisms of AE. Patients with available histopathology show variable humoral and cell-mediated autoimmune mechanisms, with cytotoxic T-cell inflammation targeting neuropil antigens, making them more similar than not, to primary CNS vasculitis. However, one important difference is the more favorable outcome in autoimmune encephalopathy and HE compared with primary CNS vasculitis, making their recognition essential in choosing appropriate immunotherapy to achieve long-lasting remission.

REFERENCES

1. Dalmau J. NMDA receptor encephalitis and other antibody-mediated disorders of the synapse: the 2016 Cotzias Lecture. Neurology 2016;87:2471–82.
2. Lancaster E, Dalmau J. Neuronal autoantigens–pathogenesis, associated disorders and antibody testing. Nat Rev Neurol 2012;8:380–90.
3. Graus F, Titulaer MJ, Balu R, et al. A clinical approach to diagnosis of autoimmune encephalitis. Lancet Neurol 2016;15:391–404.
4. Salvarani C, Brown RD, Hunder GG. Adult primary central nervous system vasculitis. Isr Med Assoc J 2017;19:448–53.
5. Elbers J, Benseler SM. Central nervous system vasculitis in children. Curr Opin Rheumatol 2008;20:47–54.
6. Matar RK, Alshamsan B, Alsaleh S, et al. New onset refractory status epilepticus due to primary angiitis of the central nervous system. Epilepsy Behav Case Rep 2017;8:100–4.
7. Torres J, Loomis C, Cucchiara B, et al. Diagnostic yield and safety of brain biopsy for suspected primary central nervous system angiitis. Stroke 2016;47:2127–9.

8. Corsellis JA, Goldberg GJ, Norton AR. "Limbic encephalitis" and its association with carcinoma. Brain 1968;91:481–96.
9. Dalmau J, Graus F, Rosenblum MK, et al. Anti-Hu associated paraneoplastic encephalomyelitis/sensory neuronopathy: a clinical study of 71 patients. Medicine 1991;71:59–72.
10. Budde-Steffen C, Anderson NE, Rosenblum MK, et al. An antineuronal autoantibody in paraneoplastic opsoclonus. Ann Neurol 1988;23:528–31.
11. Younger DS, Graber J, Hayakawa-Yano Y, et al. Ri/Nova gene-associated paraneoplastic subacute motor neuronopathy. Muscle Nerve 2013;47:617–8.
12. Greenlee JE, Brashear HR. Antibodies to cerebellar Purkinje cells in patients with paraneoplastic cerebellar degeneration and ovarian carcinoma. Ann Neurol 1983;14:609–13.
13. Dalmau J, Gultekin SH, Voltz R, et al. Ma1, a novel neuron- and testis-specific protein, is recognized by the serum of patients with paraneoplastic neurological disorders. Brain 1999;122:27–39.
14. Voltz R, Gultekin SH, Rosenfeld MR, et al. A serological marker of paraneoplastic limbic and brain-stem encephalitis in patients with testicular cancer. N Engl J Med 1999;340:1788–95.
15. Bernal F, Graus F, Pifarre A, et al. Immunohistochemical analysis of anti-Hu-associated paraneoplastic encephalomyelitis. Acta Neuropathol 2002;103:509–15.
16. Bien CG, Schulze-Bonhage A, Deckert M, et al. Limbic encephalitis not associated with neoplasm as a cause of temporal lobe epilepsy. Neurology 2000;55:1823–8.
17. Solimena M, Folli F, Denis-Donini S, et al. Autoantibodies to glutamic acid decarboxylase in a patient with stiff-man syndrome, epilepsy, and type 1 diabetes. N Engl J Med 1988;318:1012–20.
18. Murinson BB, Guarnaccia JB. Stiff-person syndrome with amphiphysin antibodies: distinctive features of a rare disease. Neurology 2008;71:1955–8.
19. Vincent A, Buckley C, Schott JM, et al. Potassium channel antibody-associated encephalopathy: a potentially immunotherapy-responsive form of limbic encephalitis. Brain 2004;127:701–12.
20. Irani SR, Gelfand JM, Al-Diwani A, et al. Cell-surface central nervous system autoantibodies: clinical relevance and emerging paradigms. Ann Neurol 2014;76:168–84.
21. Buckley C, Oger J, Clover L, et al. Potassium channel antibodies in two patients with reversible limbic encephalitis. Ann Neurol 2001;50:73–8.
22. Graus F, Saiz A, Dalmau J. Antibodies and neuronal autoimmune disorders of the CNS. J Neurol 2010;257:509–17.
23. Bien CG, Vincent A, Barnett MH, et al. Immunopathology of autoantibody-associated encephalitides: clues for pathogenesis. Brain 2012;135:1622–38.
24. Bauer J, Bien CG. Neuropathology of autoimmune encephalitides. Handb Clin Neurol 2016;133:107–20.
25. Bataller L, Dalmau J. Paraneoplastic disorders of the central nervous system: update on diagnostic criteria and treatment. Semin Neurol 2004;24:461–71.
26. Dalmau J, Gleichman AJ, Hughes EG, et al. Anti-NMDA-receptor encephalitis: case series and analysis of the effects of antibodies. Lancet Neurol 2008;7:1091–8.
27. Turner MR, Irani SR, Leite MI, et al. Progressive encephalomyelitis with rigidity and myoclonus: glycine and NMDA receptor antibodies. Neurology 2011;77:439–43.

28. Leypoldt F, Armangue T, Dalmau J. Autoimmune encephalopathies. Ann N Y Acad Sci 2015;1338:94–114.
29. Ances BM, Vitaliani R, Taylor RA, et al. Treatment-responsive limbic encephalitis identified by neuropil antibodies: MRI and PET correlates. Brain 2005;128: 1764–77.
30. Goldsmith CA, Rogers DP. The case for autoimmunity in the etiology of schizophrenia. Pharmacotherapy 2008;28:730–41.
31. Najjar S, Steiner J, Najjar A, et al. A clinical approach to new-onset psychosis associated with immune dysregulation: the concept of autoimmune psychosis. J Neuroinflammation 2018;15:40.
32. Ching KH, Burbelo PD, Carlson PJ, et al. High levels of anti-GAD65 and anti-Ro52 autoantibodies in a patient with major depressive disorder showing psychomotor disturbance. J Neuroimmunol 2010;222:87–9.
33. Kayser MS, Dalmau J. The emerging link between autoimmune disorders and neuropsychiatric disease. J Neuropsychiatry Clin Neurosci 2011;23:90–7.
34. Campbell S, MacQueen G. The role of the hippocampus in the pathophysiology of major depression. J Psychiatry Neurosci 2004;29:417–26.
35. MacQueen GM, Ramakrishnan K, Ratnasingan R, et al. Desipramine treatment reduces the long-term behavioural and neurochemical sequelae of early-life maternal separation. Int J Neuropsychopharmacol 2003;6:391–6.
36. Belmaker RH, Agam G. Major depressive disorder. N Engl J Med 2008;358: 55–68.
37. Younger DS. Autoimmune encephalitides. World J Neurosci 2017;7:327–61.
38. Gilbertson MW, Shenton ME, Ciszewski A, et al. Smaller hippocampal volume predicts pathologic vulnerability to psychological trauma. Nat Neurosci 2002; 5:1242–7.
39. McKeon A, Tracy JA. GAD65 neurological autoimmunity. Muscle Nerve 2017;56: 15–27.
40. Espay AJ, Chen R. Rigidity and spasms from autoimmune encephalomyelopathies: stiff person syndrome. Muscle Nerve 2006;34:677–90.
41. Falip M, Carreño M, Miró J, et al. Prevalence and immunologic spectrum of temporal lobe epilepsy with glutamic acid decarboxylase antibodies. Eur J Neurol 2012;19:827–33.
42. Malter M, Helmstaedter C, Urbach H, et al. Antibodies to glutamic acid decarboxylase define a form of limbic encephalitis. Ann Neurol 2010;67:470–8.
43. Gagnon M-M, Savard M. Limbic encephalitis: associated with GAD65 antibodies: brief review of the relevant literature. Can J Neurol Sci 2016;43:486–93.
44. Giometto B, Nicolao P, Macucci M, et al. Temporal lobe epilepsy associated with glutamic-acid-decarboxylase autoantibodies. Lancet 1998;352:457.
45. Bien CG, Urbach H, Schramm J, et al. Limbic encephalitis as a precipitating event in adult-onset temporal lobe epilepsy. Neurology 2007;69:1236–44.
46. Najjar S, Pearlman D, Devinsky O, et al. Neuropsychiatric autoimmune encephalitis without VGKC-complex, NMDAR, and GAD autoantibodies: case report and literature review. Cogn Behav Neurol 2013;26:36–49.
47. Najjar S, Pearlman D, Zagzag D, et al. Spontaneously resolving seronegative autoimmune limbic encephalitis. Cogn Behav Neurol 2011;24:99–105.
48. Dalmau J, Bataller L. Limbic encephalitis: the new cell membrane antigens and a proposal of clinical-immunological classification with therapeutic implications. Neurologia 2007;22:526–37.
49. Prüss H, Dalmau J, Harms L, et al. Retrospective analysis of NMDA receptor antibodies in encephalitis of unknown origin. Neurology 2010;75:1735–9.

50. Thomas L, Mailles A, Desestret V, et al. Autoimmune N-methyl-D-aspartate glutamate receptor antibodies in patient with an initial diagnosis of schizophrenia: specific relevance of IgG NR 1a antibodies for distinction from N-methyl-D-aspartate glutamate receptor encephalitis. J Infect 2014;68:419–25.
51. Granerod J, Ambrose HE, Davies NW, et al. Causes of encephalitis and differences in their clinical presentations in England: a multicenter, population-based prospective study. Lancet Infect Dis 2010;10:835–44.
52. Izuka T, Sakai F, Ide T, et al. Anti-NMDA receptor encephalitis in Japan: long-term outcome without tumor removal. Neurology 2008;70:504–11.
53. Dalmau J, Lancaster E, Martinez-Hernandez E, et al. Clinical experience and laboratory investigations in patients with anti-NMDAR encephalitis. Lancet Neurol 2011;10:63–74.
54. Sansing LH, Tuzun E, Ko MW, et al. A patient with encephalitis associated with NMDA receptor antibodies. Nat Clin Pract Neurol 2007;3:291–6.
55. Irani SR, Bera K, Waters P, et al. N-methyl-D-aspartate antibody encephalitis: temporal progression of clinical and paraclinical observations in a predominantly nonparaneoplastic disorder of both sexes. Brain 2010;133:1655–67.
56. Titulaer MJ, McCracken L, Gabilondo I, et al. Treatment and prognostic factor for long-term outcome in a patient with N-methyl-D-aspartate (NMDA) receptor encephalitis: a cohort study. Lancet Neurol 2013;12:157–65.
57. Martinez-Hernandez E, Horvath J, Shiloh-Malawsky Y, et al. Analysis of complement and plasma cells in the brain of patients with anti-NMDAR encephalitis. Neurology 2011;77:589–93.
58. Kelley BP, Patel SC, Marin HL, et al. Autoimmune encephalitis: pathophysiology and imaging review of an overlooked diagnosis. AJNR Am J Neuroradiol 2017; 38:1070–8.
59. Dalmau J, Tuzun E, Hai-Yan W, et al. Paraneoplastic anti-N-methyl-D-aspartate receptor encephalitis associated with ovarian teratoma. Ann Neurol 2007;61: 25–36.
60. Stein-Wexler R, Wootton-Gorges SL, Greco CM, et al. Paraneoplastic limbic encephalitis in a teenage girl with an immature ovarian teratoma. Pediatr Radiol 2005;35:694–7.
61. Tüzün E, Zhou L, Baehring JM, et al. Evidence for antibody-mediated pathogenesis in anti-NMDAR encephalitis associated with ovarian teratoma. Acta Neuropathol 2009;118:737–43.
62. Camdessanche JP, Streichenberger N, Cavillon G, et al. Brain immunohistopathological study in a patient with anti-NMDAR encephalitis. Eur J Neurol 2011; 18:929–31.
63. Hughes EG, Peng X, Gleichman AJ, et al. Cellular and synaptic mechanisms of anti-NMDA receptor encephalitis. J Neurosci 2010;30:5866–75.
64. Lai M, Huijbers MG, Lancaster E, et al. Investigation of LGI1 as the antigen in limbic encephalitis previously attributed to potassium channels: a case series. Lancet Neurol 2010;9:776–85.
65. Irani SR, Alexander S, Waters P, et al. Antibodies to Kv1 potassium channel-complex proteins leucine-rich, glioma inactivated 1 protein and contactin-associated protein-2 in limbic encephalitis, Morvan's syndrome and acquired neuromyotonia. Brain 2010;133:2734–48.
66. Hart IK, Waters C, Vincent A, et al. Autoantibodies detected to expressed K+ channels are implicated in neuromyotonia. Ann Neurol 1997;41:238–46.

67. Kleopa KA, Elman LB, Lang B, et al. Neuromyotonia and limbic encephalitis sera target mature Shaker-type K+ channels: subunit specificity correlates with clinical manifestations. Brain 2006;129:1570–84.

68. Granerod J, Cousens S, Davies NW, et al. New estimates of incidence of encephalitis in England. Emerg Infect Dis 2013;19:1455–62.

69. Lin JJ, Lin KL, Wang HS, et al. VGKG complex antibodies in pediatric severe acute encephalitis: a study and literature review. Brain Dev 2013;35:630–5.

70. Irani SR, Vincent A. Voltage-gated potassium channel-complex autoimmunity and associated clinical syndromes. Handb Clin Neurol 2016;133:185–217.

71. Flanagan EP, McKeon A, Lennon VA, et al. Autoimmune dementia: clinical course and predictors of immunotherapy response. Mayo Clin Proc 2010;85: 881–97.

72. Parthasarathi UD, Harrower T, Tempest M, et al. Psychiatric presentation of voltage-gated potassium channel antibody-associated encephalopathy. Case report. Br J Psychiatry 2006;189:182–3.

73. Bettcher BM, Gelfand JM, Irani SR, et al. More than memory impairment in voltage-gated potassium channel complex encephalopathy. Eur J Neurol 2014;21:1301–10.

74. Kalachikov S, Evgrafov O, Ross B, et al. Mutations in LGI1 cause autosomal-dominant partial epilepsy with auditory features. Nat Genet 2002;30:335–41.

75. Ohkawa T, Fukata Y, Yamasaki M, et al. Autoantibodies to epilepsy-related LGI1 in limbic encephalitis neutralize LGI1-ADAM22 interaction and reduce synaptic AMPA receptor. J Neurosci 2013;33:18161–74.

76. Fukata Y, Lovero KL, Iwanaga T, et al. Disruption of LGI1-linked synaptic complex causes synaptic transmission and epilepsy. Proc Natl Acad Sci U S A 2010;107:3799–804.

77. Younger DS. Limbic encephalitis associated with voltage-gated potassium channel-complex antibodies: patient report and literature review. World J Neurosci 2017;7:19–31.

78. Klein CJ, Lennon VA, Aston PA, et al. Chronic pain as a manifestation of potassium channel-complex autoimmunity. Neurology 2012;79:1136–44.

79. Lahoria R, Pittock SJ, Gadoth A, et al. Clinical-pathologic correlations in VGKC-subtyped autoimmune painful polyneuropathy. Muscle Nerve 2016. https://doi.org/10.1002/mus.25371.

80. Peñagarikano O1, Abrahams BS, Herman EI. CNTNAP2 leads to epilepsy, neuronal migration abnormalities, and core autism-related deficits. Cell 2011; 147:235–46.

81. Whalley HC, O'Connell G, Sussmann JE. Genetic variation in CNTNAP2 alters brain function during linguistic processing in healthy individuals. Am J Med Genet B Neuropsychiatr Genet 2011;156B:941–8.

82. Paterson RW, Zandi MS, Armstrong R, et al. Clinical relevance of positive voltage-gated potassium channel (VGKC)-complex antibodies: experience from a tertiary referral centre. J Neurol Neurosurg Psychiatry 2014;85:625–30.

83. Gast H, Schindler K, Z'Graggen WJ, et al. Improvement of non-paraneoplastic voltage-gated potassium channel antibody-associated limbic encephalitis without immunosuppressive therapy. Epilepsy Behav 2010;17:555–7.

84. Day BK, Eisenman L, Black J, et al. A case study of voltage-gated potassium channel antibody-related limbic encephalitis with PET/MRI findings. Epilepsy Behav Case Rep 2015;4:23–6.

85. Baumgartner A, Rauer S, Mader I, et al. Cerebral FDG-PET and MRI findings in autoimmune limbic encephalitis: correlation with autoantibody types. J Neurol 2013;260:2744–53.
86. Jarius S, Hoffman L, Clover L, et al. CSF findings in patients with voltage gated potassium channel antibody associated limbic encephalitis. J Neurol Sci 2008; 268:74–7.
87. Dunstan EJ, Winer JB. Autoimmune limbic encephalitis causing fits, rapidly progressive confusion and hyponatremia. Age Ageing 2006;35:536–7.
88. Park DC, Murman DL, Perry KD, et al. An autopsy case of limbic encephalitis with voltage-gated potassium channel antibodies. Eur J Neurol 2007;14:e5–6.
89. Khan NL, Jeffree MA, Good C, et al. Histopathology of VGKC antibody-associated limbic encephalitis. Neurology 2009;72:1703–5.
90. Bataller L, Kleopa KA, Wu GF, et al. Autoimmune limbic encephalitis in 39 patients: immunophenotypes and outcomes. J Neurol Neurosurg Psychiatry 2007;78:381–5.
91. Morante-Redolat JM, Gorostidi-Pagola A, Piquer-Sirerol S, et al. Mutations in the LGI1/Epitemprin gene on 10q24 cause autosomal dominant lateral temporal epilepsy. Hum Mol Genet 2002;11:1119–28.
92. Brain L, Jellinek EH, Ball K. Hashimoto's disease and encephalopathy. Lancet 1966;2:512–4.
93. Jellinek EH, Ball K. Hashimoto's disease, encephalopathy, and splenic atrophy. Lancet 1976;1:1248.
94. Chong JY, Rowland LP, Utiger RD. Hashimoto encephalopathy. Syndrome or myth? Arch Neurol 2003;60:164–71.
95. Ochi H, Horiuchi I, Araki N, et al. Proteomic analysis of human brain identifies α-enolase as a novel autoantigen in Hashimoto's encephalopathy. FEBS Lett 2002;528:197–202.
96. Kishitani T, Matsunaga A, Masamichi I, et al. Limbic encephalitis associated with anti-NH2-terminal of a-enolase antibodies. A clinical subtype of Hashimoto encephalopathy. Medicine 2017;96(10):e6181.
97. Inoue K, Kitamura J, Yoneda M, et al. Hashimoto's encephalopathy presenting with micrographia as a typical feature of parkinsonism. Neurol Sci 2012;33: 395–7.
98. Younger DS. Hashimoto's thyroiditis and encephalopathy. World J Neurosci 2017;7:307–26.
99. Nolte KW, Unbehaun A, Sieker H, et al. Hashimoto encephalopathy: a brainstem encephalitis? Neurology 2000;54:769–70.
100. Shibata N, Yamamoto Y, Sunami N, et al. Isolated angiitis of the CNS associated with Hashimoto's disease. Rinsho Shinkeigaku 1992;32:191–8.
101. Li M, Li J, Li Y, et al. Serum levels of anti-a-enolase activity in untreated systemic lupus erythematosus patients correlates with 24-hour protein and D-dimer. Lupus 2018. https://doi.org/10.1177/0961203317721752.
102. Pancholi V. Multifunctional alpha-enolase: its role in diseases. Cell Mol Life Sci 2001;58:902–20.

Neuroophthalmologic Aspects of the Vasculitides

David S. Younger, MD, MPH, MS[a,b,*]

KEYWORDS

- Ophthalmology • Neuroophthalmology • Primary • Secondary • Vasculitis
- Autoimmune • Nervous system

KEY POINTS

- There have been significant advances in the understanding of the vasculitides in the past several years, leading to more precise classification and nosology.
- Ophthalmologic manifestations may be the presenting feature of and a clue to the diagnosis of vasculitis.
- Neuroophthalmologic findings may develop in the course of the illness owing to a common disease mechanism.
- Precise diagnosis and prompt treatment of ophthalmologic vasculitis involvement prevents short- and long-term ophthalmologic sequel.

INTRODUCTION

Vasculitis is a term used to characterize a spectrum of diseases associated with vascular inflammation. Ophthalmologic manifestations may be the presenting features of primary and secondary systemic vasculitis and a clue to early diagnosis to prevent ischemic vascular sequela. Unrecognized and therefore untreated, the ophthalmologic and neuroophthalmologic features can be catastrophic with irreversible loss of function, particularly when visual involvement coincides with vasculitic brain infarction, hemorrhage, and aneurysm formation or ischemic involvement of the optic nerve or surrounding orbital structures. This article considers the ophthalmologic aspects of primary systemic vasculitis and primary central nervous system vasculitis (PCNSV) in children and adults.

CLASSIFICATION OF VASCULITIS

The revised Chapel Hill Consensus Conferences (CHCC) in 2012[1] provides consensus on nosology and definitions for the commonest forms of vasculitis in adults based on

Disclosure Statement: The author has nothing to disclose.
[a] Department of Neurology, Division of Neuro-Epidemiology, New York University School of Medicine, New York, NY 10016, USA; [b] School of Public Health, City University of New York, New York, NY, USA
* 333 East 34th Street, Suite 1J, New York, NY 10016.
E-mail address: youngd01@nyu.edu
Website: http://davidsyounger.com

the caliber of vessels involved. The Pediatric Rheumatology European Society and the European League against Rheumatism proposed specific classification criteria for the commonest childhood vasculitis syndrome[2] based on vessel size similar to the CHCC nomenclature. The European League against Rheumatism, Pediatric Rheumatology European Society, and the Pediatric Rheumatology International Trials Organization defined the clinical, laboratory, and radiographic characteristics of several childhood systemic vasculitides in a validated classification of pediatric vasculitis.[3] There is a continuum of vasculitic disorders, with some occurring exclusively in childhood or in older adults, and others across the age spectrum, although with differing epidemiology, clinical and laboratory manifestations, and response to treatment.

LARGE VESSEL VASCULITIS
Giant Cell Arteritis

This granulomatous large vessel vasculitis involves cranial branches of the arteries arising from the arch of the aorta. The American College of Rheumatology (ACR) 1990 criteria for the classification of giant cell arteritis (GCA)[4] identified 5 criteria from which 3 or more in a given patient was associated with a sensitivity of 93.5% and a specificity of 91.2%, for the diagnosis of GCA: age equal to or greater than 50 years at disease onset, new localized headache, temporal artery tenderness or decreased temporal artery pulse, elevated erythrocyte sedimentation rate to 50 mm/h or more, and vascular tissue biopsy sample showing necrotizing arteritis with predominance of mononuclear cells infiltration or granulomatous multinucleated giant cell inflammation. The histopathology of biopsy-positive GCA includes vessel wall infiltration by mononuclear cells, $CD4^+$ T cells, activated macrophages, and multinucleated giant cells that form granulomas close to the internal elastic lamina of involved vessels in up to one-half of specimens.[5]

A prospective study of 170 patients with biopsy-confirmed GCA[6] noted ocular involvement in 85 patients (50%), including visual loss present in 83 (97.7%), amaurosis fugax in 26 (30.6%), eye pain in 7 (8.2%), and diplopia in 5 (5.9%). Ocular ischemic lesions consisted of arteritic anterior ischemic optic neuropathy (AION) in 69 cases (81.2%), central retinal artery and cilioretinal occlusions each in 12 cases (14.1%) cases, the latter after satisfactory fundus fluorescein angiography (FFA); as well as, posterior ischemic optic neuropathy in 6 cases (7.1%), and ocular ischemia in 1 case (1.2%). Among 42 other patients in Olmsted County Minnesota studied by Huston and coworkers,[7] visual symptoms preceded the clinical and histopathologic diagnosis of GCA in 15 patients (40%). Blurred vision was noted in 6 patients (19%), followed by diplopia in 5 patients (12%), transient vision loss in 5 patients (12%), permanent partial loss in 4 patients (10%), and permanent complete loss in 3 patients (10%). A follow-up Olmsted County cohort 25 years later totaling 168 patients with GCA[8] found visual disturbances at presentation in 16 patients (9.5%) and at the time of diagnosis in 37 patients (22%), of whom 14 patients (8.3%) had transient vision loss, 18 (10.7%) had permanent vision loss, and 14 (8.3%) had diplopia.

Of 18 patients with varying visual loss and occult GCA,[9] amaurosis fugax was noted in 6 patients (33.3%), diplopia in 2 patients (11.1%), and eye pain in 1 patient (5.6%). Ocular ischemic lesions included AION in 17 patients (94.4%) and central retinal artery occlusion and cilioretinal artery occlusions each in 2 patients (11.1%) after FFA. A high index of suspicion for GCA for patients older than 50 years who develop amaurosis fugax, visual loss, or AION in the absence of constitutional and systemic symptoms (**Fig. 1**).

A finding that supports the diagnosis of arteritic AION is chalky-white optic disc swelling. A small disc and cup may be associated with both arteritis and nonarteritic

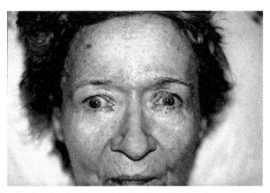

Fig. 1. Patient with giant cell arteritis and brainstem stroke demonstrating left gaze paresis.

AION, whereas a normal or large cup is highly suggestive of an underlying arteritic process. Color Doppler imaging of the central retinal and short posterior ciliary arteries is helpful in distinguishing GCA from nonarteritic AION.

The mainstay of treatment for GCA is corticosteroids (CS); however, the exact dosing regimen and mode of administration depends on the presence of visual involvement at the time of diagnosis. Salvarani and colleagues[10] used 40 to 60 mg oral prednisone for GCA, and intravenous methylprednisolone 1 g/day for 3 days for those with recent or impending visual loss. The addition of low-dose aspirin was beneficial in preventing cranial ischemic complications, including acute visual loss and cerebrovascular complications of GCA compared with CS alone. Such patients are 5-fold less likely to experience cranial ischemic complications as those who receive CS alone. Danesh-Meyer and colleagues[11] evaluated the incidence and extent of visual recovery of 34 patients with biopsy-proven GCA treated with high-dose systemic CS, noting that 27% of eyes suffered loss of visual acuity (VA) by 2 or more lines within 1 week of starting CS treatment, and 15% of eyes so treated showed an improved VA of 2 or more lines. Of the 15% of eyes that showed an improvement in VA, none showed further improvement in visual fields or color vision, leading the authors to conclude that the improvement in VA may reflect learning to view eccentrically.

Takayasu Arteritis

Takayasu arteritis (TAK) predominantly occurs in young Japanese females, typically before the age of 40 years. The ACR[12] selected 6 criteria for the classification of TAK, from which 3 or more in a given patient were associated with a sensitivity of 90.5% and a specificity of 97.8%, from among the following: age less than or equal to 40 years, claudication of an extremity, decreased brachial artery pulse, greater than 10 mm Hg difference in systolic blood pressure between arms, a bruit over the subclavian arteries or the aorta, and arteriographic evidence of narrowing or occlusion of the entire aorta, its primary branches, or large arteries in the proximal upper or lower extremities. Ocular features not formally part of the criteria of TAK occur in 35% to 68% of patients, typically owing to ischemia and hypoperfusion resulting from occlusive arteritis of the aortic arch branches, whereas those arising in the setting of hypertension result from vasculitic renal artery involvement.

The commonest ischemic ocular manifestation of TAK is retinopathy, first described by Takayasu,[13] who noted peculiar fundus changes consisting of dilated vessels around the optic disc owing to arteriovenous anastomoses in female patients without a palpable radial pulse. Less common manifestations of ocular ischemic include AION, central retinal artery occlusion, and ocular ischemic syndrome. The retinal changes in

TAK vary in symptomatology and severity depending on the location of carotid artery involvement, the rate and duration of ocular vascular hypoperfusion, and the presence of collateral blood supply to the eye. Uyama and Asayama[14] classified retinopathy into stages 1 to 4 wherein 20 patients (53%) with stage 1 had dilations of small vessels, 12 patients (32%) with stage 2 disease had microaneurysm formation, and 3 patients (8%) each with either stage 3 or 4 disease, respectively, manifested arteriovenous anastomoses or ocular complications of vitreous hemorrhages, proliferative retinopathy, and vision loss. The authors attributed retinal vascular changes to decreasing blood flow in the retinal vasculature, noting decreased intraocular pressure with disease progression. In contrast with type I TAK, hypertensive fundal changes predominated in patients with type III disease with 12 patients (86%) demonstrating hypertensive changes occurring in the fundus and 2 patients (14%) manifesting hypertensive retinopathy.

Kerr and colleagues[15] noted a 60% response rate to CS alone among 60 patients with TAK with an estimated time to remission of 22 months. Among 4 patients with TAK treated with CS described by Ishikawa,[16] one improved from stage 3 to stage 2 TAK, whereas another patient developed unilateral blindness, and 2 others, were stable. Panretinal photocoagulation is an adjunctive therapy used to treat cases of severe retinal ischemia,[17] whereas antiplatelet agents decreased the frequency of arterial ischemic events. The inflammatory process underlying ocular manifestations may lead to improvement; however, arterial stenoses require bypass surgery.

MEDIUM VESSEL VASCULITIS
Polyarteritis Nodosa

Polyarteritis nodosa (PAN) predominantly affects medium-sized arteries. The pathologic findings of PAN include a hyaline-like necrosis in the media, which rapidly spreads to the adventitia and intima, with infiltration by neutrophils, eosinophils, lymphocytes, and plasma cells. This process is followed by proliferation of fibroblasts that can thicken the intima and occlude vascular lumina.

Although ocular manifestations are not a part of the diagnostic criteria for PAN, they occur in 10% to 20% of patients[18] either owing to the direct effects of arteritis that results in vascular ischemia, or as a secondary effect of renovascular hypertension with subsequent retinal edema, transudates, hemorrhages, and cystoid body formation. The most common arteries affected are the posterior ciliary arteries and choroidal vessels, which can result in choroidal infarcts and exudative retinal detachments. Conjunctival and anterior uveal involvement may occur. In an analysis of 393 patients with PAN,[19] 42 patients (10.7%) had ophthalmologic manifestations, of which blurred vision was the most common and noted in 13 of 42 patients (31%), followed by conjunctivitis in 8 patients (19%), retinal exudates in 8 patients (19%), and retinal vasculitis in 7 patients (17%). Other less common manifestations included uveitis in 5 patients (12%), episcleritis in 4 patients (10%), thrombosis in 4 patients (10%), keratitis and optic neuropathy each in 3 patients (7.1%), retinal hemorrhages in 2 patients (5%), and oculomotor nerve palsy in 1 patient (2%).

Reports of fundoscopic examination findings in patients with PAN variably include papilledema, macular star formation, cotton-wool spots, retinal or subhyaloid hemorrhages, retinal exudates, vascular occlusion of the central retinal artery, and irregularity of the retinal arteries with or without aneurysm formation.[20] Other common features on fluorescein angiography in PAN include retinal vasculitis with multiple arteriolar and capillary occlusions.

Akova and colleagues[21] described the responsiveness of a spectrum of ocular findings including scleritis, peripheral ulcerative keratitis, nongranulomatous uveitis, retinal vasculitis, pseudotumor of the orbit, and central retinal artery occlusion in 5 patients, 4 of whom responded to combination CS and cyclophosphamide or azathioprine therapy.

Kawasaki Disease

Kawasaki disease (KD) is a common vasculitis in children. There are 6 diagnostic features of KD, 5 of which are needed for the diagnosis, including fever of unknown origin lasting 5 days or more not responding to antibiotics, bilateral conjunctival hyperemia and indurated edema that spares the limbal region, orolabial lesions, redness and edema of palms and soles followed by fingertip desquamation, an erythematous polymorphous rash, and cervical lymph node enlargement.[22]

Ocular involvement in KD is typified by bilateral conjunctival hyperemia and indurated edema that spares the limbal region and the conjunctivitis that occurs in 83% to 92% of patients. The conjunctival lesion typically develops within a day or 2 of fever onset and lasts up to several months. Burke and Rennebohm[23] noted that anterior uveitis was a predominant finding during the acute phase of illness.

Posterior segment involvement in KD was documented in 2 patients with bilateral vitreous opacities and bilateral optic disc swelling,[24] unilateral retinal exudates, and macular and disc edema with severe visual loss, as well as in a patient with bilateral inner retinal ischemia diagnosed at postmortem examination.[25] Retinal vasculitis occurs rarely in KD owing to selective inflammation of the blood–ocular barrier. Several reported patients underwent FFA for retinal vasculitis, including one with retinal exudation, macular edema, and temporal disc swelling that showed no leakage,[26] and another with bilateral acute anterior uveitis, in whom FFA showed disc edema and leakage with localized areas of perivascular sheathing suggestive of periphlebitis and vasculitis.[27]

Rennebohm and associates[28] described 6 children with KD, 5 of whom developed anterior uveitis during the acute phase of KD. Both children treated with CS and cycloplegic drugs improved, as did the other 3 untreated children. Similarly, Puglise an colleagues[29] described a 4-year-old child with KD who presented with bilateral swelling and hyperemia of the conjunctiva unresponsive to intense topical steroid therapy; however, there was a decrease in conjunctival inflammation within 1 week of 30 mg/kg of aspirin therapy and complete resolution in 4 weeks.

SMALL VESSEL ANTINEUTROPHIL CYTOPLASMIC ANTIBODY-ASSOCIATED VASCULITIS
Granulomatosis with Polyangiitis

Granulomatosis with polyangiitis (GPA) is characterized by granulomatous inflammation of the upper and lower respiratory tract, and focal necrotizing glomerulonephritis with a triad of multinucleated giant cell granulomatous inflammation, vasculitis, and necrosis.[30] The ACR[31] identified 4 diagnostic criteria for GPA, 2 of which must be present to make the diagnosis from among the following, including nasal or oral inflammation, an abnormal chest radiographic showing nodules, fixed infiltrates, or cavities, urinary sediment showing microhematuria or red cell casts, and granulomatous inflammation on biopsy. The presence of 2 or more criteria imparts a sensitivity of 88.2% and specificity of 92.0% for the diagnosis of GPA. Although the serum antineutrophil cytoplasmic antibody (ANCA) level is not part of the ACR criteria, GPA is associated with ANCA seropositivity, particularly c-ANCA, the presence of which had a

99% specificity and 96% sensitivity for generalized GPA, and 67% sensitivity for the limited form. Ocular findings are not part of the diagnostic criteria for GPA; however, among patients with vasculitis, ocular inflammation, so noted as scleritis, episcleritis, and proptosis, have a sensitivity of 27.4% and a specificity of 96.9% for the diagnosis of GPA.

Ocular manifestations occur overall in 30% to 60% of patients with GPA, and are the presenting features in up to 16% of patients.[32] Ocular symptoms can be due to primary inflammation or focal vasculitis that affects the anterior and posterior segments of the eye, causing conjunctivitis, episcleritis, and keratitis, and optic nerve vasculitis, or as a result of the contiguous spread of longstanding granulomatous sinusitis leading to proptosis, orbital pseudotumor, and nasolacrimal duct obstruction. Vascular complications such as retinal artery occlusion can occur. Frequent symptoms of orbital disease included ocular pain, epiphora, and injection, although proptosis, vision loss, diplopia, and ophthalmoplegia can also occur.

Hoffman and colleagues[32] noted ocular manifestations of GPA among 15% of 158 patients at presentation, and in 52% of those in the course of the illness. Conjunctivitis and dacrocystitis each occurred in 20% of patients; however, they are considered nonspecific features. Painful proptosis, often associated with visual loss owing to optic nerve ischemia, and diplopia resulting from extraocular muscle entrapments, so noted in up to 2% of patients at the onset of disease and in 15% throughout the course of illness, are useful diagnostic features typically caused by retroorbital pseudotumor. Fauci and colleagues[33] identified proptosis in 15 of 49 patients (31%) with ocular involvement associated with GPA owing to retroorbital mass lesions.

Akikusa and colleagues[34] found eye involvement in 13 of 25 children (52%) with GPA at presentation, and in 15 children (60%) over the course of illness. The commonest ocular manifestations in affected children were conjunctivitis in 14 patients (56%), scleritis or episcleritis in 3 patients (12%), and proptosis in 2 patients (8%). Cabral and colleagues[35] reviewed the presenting clinical features of pediatric patients with GPA in 3 single-center cohorts and 1 multicenter cohort, noting ocular manifestations as common presenting features of GPA in children, with conjunctivitis occurring in up to 44% at presentation.

Fauci and colleagues[33] recommended remission induction treatment of GPA with 2 mg/kg/d of oral cyclophosphamide and 1 mg/kg/d of prednisone, followed by a tapering of prednisone to an alternate day administration, achieving complete remission rates of 93% for a mean duration of 48.2 months. Chan and colleagues[36] reported a patient with bilateral corneal ulcers and VA that decreased to 20/200 in the right eye and 20/70 in the left eye and was treated with 2 mg/kg/d of oral cyclophosphamide and 1 mg/kg/d of prednisone. Two years later, the VA in both eyes returned to 20/40, and the peripheral corneal ulcers healed, although shallow peripheral corneal thinning remained. Foster and colleagues[37] studied a patient with GPA and progressive blurred vision, diplopia, and increased supraorbital pressure who was found to have a VA of 20/200 in the right eye, 20/40 in the left eye, 90% ophthalmoplegia in the left eye, and a normal fundoscopic examination. The patient was treated with oral cyclophosphamide and prednisone, and 1 month later the VA improved to 20/40 with complete resolution of ophthalmoplegia. Vischio and McCrary[38] reported a 70-year-old man with left eye visual change, third nerve palsy, and orbital mass compressing the optic nerve that was biopsied with proven GPA. The patient was treated with prednisone 40 mg twice daily and cyclophosphamide 125 mg/d, without visual improvement 11 weeks later. There is substantial ocular morbidity associated with GPA despite efficacious immunosuppressant therapy so noted in 3 enucleations among 140 patients.[39] Sadiq and colleagues[40] identified a subgroup of patients with GPA and orbital involvement with a poor prognosis as evidenced by permanent visual loss in 43% of patients. Patients with episcleritis, conjunctivitis, and anterior uveitis respond to topical therapy, but they should not be used because of secondary corneal thinning and perforation.[41]

Eosinophilic Granulomatosis with Polyangiitis

Eosinophilic GPA (EGPA) involves multiple organ systems, causing chronic rhinosinusitis, asthma, and eosinophilia. The ACR 1990 diagnostic criteria for EGPA[42] included 6 criteria, 4 of which were necessary from the following, including asthma, eosinophilia greater than 10%, neuropathy, pulmonary infiltrates, paranasal sinus abnormality, and extravascular eosinophils. The presence of 4 or more criteria yielded a sensitivity of 85.0% and a specificity of 99.7% for the diagnosis of EGPA. Although ANCA positivity is not part of the ACR's diagnostic criteria, it can be helpful in making the diagnosis in up to 70% of patients.[43] The characteristic changes of EGPA histopathology include necrotizing vasculitis and extravascular necrotizing granulomas with eosinophilic infiltrates; however, early cases may be characterized by tissue infiltration by eosinophils without overt vasculitis.[44]

Ocular features of EGPA can involve all parts of the eye and orbit. Takanashi and colleagues[45] classified the ocular manifestations into 2 types, pseudotumor or orbital inflammatory and ischemic vasculitis types. Patients with the pseudotumor type typically present with a chronically red eye, dacryoadenitis, mysositis, periscleritis, perineuritis, conjunctival granuloma, episcleritis, orbital abnormalities on imaging, and ANCA seronegativity. Those with the ischemic vasculitis present with sudden visual loss, amaurosis fugax, AION, central retinal artery or branch retinal artery occlusion, normal orbital imaging, and ANCA seropositivity.

Among 270 patients with EGPA,[19] 30 (11%) had ocular manifestations of which conjunctivitis was the most common, so noted in 13 patients (43.3%) followed by blurred vision in 9 patients (30%); oculomotor nerve palsy and sudden visual loss each in 4 patients (13.3%); retinal vasculitis in 3 patients (12%); orbital inflammatory disease, and retinal exudates each in 2 patients (6.7%); and episcleritis, keratitis, uveitis, retinal thrombosis, and retinal exudates present each in 1 patient (3.3%). Central retinal artery occlusion is another complication of EGPA, leading to sudden visual loss.

Among 96 patients with EGPA described by Guillevin and colleagues,[46] 3 patients (3.1%) presented with ophthalmic involvement. Two had episcleritis and 1 had bilateral exophthalmos. Jordan and colleagues[47] reported 2 patients with EGPA who presented with dacryoadenitis and diffuse orbital inflammation. Takanashi and colleagues[45] recommended enhanced orbital imaging to look for inflammatory lesions. Fundoscopy is useful in identifying patients with central retinal artery occlusion. There are no randomized, controlled studies of the efficacy of treatment on the ocular manifestations of EGPA.

Microscopic Polyangiitis

Microscopic polyangiitis (MPA) typically affects the kidney causing a pauci-immune focal necrotizing crescentic glomerulonephritis and pulmonary capillaritis. The histopathology of MPA is similar to GPA and EGPA; however, the absence of granulomatous inflammation distinguishes MPA from GPA, as does absence of asthma and eosinophilia from EGPA. Ocular findings are not part of the diagnostic criteria for MPA, and are much less common in MPA than other ANCA-associated vasculitis (AAV). Nevertheless, ocular involvement can occur in up to 24% of patients with MPA, most often presenting as episcleritis or conjunctivitis. Of those with ocular manifestations, the most common was conjunctivitis occurring in 7 (28%), episcleritis occurring in 5 (20%), and blurred vision occurring in 4 (16%). Other less frequent ocular manifestations included retinal vasculitis in 3 patients (12%), retinal exudates, optic neuropathy, sudden visual loss and oculomotor nerve palsy in 2 patients (8%) patients each, and scleritis, keratitis, uveitis, retinal hemorrhage in 1 patient (4%) each.

Because ocular features in MPA are rare, the effects of treatment on ocular disease have been documented through single patient reports or small series. Mihara and colleagues[48] described 2 patients, one of whom had hypopyon iridocyclitis in the right eye, and ophthalmoscopy with retinal cotton-wool spots in the left eye, both of which responded to oral prednisolone, topical instillation of 1% atropine sulfate, and subconjunctival injections of betamethasone.

SMALL VESSEL IMMUNE COMPLEX-MEDIATED VASCULITIS
C1q-Associated Hypocomplementemia Urticarial Vasculitis

C1q/hypocomplementemia urticarial vasculitis (HUV) is a rare severe systemic form of urticarial vasculitis characterized by chronic nonpruritic urticarial lesions, angioedema, ocular inflammation, arthritis or arthralgia, obstructive lung disease, and glomerulonephritis. Its exact incidence is unknown, but it is two times more common in women than in men, and its peak incidence is seen in the fifth decade of life.[49] The histopathology of HUV is characterized by an interstitial neutrophilic infiltrate of the dermis, and a necrotizing vasculitis with immunoglobulin or C3 deposits in the blood vessels on immunofluorescence.

The diagnostic criteria for C1q/HUV were first described by Schwartz and colleagues.[50] The major criteria are urticaria for more than 6 months' duration and hypocomplementemia. The minor criteria, 2 of which are required for diagnosis, are dermal venulitis on biopsy, arthralgia or arthritis, uveitis or episcleritis, mild glomerulonephritis, recurrent abdominal pain, and a positive C1q precipitin test by immunodiffusion, with a decreased circulating C1q level. Exclusion criteria included significant cryoglobulinemia, elevated anti-DNA antibody titer, high titer of antinuclear antibody, hepatitis B virus antigenemia, decreased C-esterase inhibitor levels, and inherited complement deficiency. C1q/HUV and systemic lupus erythematosus share many clinical features; thus, it is important to note that uveitis is typically found in C1q/HUV, but not systemic lupus erythematosus.[51]

Ocular manifestations of C1q/HUV are found in up to 60% of patients. A study by Wisnieski and colleagues[51] in 18 patients with C1q/HUV found that 11 patients (61%) had ocular manifestations; 8 (44%) had conjunctivitis, episcleritis, and/or inflammation of the uveal tract; and 3 (16.6%) had scleral inflammation and photophobia. The treatment of C1q/HUV consists of dapsone and systemic CS and nonsteroidal antiinflammatory drugs.

Cryoglobulinemic Vasculitis

Cryoglobulinemic vasculitis (CV) is an small vessel vasculitis (SVV) that involves the skin, joints, peripheral nervous system, and kidneys. The histopathology of CV is characterized by a leukocytoclastic vasculitis, B-lymphocyte expansion, and tissue B-cell infiltrates. The 2012 CHCC defined CV as a vasculitis with cryoglobulin immune deposits affecting small vessels associated with serum cryoglobulins. Skin, glomeruli, and peripheral nerves are often involved. Ocular signs and symptoms are neither part of the diagnostic criteria for CV, nor are they very common.

The first ocular manifestation of CV was likely described by Wintrobe and Buell[52] in a patient suffering from multiple myeloma that had bilateral thrombosis of the central retinal veins and visual impairment. Other ocular manifestations included anterior uveitis, scleritis, and peripheral ulcerative keratitis. Purtscher-like retinopathy was described by Myers and colleagues[53] in a 44-year-old man with chronic hepatitis C virus (HCV)-associated CV who developed sudden loss of vision in his left eye and abdominal pain. Fundoscopy revealed peripapillary cotton-wool spots and superficial retinal whitening in the macula. FFA revealed retinal vascular nonperfusion in the left macular and peripapillary region, but not in the periphery, consistent with Purtscher retinopathy. The authors proposed that retinopathy developed as a result of complement-mediated microembolism leading to vasoocclusion. Sauer and coworkers[54] documented a patient with Purtscher-like retinopathy associated with HCV-associated CV with complaints of visual loss.

Central serous chorioretinopathy is an ocular complication of CV reported in 2 patients by Cohen and colleagues.[55] These patients presented with serous retinal and retinal pigment epithelial detachments resembling central serous chorioretinopathy. The authors postulated that the increased protein content of the choroid in patients with CV caused an abnormal excess of interstitial fluid to accumulate in the subretinal pigment epithelium or subretinal space resulting in retinal pigment epithelial detachment.

The treatment of CV that consists of CS plus an alkylating agent is associated with induction of remission in up to 62% of patients compared with rituximab plus CS in promoting induction of remission in up to 64% of patients; in those with HCV-associated CV, treatment of HCV with pegylated interferon and ribavirin in addition to rituximab optimally treats most patients.[56] Myers and colleagues[53] described successful treatment of Purtscher retinopathy with plasmapheresis, prednisone and cyclophosphamide leading to improvement of left eye VA from 1/200 to 20/200, and resolution of retinal whitening, cotton-wool spots, and retinal hemorrhages observed on fundoscopy in 6 months. Central serous chorioretinopathy, another ocular manifestation of CV, responds to treatment with laser photocoagulation.

IgA Vasculitis/Henoch-Schönlein Purpura

IgA vasculitis (IgAV)/Henoch-Schönlein purpura (HSP) is characterized by IgA immune complex deposition, in addition to nonthrombocytopenic palpable purpura, abdominal pain, and arthritis. The pathology of IgAV/HSP includes infiltration of small blood vessels with polymorphonuclear leukocytes and leukocytoclasia. The ACR diagnostic criteria have found that the presence of 2 or more of the following criteria were 89.4% diagnostically sensitive and 88.1% specific for IgAV/HSP, including age at onset before 20 years, palpable purpura, acute abdominal pain, and biopsy showing granulocytes around arterioles or venules.[57]

Ocular manifestations of IgAV/HSP are rare, but case reports document a range of ophthalmologic complications. Recurrent episcleritis was one of the first ocular complications of IgAV/HSP in a 14-year-old girl who developed photophobia and intermittent ocular pain 5 weeks after the onset of joint symptoms,[58] ophthalmologic evaluation of whom revealed episcleritis and engorgement of the episcleral vessels.

The association between anterior uveitis and IgAV/HSP was first described by Yamabe and colleagues[59] in the description of a patient with nephritis, anterior uveitis, and keratitis later found to have IgAV/HSP. Muqit and colleagues[60] reported a 42-year-old man with IgAV/HSP complicated by keratitis and granulomatous anterior uveitis. Erer and colleagues[61] reported a 39-year-old man who presented with 3 episodes of anterior uveitis, one of which was bilateral, and unilateral episodes of each eye. Kaur and colleagues[62] documented bilateral anterior uveitis associated in an 11-year-old boy with IgAV/HSP and a 4-year history of eye pain and photosensitivity. Uveitis in IgAV/HSP is due to circulating immune complexes, which reach the eye and deposit in uveal tissues. Immune complexes can deposit in vascular endothelial cells, pigmented epithelial cells, and corneal endothelial cells, expressing adhesion molecules that allows leukocytes to migrate to the uveal tissue and cornea causing injury.

Other rare ocular manifestations include AION[63] and acute visual loss owing to bilateral cystoid macular edema and cotton wool spots. The treatment of IgAV/HSP varies with disease severity with milder cases of IgAV/HSP responsive to supportive therapy and self-resolve in 6 to 16 weeks, and more severe involvement requiring systemic CS and intravenous immune globulin. Ocular manifestations of IgAV/HSP resolve with a combination of systemic and topical CS.

VARIABLE VESSEL VASCULITIS
Behçet Disease

Behçet disease (BD) is characterized by relapsing aphthous ulcers of the mouth, eye, and genitalia. The most widely used diagnostic criteria of BD were formulated by the International Study Group[64] and included recurrent oral ulcerations plus any 2 of genital ulceration, typical defined eye lesions, typical skin lesions, or a positive pathergy. Citirik and colleagues[65] described ocular findings in 34 pediatric patients that included panuveitis, and posterior and anterior uveitis in 53%, 32%, and 15% of patients, respectively. Other ocular findings included cataracts in 59%, posterior synechiae in 24%, postoperative capsular opacification 24%, vitreous condensation after vitritis in 50%, optic atrophy in 30%, cystoid macular edema 15%, narrowed or occluded retinal vessels after retinal phlebitis and branched retinal occlusions in 6%, and neovascularization of the disk and phthisis bulbi each in 3% of patients. Arai and colleagues[66] described the postmortem findings in a young man with BD with relapsing unilateral uveitis, sensorineural hearing loss, slight fever, and progressive CNS and autonomic nervous system involvement that included multifocal brainstem and cerebellar necrotic foci, perivascular neutrophilic inflammation, and perivasculitis.

Cortical venous sinus thrombosis in BD most commonly presents with symptoms and signs of increased intracranial pressure with a rarity of venous infarcts. Prothrombosis, when present, is presumed to commence as an endothelial disturbance. The treatment of BD-related cortical venous sinus thrombosis includes consideration of anticoagulation and CS alone or in association with another immunosuppressive agent.

Cogan Syndrome

Cogan syndrome was first described in a 26-year-old man with recurrent pain, spasm, and redness of the left eye with photophobia, excessive tearing, and marked conjunctival injection, followed by severe attack of dizziness, tinnitus, vertigo, nausea, vomiting, ringing in the ears, profuse perspiration, deafness, and nonsyphilitic interstitial keratitis.[67] Such symptoms tended to recur periodically for years before becoming quiescent. Vestibuloauditory dysfunction was manifested by sudden onset of Menière-like attacks of nausea, vomiting, tinnitus, vertigo, and frequently progressive hearing loss that characteristically occurred before or after the onset of interstitial keratitis. However, within 1 to 6 months of the onset of eye symptoms, auditory symptoms progressed to deafness over a period of 1 to 3 months, and certainly no longer than 2 years.

Gluth and associates[68] reviewed a cohort of patients with Cogan syndrome seen at the Mayo Clinic between 1940 and 2002. The commonest symptoms at presentation were sudden hearing loss in 50%, balance disturbance in 40%, ocular irritation in 32%, photophobia in 23%, tinnitus in 13%, and blurred vision in 10% of cases.

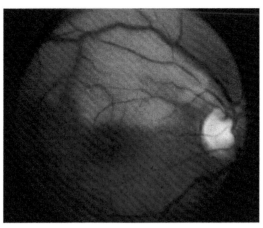

Fig. 2. Branch retinal artery occlusion in a patient with isolated central nervous system vasculitis.

Inflammatory eye findings that occurred in the course of disease included interstitial keratitis in 77%, iritis or uveitis in 37%, oscillopsia in 25%, scleritis or episcleritis in 23%, and conjunctivitis in 10%.

Most patients with Cogan syndrome (58%) are treated with CS with an overall favorable response in both vestibuloauditory and ophthalmologic manifestations, with the remainder demonstrating only ophthalmologic (23%) or vestibuloauditory improvement (19%) alone. Other therapies include methotrexate, cyclophosphamide, azathioprine, entanercept, hydroxchloroquine, and intravenous immune globulin therapy. Surgical cochlear implantation can led to objective and subjective benefits with improved hearing recognition.

Primary Central Nervous System Vasculitis

Primary angiitis of the CNS[69] and PCNSV[70] and granulomatous angiitis of the brain[73] are equivalent terms for a prototypical primary vasculitic disorder restricted to the CNS of diverse causes and clinicopathologic expressions. The diagnosis relies on the presence of the classic angiographic features of beading in cerebral angiographic studies and the histopathologic features of angiitis in brain and meningeal vessels in the absence of systemic vasculitis or another cause for the observed findings. Younger and colleagues[73] described symptoms and signs in 4 patients with granulomatous angiitis of the brain among whom visual symptoms included diplopia, amaurosis fugax, and blurring of vision. The one patient with granulomatous angiitis of the brain and herpes zoster ophthalmicus had contiguous involvement of the eye in in association with V1 dermatomal varicella zoster virus lesions. Among 4 patients described by Cupps and colleagues,[74] neuroophthalmologic involvement was noted in 2 patients. Patient 1 had transient hemifield visual loss accompanied by headaches before the angiographic diagnosis of isolated angiitis of the central nervous system with the involvement of named cerebral vessels, followed several months later after the commencement of a combination immunosuppressant therapy by a 1-week period of altered VA. Patient 3 had a unilateral fundus Roth spot, with markedly decreased VA and normal pupillary response before diagnostic cerebral angiography of isolated angiitis of the central nervous system showed narrowing of named cerebral vessels, followed months later after commencement of combination immunosuppressant therapy by occipital headaches, transient decreased VA, and a starburst image of the central visual field.

Calabrese and Mallek[69] reported eye signs in 15% of literature cases with angiographically or pathologically defined primary angiitis of the CNS, but in none of the 8 Cleveland Clinic patients. Among 70 patients with angiographically defined PCNSV and 31 patients with pathologically verified proven PCNSV described by Salvarani and colleagues,[70] blurred vision and decreased acuity were most common in those with angiographically defined PCNSV overall in 68% of patients. Lanthier and coworkers,[71] who described histologically proven isolated angiitis of the central nervous system in 2 children, described 1 child with bilateral optic disk swelling and persistent conjugated gaze-evoked nystagmus at presentation. Among 4 children with angiographically negative childhood primary angiitis of the CNS described by Benseler and colleagues,[72] 1 child was noted to have gaze-evoked nystagmus (**Fig. 2**).

SUMMARY

Ophthalmologic and neuroophthalmologic manifestations of primary systemic and isolated CNS vasculitis typically arise in association with ischemic vascular disease of the CNS. Although uncommon, such manifestations may be the first clue to underlying ischemic disease owing to primary or secondary involvement of visual and eye movement pathways warranting further evaluation for CNS vasculitis.

REFERENCES

1. Jennette JC, Falk RJ, Bacon PA. 2012 revised international Chapel Hill Consensus Conference nomenclature of vasculitides. Arthritis Rheum 2013;65: 1–11.
2. Ozen S, Ruperto N, Dillon MJ, et al. EULAR/PRES endorsed consensus criteria for the classification of childhood vasculitides. Ann Rheum Dis 2006;65:936–41.
3. Ruperto N, Ozen S, Pistorio A, et al. EULAR/PINTO/PRES criteria for Henoch-Schönlein purpura, childhood polyarteritis nodosa, childhood Wegener granulomatosis and childhood Takayasu arteritis: Ankara 2008. Part I: overall methodology and clinical characterization. Ann Rheum Dis 2010;69:790–7.
4. Hunder GG, Bloch DA, Michel BA, et al. The American College of Rheumatology 1990 criteria for the classification of giant cell arteritis. Arthritis Rheum 1990;33: 1122–8.
5. Weyand CM, Goronzy JJ. Medium-and large-vessel vasculitis. N Engl J Med 2003;349:160–9.
6. Hayreh SS, Podhajsky P, Zimmerman B. Ocular manifestations of giant cell arteritis. Am J Ophthalmol 1998;125:509–20.
7. Huston KA, Hunder GG, Lie JT, et al. Temporal arteritis: a 25-year epidemiologic, clinical, and pathologic study. Ann Intern Med 1978;88:162–7.
8. Nuenninghoff DM, Hunder GG, Christianson TJ, et al. Incidence and predictors of large-artery complication (aortic aneurysm, aortic dissection, and/or large-artery stenosis) in patients with giant cell arteritis. Arthritis Rheum 2003;48:3532–7.
9. Hayreh SS, Podhajsky PA, Zimmerman B. Occult giant cell arteritis: ocular manifestations. Am J Ophthalmol 1998;125:521–6.
10. Salvarani C, Cantini F, Boiardi L, et al. Medical progress: polymyalgia rheumatic and giant cell arteritis. N Engl J Med 2002;347:261–71.
11. Danesh-Meyer H, Savino PJ, Gamble GG. Poor prognosis of visual outcome after visual loss from giant cell arteritis. Ophthalmology 2005;112:1098–103.

12. Arend WP, Michel BA, Bloch DA, et al. The American College of Rheumatology 1990 criteria for the classification of Takayasu arteritis. Arthritis Rheum 1990;33: 1129–34.

13. Takayasu M. A case with peculiar changes of the central retinal vessels. Acta Soc Ophthalmol Jpn 1908;12:554–7.

14. Uyama M, Asayama K. Retinal Vascular Changes in Takayasu's Disease (Pulseless DIsease), Occurence and Evolution of the Lesion. In: De Laey JJ, editor. International Symposium on Fluorescein Angiography Ghent 28 March 1, April 1976. Documenta Ophthalmologica Proceedings Series, vol 9. Springer, Dordrecht.

15. Kerr GS, Hallahan CW, Giordana J, et al. Takayasu arteritis. Ann Intern Med 1994; 120:919–29.

16. Ishikawa K. Natural history and classification of occlusive thromboaortopathy (Takayasu's disease). CIrculation 1978;57:27–35.

17. Chun YS, Park SJ, Park IK, et al. The clinical and ocular manifestations of Takayasu arteritis. Retina 2001;21:132–40.

18. Nanjiani MR. Ocular manifestations of polyarteritis nodosa. Br J Ophthalmol 1967; 51:696–7.

19. Rothschild PR, Pagnoux C, Seror R, et al. Ophthalmologic manifestations of systemic necrotizing vasculitides at diagnosis: a retrospective study of 1286 patients and review of the literature. Semin Arthritis Rheum 2013;43:507–14.

20. Morgan C, Foster S, D'Amico D, et al. Retinal vasculitis in polyarteritis nodosa. Retina 1986;6:205–9.

21. Akova YA, Jabbur NS, Foster CS. Ocular presentation of polyarteritis nodosa. Clinical course and management with steroid and cytotoxic therapy. Ophthalmology 1993;100:1775–81.

22. Ayusawa M, Sonobe T, Uemura S, et al. Revision of diagnostic guidelines for Kawasaki disease (the 5th revised edition). Pediatr Int 2005;47:232–4.

23. Burke MJ, Rennebohm RM. Eye involvement in KD. J Pediatr Ophthalmol Strabismus 1981;18:7–11.

24. Ohno S, Miyajima T, Higuchi M, et al. Ocular manifestations of Kawasaki's disease (mucocutaneous lymph node syndrome). Am J Ophthalmol 1982;93:713–7.

25. Font RL, Mehta RS, Streusand SB, et al. Bilateral retinal ischemia in Kawasaki disease. Postmortem findings and electron microscopic observations. Ophthalmology 1983;90:569–77.

26. Verghote M, Roussea E, Jacob J, et al. An uncommon clinical sign in mucocutaneous lymph node syndrome. Acta Paediatr Scand 1981;70:591–3.

27. Anand S, Yang TC. Optic disc changes in KD. J Pediatr Ophthalmol Strabismus 2004;41:177–9.

28. Rennebohm RM, Burke MJ, Crowe W, et al. Anterior uveitis in Kawasaki's disease. Am J Ophthalmol 1981;91:535–7.

29. Puglise J, Rao N, Weiss R, et al. Ocular features of Kawasaki's disease. Arch Ophthalmol 1982;100:1101–3.

30. McDonald J, Edwards R. Wegener's granulomatosis- a triad. JAMA 1960;173: 1205–9.

31. Leavitt R, Fauci A, Bloch D, et al. The American College of Rheumatology 1990 criteria for the classification of Wegener's granulomatosis. Arthritis Rheum 1990;33:1101–7.

32. Fauci AS, Haynes BF, Katz P, et al. Wegener's granulomatosis: prospective clinical and therapeutic experience with 85 patients for 21 years. Ann Intern Med 1983;98:76–85.

33. Hoffman G, Kerr G, Leavitt R, et al. Wegener granulomatosis: an analysis of 158 patients. Ann Intern Med 1992;116:488–98.
34. Akikusa JD, Schneider R, Harvey EA, et al. Clinical features and outcome of pediatric Wegener's granulomatosis. Arthritis Rheum 2007;57:837–44.
35. Cabral D, Uribe A, Benseler S, et al. Classification, presentation, and initial treatment of Wegener's granulomatosis in childhood. Arthritis Rheum 2009;60:3413–24.
36. Chan A, Li E, Choi P, et al. Unusual eye signs in Wegener's granulomatosis. Hong Kong Med J 2007;13:241–2.
37. Foster W, Greene S, Millman B. Wegener's granulomatosis presenting as ophthalmoplegia and optic neuropathy. Otolaryngol Head Neck Surg 1995;112:758–62.
38. Vischio J, McCrary C. Orbital Wegener's granulomatosis: a case report and review of the literature. Clin Rheumatol 2008;27:1333–6.
39. Bullen CL, Liesegang TJ, McDonald TJ, et al. Ocular complications of Wegener's granulomatosis. Ophthalmology 1983;90:279–90.
40. Sadiq SA, Jenning CR, Jones NS, et al. Wegener's granulomatosis: the ocular manifestations revisited. Orbit 2000;19:253–61.
41. Pakrou N, Selva D, Leibovitch I. Wegener's granulomatosis: ophthalmic manifestations and management. Semin Arthritis Rheum 2006;35:284–92.
42. Masi AT, Hunder GG, Lie JT, et al. The American College of Rheumatology 1990 criteria for the classification of Churg-Strauss syndrome (allergic granulomatosis and angiitis). Arthritis Rheum 1990;33:1094–100.
43. Mahr A, Guillevin L, Poissonnet M, et al. Prevalences of polyarteritis nodosa, microscopic polyangiitis, Wegener's granulomatosis, and Churg-Strauss syndrome in a French urban multiethnic population in 2000: a capture-recapture estimate. Arthritis Rheum 2004;51:92–9.
44. Churg A. Recent advances in the diagnosis of Churg-Strauss syndrome. Mod Pathol 2001;14:1284.
45. Takanashi T, Uchida S, Arita M, et al. Orbital inflammatory pseudotumor and ischemic vasculitis in Churg-Strauss syndrome. Report of two cases and review of the literature. Ophthalmology 2001;108:1129–33.
46. Guillevin L, Cohen P, Gayraud M. Churg-Strauss syndrome. Clinical study and long-term follow-up of 96 patients. Medicine 1999;78:26–37.
47. Jordan N, Verma H, Ekbote A. Dacryoadenitis and diffuse orbital inflammation: unusual first presentation of Churg-Strauss syndrome. Orbit 2011;30:160–1.
48. Mihara M, Hayasaka S, Watanabe K, et al. Ocular manifestations in patients with microscopic polyangiitis. Eur J Ophthalmol 2004;15:138–42.
49. Grotz W, Baba H, Becker J, et al. Hypocomplementemic urticarial vasculitis syndrome. An interdisciplinary challenge. Dtsch Arztebl Int 2009;106:756–63.
50. Schwartz HR, McDuffie FC, Black LF, et al. Hypocomplementemic urticarial vasculitis: association with chronic obstructive pulmonary disease. Mayo Clin Proc 1982;57:231–8.
51. Wisnieski JJ, Baer AN, Christensen J, et al. Hypocomplementemic urticarial vasculitis syndrome: clinical and serologic findings in 18 patients. Medicine (Baltimore) 1995;74:24–41.
52. Wintrobe M, Buell M. Hyperproteinemia associated with multiple myeloma. With report of a case in which an extraordinary hyperproteinemia was associated with thrombosis of the retinal veins and symptoms suggesting Raynaud's disease. J Am Med Assoc 1932;99:1411–4.
53. Myers JP, Di Bisceglie AM, Mann ES. Cryoglobulinemia associated with Purtscher-like retinopathy. Am J Ophthalmol 2001;131:802–4.

54. Sauer A, Nasic X, Zorn F, et al. Cryoglobulinemia revealed by a Purtscher-like retinopathy. Clin Ophthalmol 2007;1:555–7.
55. Cohen SM, Kokame GT, Gass JD. Paraproteinemias associated with serous detachments of the retinal pigment epithelium and neurosensory retina. Retina 1996;16:467–73.
56. Terrier B, Cacoub P. Cryoglobulinemia vasculitis: an update. Curr Opin Rheumatol 2013;25:10–8.
57. Mills JA, Michel BA, Bloch DA, et al. The American College of Rheumatology 1990 criteria for the classification of Henoch-Schönlein purpura. Arthritis Rheum 1990;33:1114–21.
58. Lorentz WB, Weaver RG. Eye involvement in anaphylactoid purpura. Am J Dis Child 1980;134:524–5.
59. Yamabe H, Ozawa F, Fukushi K, et al. IgA nephropathy and Henoch-Schönlein purpura nephritis with anterior uveitis. Nephron 1988;50:368–70.
60. Muqit MMK, Gallagher MJ, Gavin M, et al. Henoch-Schonlein purpura with keratitis and granulomatous anterior uveitis. Br J Ophthalmol 2005;89:1221–2.
61. Erer B, Kamali S, Cingu K, et al. Recurrent anterior uveitis in Henoch Schonlein's vasculitis. Rheumatol Int 2010;30:1377–9.
62. Kaur S, Maheshwari A, Aneja S, et al. Henoch-Schönlein purpura with uveitis: an unusual case and review of literature. Rheumatol Int 2012;32:4057–9.
63. Chuah J, Meaney T. Anterior ischaemic optic neuropathy secondary to Henoch-Schönlein Purpura. Eye 2005;19:1028.
64. Criteria for diagnosis of Behçet's disease. International Study Group for Behçet's Disease. Lancet 1990;335:1078–80.
65. Citirik M, Berker N, Songur MS, et al. Ocular findings in childhood-onset Behcet disease. J AAPOS 2009;13:391–5.
66. Arai Y, Kohno S, Takahashi Y, et al. Autopsy case of neuro-Behcet's disease with multifocal neutrophilic perivascular inflammation. Neuropathology 2006;26: 579–85.
67. Morgan RF, Baumgartner CJ. Meniere's disease complicated by recurrent interstitial keratitis: excellent results following cervical ganglionectomy. West J Surg 1934;42:628.
68. Gluth MB, Baratz KH, Matteson EL, et al. Cogan syndrome: a retrospective review of 60 patients throughout a half century. Mayo Clin Proc 2006;81:483–8.
69. Calabrese HL, Mallek JA. Primary angiitis of the central nervous system: report of 8 new cases, review of the literature, and proposal for diagnostic criteria. Medicine (Baltimore) 1988;67:20–39.
70. Salvarani C, Brown RD Jr, Calamia KT, et al. Primary central nervous system vasculitis: analysis of 101 patients. Ann Neurol 2007;62:442–51.
71. Lanthier S, Lortie A, Michaud J, et al. Isolated angiitis of the CNS in children. Neurology 2001;56:837–42.
72. Benseler SM, deVeber G, Hawkins C, et al. Angiography-negative primary central nervous system vasculitis in children. Arthritis Rheum 2005;52:2159–67.
73. Younger DS, Hays AP, Brust JCM, et al. Granulomatous angiitis of the brain. An inflammatory reaction of diverse etiology. Arch Neurol 1988;45:514–8.
74. Cupps TR, Moore PM, Fauci AS. Isolated angiitis of the central nervous system. Prospective diagnostic and therapeutic experience. Am J Med 1983;74:97–105.

Treatment of Vasculitis of the Nervous System

David S. Younger, MD, MPH, MS[a,b],*

KEYWORDS

• Immune suppression • Vasculitis • Nervous system • Clinical trials

KEY POINTS

- There is general agreement on 5 principles in the diagnosis and treatment of nervous system vasculitides.
- Vasculitides of the nervous system is a potentially serious disorder with a propensity for permanent disability owing to tissue ischemia and infarction.
- Undiagnosed and therefore untreated, there is a likelihood of excess morbidity and mortality.
- A favorable response to an empiric course of immunosuppressive and immunomodulating therapy should never be considered a substitute for the absolute proof of the laboratory diagnosis of vasculitis.
- Histopathologic confirmation of vasculitis is essential for accurate diagnosis.
- Treatments are initially guided toward stabilization of the blood-brain or blood-nerve barriers, followed by maintenance immunosuppressive therapy directed at the humoral and cell-mediated autoimmune inflammatory mechanisms.

INTRODUCTION

The Revised International Chapel Hill Consensus Conference (CHCC) nomenclature[1] provides a useful framework for the distinction of specific vasculitides based on the caliber of the vessels involved, both arteries and veins. So defined, small vessel vasculitis (SVV) includes granulomatosis with polyangiitis (GPA) (Wegener type), microscopic polyangiitis (MPA), and eosinophilic granulomatosis with polyangiitis (EGPA) (Churg-Strauss syndrome [CSS]), known collectively as antineutrophil cytoplasmic antibody (ANCA)–associated vasculitides (AAV). Vasculitic disorders associated with immune complexes (ICs) include immunoglobulin (Ig) A vasculitis (IgAV) (Henoch-Schönlein purpura [HSP]), cryoglobulinemic vasculitis (CV), and hypocomplementemic urticarial vasculitis (HUV) associated with C1q antibodies. Vasculitis without a

Disclosure: The author has nothing to disclose.
a Department of Neurology, Division of Neuro-Epidemiology, New York University School of Medicine, New York, NY, USA; b School of Public Health, City University of New York, New York, NY, USA
* 333 East 34th Street, Suite 1J, New York, NY 10016.
E-mail address: youngd01@nyu.edu
Website: http://www.davidsyounger.com

Neurol Clin 37 (2019) 399–423
https://doi.org/10.1016/j.ncl.2019.01.014
0733-8619/19/© 2019 Elsevier Inc. All rights reserved.

predominant vessel size and caliber, respectively from small to large, involving arteries, veins, and capillaries, comprises the category of variable vessel vasculitis (VVV), characteristic of Behçet disease (BD) and Cogan syndrome. Medium vessel vasculitides (MVV) includes polyarteritis nodosa (PAN) and Kawasaki disease (KD). Large vessel vasculitides (LVV) are represented by giant cell arteritis (GCA) and Takayasu arteritis (TAK). Vascular inflammation confirmed to a single organ system, such as vasculitis restricted to the central nervous system (CNS) and peripheral nervous system (PNS), and IgG4-related aortitis (IgG4-related disease [RD]), are collectively referred to as single organ vasculitides (SOV).

At the turn of the twentieth century, granulomatous angiitis of the nervous system[2] was the prototypical form of a vasculitis restricted to the CNS, recognized not only for its clinical heterogeneity in association with a variety of comorbid illnesses such as cancer, sarcoidosis, amyloid, human immunodeficiency virus, and zoster varicella virus infection, but also for the predilection for cerebral vessels of varying caliber from small meningeal to named cerebral vessels. Decades later,[3] recognition of the caliber of cerebral vessels involved by cerebral angiography and histopathologic examination of brain and meningeal tissue provided valuable clues to effective treatment and prognosis of primary CNS vasculitides (PCNSV). Adult[4] and childhood isolated CNS angiitis,[5] primary angiitis of the CNS (PACNS),[6] granulomatous angiitis of the brain (GAB),[7] and granulomatous angitis of the nervous system (GANS)[2]; and adult[8] and childhood PACNS (cPACNS)[9] are equivalent terms for a prototypical primary vasculitic disorders restricted to the CNS.

Similarly, identification of necrotizing arteritis in arteriae nervorum was synonymous with peripheral nerve vasculitis (PNV), whereas inflammatory involvement in or around smaller epineurial blood vessels defined microvasculitis (MV) and perivasculitis (PV).[10] Although diabetes was not been considered a predisposing factor in PNV, MV became a defining feature in lumbosacral radiculoplexus neuropathy (LSRPN)[11,12] with or without diabetes, and the classification and treatment of patients with systemic and nonsystemic PNV (NPNV) expanded in parallel with systemic vasculitides, incorporating the electrodiagnostic and clinicopathologic features in well-defined observational cohorts and subsets of patients determined in large part by the caliber of vessels involved.[13]

The Pediatric Rheumatology European Society (PRES), the European League against Rheumatism (EULAR), and the Pediatric Rheumatology International Trials Organization (PRINTO) reported methodology and overall clinical, laboratory, and radiographic characteristics for several childhood systemic vasculitides[14] followed by a final validated classification[15] also based on vessel size, similar to the CHCC nomenclature.[1]

Insight into effective therapies of systemic vasculitides have been guided by collaborative evidence-based randomized controlled trials (RCTs) or observational cohorts by the French Vasculitis Study Group (FVSG) database, United States–Canadian Vasculitis Clinical Research Consortium, European Vasculitis Study Society (EUVAS), EULAR, The French Vasculitis Cohort of Patients with Primary Vasculitis of the Central Nervous System (COVAC), Diagnostic and Classification Criteria in Vasculitis Study (DCVAS), the Pediatric Vasculitis Initiative (PedVas), DCVAS, and the Web-based network BrainWorks.

Physicians treating patients with clinically definite CNS vasculitides, whether primary or secondary, must now choose the sequence and combination of induction and maintenance immunosuppression available from available corticosteroid (CS) preparations, cyclophosphamide (CYC), azathioprine (AZA), methotrexate (MTX), mycophenolate mofetil (MMF), the pyrimidine synthesis inhibitor leflunomide (LEF), plasma exchange (PE), high-dose intravenous immunoglobulin (IVIg), and diverse biologic therapies using humanized monoclonal antibodies (mAbs), including the anti-CD20 mAb rituximab (RTX); anti–tumor necrosis factor (TNF) alpha agents inflix-imab, etanercept, and adalimumab; and anti–interleukin (IL)-6 receptor agents such as tocilizumab (TCZ). Other drugs contemplated for use, but not rigorously used, such as antithymocyte globulin, fusion protein of cytotoxic T-lymphocyte antigen-4 (CTLA4)–Ig, the B-cell-activating factor of the TNF family (BAFF) belimumab, the anti-CD52 mAb alemtuzumab, and the anti–interleukin 5 mAb mepolizumab are not reviewed.

Since the first RCT in tuberculosis,[16] the design and complexity have evolved to include various study designs, often large numbers of study subjects, and an emphasis on multicenter studies. The past 2 decades have witnessed extraordinary progress in the conduct of RCTs in vasculitides. This progress has occurred because of several factors. First, the widespread adoption of standardized nosology, classifica-tion criteria, and improved standardization leading to eligibility criteria for participating in RCTs. Second, the use of validated outcome measures for vasculitis.[17,18] However, many forms of vasculitis still lack well-validated measures of disease activity or state for use in clinical trials. Advances in standardized approaches to conducting clinical trials are advocated by EULAR.[19]

The Vasculitis Working Group of the Outcome Measures in Rheumatology (OMER-ACT) initiative actively pursues a variety of projects to advance development of valid measures in the vasculitides.[20] Disease-specific self-reported patient-related out-comes applicable to AAV can distinguish treatments of varying efficacy, including health-related quality-of-life (HRQoL) measures, further separable by the caliber of vessels involved.[21,22] Children's self-reported HRQoL measured by the Pediatric Quality of Life Inventory Version 4.0 (PedsQL) generic scores scales repeatedly measured over time in pediatric inflammatory brain diseases (IBrainDs)[23] including cPACNS that reflected poor HRQoL in more than half of patients at diagnosis seemed to correlate with cognitive dysfunction as the most presenting symptom and small vessel cPACNS (SV-cPACNS) as the most common diagnosis.[24] The inclusion of on-line resources such as the UK Biobank that foster research in the genetic predisposi-tion and environmental exposures relevant to development of disease has widened the prospects for public health awareness and applicable research in the prevention and predisposition to vasculitic illnesses.

One other important advance in vasculitis has been the recognition of predictive clinical factors that are associated with disease course. For example, the clinical pattern, disease phenotype, and history of relapse in patients with GPA and MPA are each predictive of prognosis with treatment. Patients seropositive for anti–proteinase 3 (PR3) or c-ANCA are at substantially higher risk of relapse than patients with antimyeloperoxidase (MPO) or p-ANCA,[25] although patients with GPA are more likely to relapse than patients with MPA, a finding that is not surprising given the much higher prevalence of anti-PR3 c-ANCA among patients with GPA. A history of relapse in AAV is highly predictive of future relapse. Thus, these prognostic factors are taken into consideration when developing a treatment regimen for patients with AAV, including duration of therapy.

The Five-Factor Score (FFS), a prognostic tool created by the FVSG,[26] exemplifies how severity and specific organ involvement serves not only as a prognostic tool but also helps direct the therapeutic choice in systemic necrotizing vasculitis. The revised FFS comprises age greater than or equal to 65 years, cardiac involvement, gastroin-testinal involvement, renal insufficiency (stabilized peak creatinine level $\geq$150 μmol/L), and absence of ear-nose-throat involvement.[26]

This article examines the treatment of systemic, CNS, and PNS vasculitides, and the specific agents used. Whenever possible, it informs the reader of the underlying concepts guiding treatment of vasculitides, clinical trial standards and individualization of therapy, and the results of clinical studies where applicable with detailed references to the literature. **Box 1** summarizes the recommended approach to the treatment of vasculitides.

Systemic Vasculitides

Corticosteroids

CSs are used alone or in combination and are the single most commonly used therapeutic agent for the treatment of systemic vasculitides. The clinical benefit of CSs

---

Box 1
Recommendations for the treatment of vasculitides

Large vessel vasculitis
  GCA, TAK: CS, AZA, RTX, infliximab, anti-TNF-α, anti-IL-6R, tocilizumab, and MMF
  Adjunctive therapy: ASA and AC

Medium vessel vasculitis
  PAN, KD: CS and CYC; MMF.

SVV, AAV type
  GPA, EGPA, MPA: induction with CS + CYC, CS + RTX or CS + MMF and maintenance RTX, AZA, or MMF

SVV, IC type
  CV: MMF; INF-alfa, and PegINF-alfa plus ribavirin or RTX in HCV-associated MC
  IgAV: CS and/or MMF, and supportive care

Hypocomplementic-C1q: antihistamines, IVIg, PE

Variable vessel vasculitis
  Cogan syndrome: CS
  BD: CS, MMF; colchicine or anti-TNF-α

Single organ vasculitis-isolated aortitis, PACNS
  Isolated aortitis: CS, AZA, MMF, MTX
  PCNSV: induction with CS, CS + CYC, followed by maintenance with AZA, MTX, or MMF
  cPACNS: induction with CS, CS + CYC, followed by maintenance with AZA, MTX, or MMF

Vasculitis associated with systemic collagen vascular disease: SLE, RAV
  SLE: CS, MMF; and AC
  RAV: CS, RTX, infliximab, and AZA or MTX

Vasculitis associated with illicit substance abuse
  Avoid illicit substance

Vasculitis associated with infection
  Antimicrobial agents chosen specifically to treat a given causal organism

Abbreviations: AC, anticoagulation; ASA, aspirin; AZA, azathioprine; BD, Behçet disease; cPACNS, childhood primary angiitis of the central nervous system CS, corticosteroids, CV, cryoglobulinemic vasculitis; CYC, cyclophosphamide; EGPA, eosinophilic granulomatosis with polyangiitis; GCA, giant cell arteritis; GPA, granulomatosis with polyangiitis; HCV, hepatitis C virus; IC, Immune complex; IgAV, IgA vasculitis; INF, interferon; IL, interleukin; IVIg, intravenous immune globulin; KD, Kawasaki disease; MC, mixed cryoglobulinemia; MMF, mycophenolate mofetil; MPA, microscopic polyangiitis; MTX, methotrexate; PAN, polyarteritis nodosa; PCNSV, primary central nervous system vasculitis; PE, plasma exchange; RAV, rheumatoid arthritis vasculitis; RTX, rituximab; SLE, systemic lupus erythematosus; TAK, Takayasu arteritis; TNF, tumor necrosis factor.

stems from their inhibitory properties on inflammatory and immune responses. Their broad antiinflammatory properties include the ability to decrease vascular permeability, inhibit the migration of inflammatory cells to sites of injury or untoward inflammation, inhibition of polymorphonuclear and mononuclear cell function, and a variety of mediators important in the inflammatory response, such as kinins, histamine, and prostaglandins. They are potent inhibitors of the immune response with broad effects on antigen processing and immune activation, including lymphocyte proliferation mediator release, as well as lymphocyte trafficking.

There is general agreement on the beneficial and deleterious effects of differing CS dosing schedules. First, therapeutic efficacy and toxicity are related to the administered dose, duration of therapy, and frequency of administration, with more serious side effects during sustained daily long-term therapy without tapering. Second, divided doses of daily prednisone are probably more potent than a single high morning dose of greater than 80 mg of prednisone. Third, daily low doses of 15 mg or less of prednisone incur many of the same problems as high-dose therapy, in particular hypothalamic pituitary adrenal (HPA) axis suppression with incipient adrenal failure. Fourth, pulse therapy of 1000 mg of methylprednisolone daily for several days is generally well tolerated and is associated with fewer effects than long-term therapy with an equivalent degree of immunosuppression and short-term antiinflammatory benefit. Fifth, alternate day therapy, typically reserved for patients whose disease activity is under good control, reduces long-term toxicity, in particular HPA suppression, CS myopathy, and osteoporosis. Sixth, although the different therapeutic options for CS administration generally relate to the best ratio of benefits to risk, when the disease is life threatening or fulminant, as in systemic vasculitides, it would be most reasonable to institute pulse therapy followed by daily high doses if monotherapy is used, whereas the inverse may be more applicable if CSs are combined with an alkylating cytotoxic agent such as CYC.

Early intensive therapy has been suggested in patients with LVV, including TAK and GCA (also known as large vessel GCA [LV-GCA]), to induce remission. CSs are the mainstay of therapy in GCA; however, their use is associated with predictable and occasionally serious side effects even with an initial dose of 0.5 to 0.7 mg/kg/d of prednisone in the absence of eye involvement, or 1 mg/kg/d in the presence thereof, both of which are continued for 1 month before gradual tapering.[27,28]

There are no clinical trials of the efficacy of CSs in patients with MVV and SVV.[29] CSs used in almost all clinical trial and cohort studies to obtain remission or induce cure alone or in association with other agents for AAV are given at the dose of 1 mg/kg/d of prednisone for 3 to 4 weeks according to the EUVAS study group.[30] The FSVG[31] recommends pulse methylprednisolone for life-threatening organ involvement because of its rapid onset of action and favorable safety index.

The use of CS in the treatment of many types of vasculitides other than LVV and systemic necrotizing vasculitides is controversial. Pulse methylprednisolone was alternative therapy given over 1 to 3 days in children with KD compared with 1 or more IVIg infusions to alleviate fever and acute inflammation.[32] A prospective randomized open-label Japanese study of KD[33] that used IVIg therapy plus CSs showed significantly less coronary artery abnormality than those treated with IVIg and aspirin. Side effects of CSs in PAN and associated chronic hepatitis B virus (HBV) infection included enhancement of viral replication and progressive cirrhosis. Such patients treated with PE and antiviral therapy in addition to CSs to avert severe life-threatening manifestations allows discontinuation of CSs. They are safely administered with IFN-α to treat hepatitis C virus (HCV)–related cryoglobulinemia.[34]

Cyclophosphamide

CYC is a member of the alkylating class of cytotoxic drugs that covalently binds cross-linked DNA strands and interferes with mitosis and cell replication. The immunosuppressive effects of CYC include absolute suppression of B- and T-cells as well as suppression of both cell-mediated and humoral immunity. Interest in the use of CYC emerged in early studies by Fauci and Wolff[35] of GPA so treated with combination prednisone and oral CYC at doses of 2 mg/kg/d, showing improved long-term benefit despite severe kidney disease and treatment-related morbidity. The latter included increased propensity for infection, hemorrhagic cystitis, bladder fibrosis, bone-marrow suppression, ovarian failure, bladder cancer, and hematologic malignancies.[36] A prospective, multicenter, randomized trial comparing steroids and pulse CYC versus steroids and oral CYC in GPA[37] showed equal efficacy of pulse CYC in achieving initial remission of GPA, with fewer side effects and lower mortality. However, treatment with pulse CYC did not maintain remission or prevent relapses as well as oral CYC.

A meta-analysis by EULAR[29] concluded that pulsed CYC was more likely to result in remission status than continuous oral therapy, with a lower risk of side effects. A meta-analysis of 3 studies of intravenously pulsed CYC[38] showed that pulsed regimens reduced cumulative CYC exposure by 50%, and were at least as effective at inducing remission, with fewer infective and myelosuppressive side effects; however, there was possible increased risk of relapse.

The recommended initial dose of CYC varies from 0.5 to 0.7 g/m^2 at 2-week intervals given initially on days 1, 15, and 30, and continued every 3 weeks until remission is obtained, followed later by maintenance therapy. CYCLOPS, a randomized trial of daily oral versus pulse cyclophosphamide as therapy for ANCA-associated systemic vasculitis, enrolled 149 patients with generalized AAV to receive either pulse CYC 15 mg/kg at 2-week intervals for the first 3 doses and every 3 weeks thereafter, or daily oral CYC 2 mg/kg/d,[39] noting that pulse therapy was equally effective as daily oral CYC with a lower cumulative dose and fewer instances of leukopenia. Patients age 65 years and older with newly diagnosed PAN, GPA, MPA, and EGPA who receive low-dose intravenous pulse CYC with faster CS dose tapering have reduced rates of severe adverse events and similar remission and relapse rates.

Apart from AAV, CYC has been used in other systemic vasculitides, including severe IgAV and CV, although these indications are controversial. A multicenter, prospective, randomized, open-label trial[40] found that the addition of CYC to CS provided no further benefit compared with steroids alone in treating adult patients with severe IgAV. In patients with HBV-related PAN and HCV-related CV, treatment with PEG-IFN-α plus ribavirin was associated with a good prognosis, whereas immunosuppressive agents, including CS, were associated with a poor outcome and increased mortality.[41]

Azathioprine

Azathioprine is an antimetabolite and purine analogue that interferes with DNA synthesis. Long-term AZA immunosuppression leads to decreased numbers of B- and T-cells, as well as decreased B-cell proliferative responses and antibody synthesis. It also inhibits natural killer cell activity.[42] The Cyclophosphamide versus Azathioprine for Early Remission Phase of Vasculitis (CYCAZAREM) trial[30] studied patients with a new diagnosis of GPA and MPA and a serum creatinine concentration of 5.7 mg/dL (500 μmol/L) or less. All patients received at least 3 months of therapy with oral CYC and prednisolone. After remission, patients were randomly assigned to continued CYC therapy of 1.5 mg/kg of body weight per day or a substitute regimen of AZA of 2 mg/kg/d. Both groups continued to receive prednisolone and were followed for 18 months from study entry. Relapse was the primary end point. It concluded that patients with at least 3 months of oral CYC and prednisolone for AAV, and randomly assigned to continued CYC therapy at the dose of 1.5 mg/kg of body weight per day or a substitute regimen of AZA of 2 mg/kg/d, in addition to prednisolone, and followed 18 months from study entry, with an end point of relapse, showed no increase in the rate of relapse. The relapse rate was lower among the patients with MPA than among those with GPA (P = .03) and the withdrawal of CYC and the substitution of AZA after remission did not increase the rate of relapse. Thus, the duration of exposure to CYC may be safely reduced with the addition of AZA after initial remission in AAV.

Methotrexate

MTX is an antimetabolite that inhibits folic acid and has been used in LVV and AAV. A meta-analysis by Mahr and colleagues[43] assessed 3 randomized placebo-controlled trials in patients with newly diagnosed GCA[44–46] in whom treatment consisted of initial high-dose CS and randomly assigned oral MTX therapy of 7.5 to 15 mg/wk versus placebo, and a comparison of time to event, and continuous outcomes. Adjunctive treatment of GCA with MTX lowered the risk of relapse and reduced exposure to CS, thus MTX could be considered as a therapeutic option in addition to standard-of-care treatment with CS.[43]

A randomized, multicenter trial that enrolled 98 patients from 16 with newly diagnosed GCA to determine whether MTX reduced relapses and cumulative CS requirements and diminished disease-related and treatment-related morbidity did not support the adjunctive use of MTX to control disease activity or to decrease the cumulative dose and toxicity of CS in patients with GCA.[44]

Findings from the Wegener's granulomatosis-Entretien Trial (WEGENT) in 2008[47] suggested that AZA or MTX could effectively maintain remission of GPA or MPA. A subsequent long-term study with 10 years of follow-up for 112 of the 126 original trial participants found no between-treatment differences with regard to rates of relapse, adverse events, damage, survival without severe side effects, and survival without relapse and severe side effects. Thus, AZA and MTX are comparable treatment options for maintaining remission of GPA or MPA.

Mycophenolate mofetil

Mycophenolate mofetil is a prodrug of mycophenolic acid that inhibits inosine monophosphate dehydrogenase (required for the synthesis of DNA), thereby affecting proliferating T- and B-cells.[48] The open-label RCT, International Mycophenolate Mofetil Protocol to Reduce Outbreaks of Vasculitides (IMPROVE) trial[49] randomly assigned 156 patients to AZA starting at 2 mg/kg/d or MMF starting at 2000 mg/d after induction of remission with CYC and CS. The patients were followed for a median of 39 months. Relapses were more common in the MMF group compared with the AZA group; however, severe adverse events did not differ significantly between groups. Thus, among patients with AAV, MMF was less effective than azathioprine for maintaining disease remission, but both had similar adverse event rates.

Between 2007 and 2013, the Clinical Trial of Mycophenolate versus Cyclophosphamide in ANCA Vasculitis (MYCYC) evaluated MMF compared with intravenous CYC in the induction of remission in new cases of AAV, noting that MMF was not inferior to CYC. However, the inferiority of MMF to AZA in maintenance therapy will probably reduce the use of MMF only in patients with AAV refractory to intravenous and oral CYC, and RTX. A recent comparison of guidelines and recommendations on managing AAV[50] found that patients with nonsevere and non–organ-threatening disease should be recommended a milder regimen than CYC or RTX, with the British Society for Rheumatology (BSR), British Health Professionals for Rheumatology (BHPR),[51] and EULAR[52] including CS with either MTX or MMF (grade B recommendation for MTX and grade C recommendation for MMF, where grade A is highest and D is lowest).[53]

Leflunomide

The pyrimidine synthesis inhibitor LEF was evaluated in an open-label study to show improvement in disease activity and acute phase reactants with 20 mg/d of leflunomide in patients with TAK who were refractory or intolerant to conventional therapy with CSs and immunosuppressive agents,[54] noting that LEF was safe with a steroid-sparing effect. A multicenter, prospective, randomized controlled clinical trial[55] treated patients with GPA either with oral LEF 30 mg/d or oral MTX (starting with 7.5 mg/wk reaching 20 mg/wk after 8 weeks) for 2 years following induction of remission with CYC. The primary end point was the incidence of relapses. The investigators concluded that LEF was effective in the prevention of major relapses in GPA; however, this was associated with an increased frequency of rapidly progressive glomerulonephritis, pulmonary hemorrhage, and cerebral granuloma adverse events.

Plasma exchange

PE was initially used in systemic vasculitides considering the contributory pathogenic role of ANCA and anti–glomerular basement membrane (GBM) antibodies, cryoglobulins, cytokines, and ICs. It is presently used as a second-line agent in the treatment of PAN refractory to conventional regimens. PE improves renal survival in patients with severe renal disease as defined by a serum creatinine level greater than 500 μmol/L when used as an adjunct to daily oral CYC and CS in the prospective randomized Plasma Exchange for Renal Vasculities (MEPEX) trial.[56] A total of 137 patients with a new diagnosis of AAV confirmed by renal biopsy and serum creatinine level greater than 500 μmol/L (5.8 mg/dL) were randomly assigned to receive 7 PEs or 3000 mg of intravenous methylprednisolone; both groups received oral CYC and oral prednisolone. The primary end point was dialysis independence at 3 months. PE was associated with a reduction in risk for progression to end-stage renal disease (ESRD) of 24% at 12 months compared with methylprednisolone (95% confidence interval [CI], 6.1%–41%). Patient survival and severe adverse event rates at 1 year were 76% and 48% in the intravenous methylprednisolone group compared with 73% and 50% in the PE group. The risk reduction of 24% for ESRD with PE was clinically important in view of the cost, morbidity, and mortality of end-stage renal failure, such that the additional costs of PE were outweighed by these savings. The improvement in renal recovery rates with PE was consistent with the hypothesis that PE was most likely to be of benefit in those with the most severe disease. This study excluded patients who had been dialysis dependent for more than 2 weeks because they were considered to have little chance of renal recovery.

The protocol of the Plasma Exchange and Glucocorticoid Dosing in the Treatment of Anti-Neutrophil Cytoplasm Antibody Associated Vasculitis (PEXIVAS) Trial[57] is a 2-by-2 factorial randomized trial begun in 2013 that has been evaluating adjunctive PE and 2 oral CS regimens in severe AAV. Patients receive PE or not and a standard or reduced oral CS dosing regimen. All patients receive immunosuppression with either CYC or RTX. The primary outcome is the time to the composite of all-cause mortality and ESRD. The PEXIVAS study was due to report its findings in 2018. The primary composite outcome, death from any cause or ESRD, occurred in 28% of patients receiving PE compared with 31% in the no-PE group (hazard ratio, 0.86; 95% CI, 0.65–1.13; $P = .27$). The primary outcome occurred in 28% of patients in the reduced CS group and 26% in the standard CS group (absolute risk difference, 2.3%; 90% CI, –3.4% to 8.0%), meeting the noninferiority hypothesis. Serious infections in the first year occurred less often in the reduced CS group compared with the standard group (incidence rate ratio, 0.70; 95% CI, 0.52–0.94; $P = .02$). The investigators concluded that, in the largest ever trial in AAV, a reduced dose of CS was noninferior to a standard dose and resulted in fewer serious infections.

Levy and colleagues[58] examined the long-term outcome of severe anti-GBM antibody disease in patients who received PE, prednisolone, and CYC. Those with a serum creatinine level less than 5.7 mg/dL had patient and renal survival respectively of 100% and 95%, and patient and renal survival of 84% and 74% at last follow-up. Those with a creatinine level greater than or equal to 5.7 mg/dL but did not require immediate dialysis, and were treated with PE, prednisolone, and CYC, had comparative patient and renal survival of 83% and 82% at 1 year, and 62% and 69% at last follow-up. Patients with the anti-GBM disease and severe renal failure should be considered for urgent immunosuppression therapy, including PE, to maximize the chance of renal recovery.

Intravenous immunoglobulin

High-dose IVIg is a safe and well-tolerated therapy compared with standard CS and immunosuppressive therapy. Its use in systemic vasculitides was first established in the prevention of coronary artery aneurysms and in the reduction of systemic inflammation in children with KD.[59,60] A later study[61] showed the superiority of a single infusion of IVIg compared with 4 infusions in the treatment of acute KD. Improvement of patients with AAV was associated with a mean reduction in pretreatment ANCA levels by 51% in patients so treated.[62] It was alternative treatment in patients with GPA and MPA without threatened systemic organ involvement,[63] leading to full clinical remission lasting 1 year before commencing conventional immunosuppressive therapy. A placebo-controlled trial of a single course of 2 g/kg per kg of IVIg in AAV with persistent disease activity[64] noted reduced disease activity as judged by a reduction in the Birmingham Vasculitis Activity Score (BVAS), along with C-reactive protein and ANCA levels in subjects randomized to IVIg compared with placebo. However, the effect of a single course of IVIg was not maintained beyond 3 months, and mild reversible side effects following therapy were frequent. A multicenter, prospective, open-label study[65] for relapses of GPA and MPA during treatment or in the year following discontinuation of CS or immunosuppressive therapy led to complete remissions, some lasting up to 2 years after treatment with high-dose IVIg for up to 6 months.

Rituximab

Rituximab is a genetically engineered chimeric murine-human monoclonal IgG1k that is directed against the CD20 antigen expressed on the surface of B-cells. In 2010, 2 randomized clinical trials, RTX in ANCA-associated Vasculitides (RAVE)[66] and RTX versus CYC for ANCA-associated Vasculitides (RITUXVAS),[67] provided initial RCT evidence that, at 6 to 12 months of follow-up respectively, RTX was as safe and effective as conventional immunosuppressive therapy to control active MPA and GPA. A subgroup of 63 of 197 enrolled patients in RAVE with either GPA or MPA[66] treated with 375 mg/m^2 of body surface area per week for 4 weeks, compared with 2 mg/kg/d of CYC in those who reached the primary end point of remission of disease without use of prednisone at 6 months, showed that RTX was not inferior to daily CYC for induction of remission in severe AAV, and might even be superior to CYC in relapsing disease. A single course of RTX was as effective as continuous conventional immunosuppressive therapy with CYC followed by AZA for the induction and maintenance of remission of patients with severe organ-threatening AAV over the course of 18 months in the Rituximab in ANCA-Assocated Vasculitis (RAVE) Trial.[25] The primary outcome was complete remission of disease by 6 months, with remission maintained through 18 months. Guillevin and colleagues[68] studied 115 patients with newly diagnosed or relapsing GPA, MPA, and renal-limited AAV in complete remission after a CYC-CS regimen who were randomly assigned to receive either 500 mg of RTX on days 0 and 14 and at months 6, 12, and 18 after study entry or daily AZA until month 22. The primary end point at month 28 was the rate of major relapse (the reappearance of disease activity or worsening, with a BVAS >0, and involvement of 1 or more major organs, disease-related life-threatening events, or both). More patients with AAV had sustained remission at month 28 with RTX than with AZA. At month 28, major relapses had occurred in 29% of the AZA group compared with 5% in the RTX group, with similar frequencies of severe adverse events.

In a 24-month phase III RCT of 115 patients over time who received RTX or AZA for AAV maintenance therapy and completed a Health Assessment Questionnaire (HAQ),[69] there were mean improvements of HAQ scores, from baseline to month 24, that were significantly better for the RTX than the azathioprine group.

Zaja and colleagues[70] found that RTX was a safe and effective alternative to standard immunosuppressive therapy for type II mixed cryoglobulinemia (MC). Sansonno and colleagues[71] studied patients with MC and HCV-positive chronic active liver disease resistant to interferon alfa (INFα) therapy, noting that 80% of patients treated with an intravenous infusion of 375 mg/m² of RTX once a week for 4 consecutive weeks showed a complete response characterized by rapid improvement of clinical signs and decline of the cryocrit and anti-HCV antibody titers. Roccatello and colleagues[72] found that RTX was a safe and effective option in symptomatic patients with HCV-associated MC and glomerulonephritis and signs of systemic vasculitis. Saadoun and colleagues[73] found that 94% of patients with severe refractory HCV-related MC vasculitis showed clinical improvement, 63% of whom were complete responders with undetectable HCV RNA and serum cryoglobulins. Terrier and colleagues[74] found that RTX combined with PEG-INFα-2b plus ribavirin induced a complete and partial clinical response respectively in 80% and 15%; a complete and partial immunologic response was respectively noted in 67% and 33% of patients, and a sustained virologic response in 55% of patients so treated, making RTX combined with PEG-INFα-2b plus ribavirin safe and effective treatment in severe refractory HCV-associated mixed CV.

Ignatova and colleagues[75] studied the efficiency of traditional CS and CYC and selective RTX therapy for HCV-associated CV over an average follow-up period of 2.8 years, noting that combined therapy for RTX and antiviral therapy was most effective in patients with severe forms of vasculitis.

Anti–tumor necrosis factor alpha

The anti-TNF-α monoclonal antibody infliximab or the analogue of its receptor, etanercept, has been proposed to treat primary systemic vasculitides. Infliximab, a chimeric anti–TNF-α monoclonal antibody in combination with conventional therapy led to clinical remission in 88% of the patients with acute or persistently active AAV enrolled in an open, prospective trial.[76] In 2002, Bartolucci and colleagues[77] reported their findings of infliximab treatment in 7 patients with severe refractory GPA, all of whom obtained complete or partial remissions, with cutaneous eruption being the only adverse effect.

Etanercept, another TNF-α blocker, composed of a soluble protein derived from the p75 TNF receptor fused to the Fc portion of IgG, has been tested in AAV and in conjunction with conventional therapy to reduce relapse rate. The Wegener's Granulomatosis Etanercept (WGET) trial[78] compared etanercept with placebo in addition to receiving standard therapy of CS plus CYC or MTX. After sustained remission, the primary outcome was defined as a BVAS of 0 for at least 6 months and tapering of standard medications according to an established protocol. Of 174 patients, 72% had a sustained remission; however, there were no significant differences between the etanercept and control groups in the rates of sustained remission (69% vs 75%; $P = .39$) or in the relative risk of disease flares per 100 person-years of follow-up. The Infliximab versus Ritaximab in Systemic Necrotizing Vasculitides with Positive ANCA after Relapse or Resistant Immunosuppressant Therapies (RATTRAP) trial,[79] which compared efficacy and tolerance of infliximab versus RTX to treat refractory GPA, showed the usefulness of infliximab to obtain remission of refractory GPA, with a trend at 12 months favoring RTX. During long-term follow-up, RTX was better able to obtain and maintain remission.

Seror and colleagues[80] studied the effect of adding a 10-week course of 40 mg on alternate weeks of subcutaneous adalimumab for 10 weeks to a standard treatment of 0.7 mg/kg/d of prednisone, with a primary end point of the percentage of patients in remission on less than 0.1 mg/kg of prednisone at week 26. Among near-equal numbers of study and control subjects, there was no difference between adalimumab and prednisone in increasing the number of patients in remission on less than 0.1 mg/kg of CS at 6 months. Mekinian and colleagues,[81] who reported the findings of a multicenter retrospective tolerance study of infliximab in refractory TAK, noted a significant decrease in clinical biological activities within 3 months, with a decrease in the median CS dose at 12 months.

Tocilizumab

Tocilizumab, a humanized monoclonal antibody against the IL-6 receptor, was evaluated in retrospective series in patients with refractory LVV showing evidence of clinical and serologic improvement in patients with refractory and relapsing disease. The multicenter, randomized, double-blind, placebo-controlled study, Giant-Cell Arteritis Actemra (GiACTA) trail, began recruiting patients with GCA for evaluation of the safety and efficacy of 162 mg of subcutaneous TCZ administered weekly or every 2 weeks versus placebo for 52 weeks, with tapering of the oral daily dose of prednisone over 26 weeks compared with placebo with 52 weeks of prednisone (NCT01791153). The primary outcome measure is the proportion of patients in sustained remission at week 52, comparing TCZ plus 26 weeks of prednisone taper with placebo plus 26 weeks of prednisone taper.

Insights into treatment of antineutrophil cytoplasmic antibody–associated vasculitis

Fifty years ago, AAV had a mortality of 93% within 2 years, primarily caused by renal and respiratory failure.[82] The introduction of CSs in 1948 and CYC in the 1960s, together with adjunctive therapies such as antihypertensive and renal replacement therapies, transformed the outcome of AAV, with 5-year rates approaching 80%.[83] This therapeutic revolution transformed AAV into a chronic relapsing disorder with progressive organ damage and disability. The cumulative exposure to CS and immunosuppressive drugs, which contributes to organ damage, has raised concerns of CYC-related toxicity involving chronic myelosuppression, infection, urothelial malignancy, and infertility.[36,84] The equivalence of RTX to CYC in the induction of remission of AAV,[66,67] and the licensing of RTX for treatment of AAV, have been significant achievements. The optimal treatment strategy following RTX induction still needs to be addressed. Rates of cardiovascular disease and malignancy in AAV were increased as well as underlying patterns of disease such as accelerated atherosclerosis,[85] raising concerns that there may be nontraditional risk factors such as endothelial activation and excessive vascular remodeling to take into account as predominant causes of death, rather than uncontrolled vasculitis.[86] It is uncertain whether increasing use of RTX can remedy these unforeseen problems.

Insights into disease pathogenesis have influenced the approach to treatment. Genetic susceptibility and environmental exposures are now known to contribute to the autoimmune etiopathogenesis of AAV. Animal models of AAV show that the transfer of murine MPO-ANCA IgG without functioning B or T-cells results in a pauci-immune, necrotizing crescentic glomerulonephritis similar to that seen in AAV in humans.[87] There are also several lines of investigation linking infections to ANCA formation through molecular mimicry.[88] Fimbriated bacteria induce novel ANCA antibodies to human lysosome membrane protein-2 (LAMP-2), which in turn leads to crescentic glomerulonephritis in animals,[89] and infection with Staphylococcus aureus is associated with relapse of GPA.[90] Proteinase 3 ANCA binding levels are predictive of outcome with an increase in antibody titers before clinical relapse. However, patients who are consistently ANCA seronegative fit the clinical phenotype of AAV, and the efficacy of B-cell depletion with rituximab is not associated with ANCA status. Despite the pauci-immune nature of the histology in ANCA vasculitis, there is increasing evidence for the role of both cell and humoral immunity, with immune complex deposition and complement activation in renal involvement. Components of the alternative pathway are detected in glomeruli and small blood vessels in kidney biopsy tissue specimens from patients with AAV, which colocalize with C3d and the membrane attack complex.[91] The contribution of cell-mediated immunity is exemplified by activation of circulating T- and B-cells, with infiltration of plasmoblasts into affected tissues.[92] Autoreactive B-cells, necessary for the development of autoantibody producing cells, seem to play the important role of supporting autoreactive T-cell activity through antigen presentation, costimulation, and direct production of proinflammatory cytokines, including IL-6 and TNF-α. In view of their role as precursors of ANCA-secreting plasma cells, B-cells are a therapeutic target in AAV and T-cells play an important role in the eventual pathogenesis of AAV.[93] Class-switched IgG autoreactive antibodies receive cognate T-cell help, and T-cells cause damage via direct cytotoxicity and recruitment and activation of macrophages.[94]

Current and future treatment strategies in AAV are addressing optimization of existing therapies and the introduction of novel agents. With a greater understanding of the disease pathogenesis, and the advent of highly specific biological molecules, a targeted approach is now possible, with the ultimate goal of controlling the underlying disease process while eliminating or minimizing disease side effects associated with broad-spectrum immunosuppression. The desire to minimize CYC exposure has dominated clinical studies for the last 20 years.[36] Nonetheless, CYC remains a relatively safe and effective induction agent in AAV and is a component of the standard of care in consensus guidelines for the treatment of generalized disease.[29] Between 2003 and 2009, 3 adjustments in the administration of CYC in clinical trials showed that it could be given even more safely. First, the sequential replacement of CYC by AZA once remission was achieved, as in the CYCAZAREM study.[30] Second, the replacement of CYC by MTX for early systemic disease without critical organ manifestations in the Nonrenal Wegener's Alternatively Treated with Methotrexate (NORAM) study.[95] Third, the use of pulsed intravenous CYC with dose reductions for patients aged more than 60 years and renal impairment rather than daily oral CYC in the CYCLOPS study,[39] enabling a cumulative dose reduction of approximately one-half.). In long-term follow-up of patients in the CYCLOPS study,[96] reduced CYC was associated with a higher risk of relapse, whereas MTX was associated with less effective disease control than CYC induction therapy in the NORAM study.[97] However, in neither were long-term morbidity and mortality increased.

However, early outcome results for the treatment of childhood AAV, in particular GPA, reported by Morishita and colleagues[98] on behalf of A Registry for Childhood Vasculitis (ARChiVe) Investigators Network and the Pediatric Vasculitis (PedVas) Initiative were less encouraging. Among 105 children with AAV, mainly GPA, who received CS, CYC, MTX, or RTX for remission induction, and PE in conjunction with CYC and/or RTX, 42% achieved remission at 12 months (Pediatric Vasculitis Activity Score of 0, CS dose <0.2 mg/kg/d), 21 (48%) of whom discontinued CS by 12 months; all but 3 remained on maintenance treatment at 12 months receiving AZA, MTX, RTX, MMF, and CYC. However, up to 63% had a Pediatric Vasculitis Damage Index score of 1 or more by 12 months, with the presence of renal; ear, nose and throat; or pulmonary damage. Moreover, 41% of children reported hospitalizations. Thus, a significant proportion of patients were not in remission at 12 months, and more than one-half of the patient cohort experienced damage early in the disease course. The 12-month remission rate of 42% in the cohort was significantly lower than that found by Sacri and colleagues,[99] who reported 73% remission at postinduction and 90% overall remission rate (including secondary remissions after a median time of 6.7 months). Disappointing early outcomes in the PedVas treatment study for GPA[98] may pose some difficulty in applying the same immunosuppressant treatment strategy to cPACNS, pediatric IBrainDs, pediatric autoinflammatory diseases,[100] neuroimmune disorders,[101] and childhood autoimmune encephalitides.[102]

Primary central nervous system vasculitides

Adult As originally defined, PACNS,[6] like IACNS,[4] relied on either classic angiographic or histopathologic features of angiitis within the CNS in the absence of systemic vasculitis or another cause for the observed findings. Younger and colleagues[2,7] emphasized the etiologically diverse associations with comorbid disorders and the prototypical histopathology of granulomatous giant cell and epithelioid cell infiltration involving the walls of arteries of various caliber, from named cerebral vessels to small arteries and veins, which, when present in combined meningeal and brain biopsy, predicted similar widespread features at postmortem examination.

Patients with PCNSV typically present with headache of gradual onset, often accompanied by the signs and symptoms of dementia, and only later develop focal neurologic symptoms and signs. The clinical course may be rapidly progressive over days to weeks, or insidious over many months with prolonged periods of stabilization. By comparison with PCNSV, patients with granulomatous angiitis[2,7] present with headache, mental change, and increased cerebrospinal fluid (CSF) protein content with or without pleocytosis. Hemiparesis, quadriparesis, and lethargy, associated with a poor prognosis, mandate the need for prompt diagnosis combining brain neuro-imaging and cerebral angiography to choose the best site for meningeal and brain biopsy in an effort to establish the diagnosis with certainty. Nonetheless, 38% of adults with clinically definite PCNSV[3] and 8% of CNS tissue biopsies in children with SV-cPACNS[103] may show negative or nonspecific inflammation, which may be caused by prolonged time to biopsy, nonlesional biopsy, prior CS treatment, or inadequate specimen sampling. Among 79 cases of suspected PACNS at the Hospital of the University of Pennsylvania from 2005 to 2013,[104] 9 (11%) leptomeningeal and/or cortical brain biopsies were diagnostic of PACNS, 14 (18%) showed nondiagnostic perivascular inflammation, and 24 (30%) showed alternative diagnoses (cerebral amyloid angiopathy [CAA], lymphoma, demyelination, Alzheimer disease, tauopathy, posterior reversible encephalopathy syndrome, small vessel vasculopathy, and progressive multifocal leukoencephalopathy), and the remainder were negative. Moreover, 13 patients (16%) experienced postbiopsy complications: 6 (8%) had intracerebral hemorrhage, 2 (3%) had seizures, 3 (4%) experienced transient altered mental status, and 1 each sustained cerebral infarction and CSF leak.

Physicians treating childhood and adult PCNSV should proceed with caution in choosing the sequence and mode of immunosuppressive therapies, for the present, based on a single historical survey of clinicopathologically verified adult cases, and 2 cohort observational studies in North America and France. The only historical survey of histologically confirmed granulomatous angiitis including 54 diagnosed antemortem (30 cases) or postmortem (24 cases) reported by Younger and colleagues[2] more than 2 decades ago, had a selection bias of the most severe form of PCNSV. Twenty-eight were treated with CS alone (11 patients) or with oral CYC (in 16 patients), or AZA (in 1 patient), and followed for up to 1 year, of whom 18 (64%) improved, 7 (25%) were unchanged, and 3 (11%) died with roughly equally satisfactory outcomes after treatment with CS with or without CYC. Three patients diagnosed antemortem died while taking CS and CYC, and 2 had serious sequelae of the therapy, including fatal lymphoma, immunosuppression and opportunistic infection, or pneumonia and leukopenia. Of 24 patients diagnosed postmortem, 7 (29%) received treatment with CS alone (in 6 patients) or with CYC (in 1 patient) and 17 (71%) were untreated. Thus, 17 of 18 (94%) untreated patients died, indicating that, without therapy, the disease was usually fatal. Treatment with CS, alone or in combination with CYC, was associated with a considerable reduction in mortality; 24 of 34 (70%) so treated that survived either improved (50%) or were clinically unchanged. In this historical survey, there was no appreciable benefit in the addition of CYC; however, the numbers were small; unmatched for age, disease activity, or other factors; and follow-up was not uniform. Based on this historical survey, the investigators suggested that CYC be reserved for histologically confirmed cases of PCNSV, especially those patients who continue to progress or fail to improve on CS alone, and who can be monitored closely for serious medication side effects.

Two cohorts, one retrospective[3] and the other prospective,[105] have stratified cases based on clinical, neuroradiographic, and histopathologic laboratory features, offering additional insights into the management of CNS vasculitis. Over nearly 3 decades from 1983 to 2011, 163 patients at the Mayo Clinic with PCNSV were retrospectively analyzed by Salvarani and colleagues,[3] enrolling 105 patients (64%) who met inclusion criteria similar to those used by Calabreses and Mallek[6] and the proposed changes thereof by Birnbaum and Hellmann[106] for the diagnosis of probable CNS vasculitis based on cerebral angiography manifesting areas of smooth-wall segmental narrowing or dilatation, and occlusions that affected multiple cerebral arteries without the proximal vessel changes of atherosclerosis (or other causes); 58 patients (36%) met the definite diagnosis based on a CNS tissue biopsy showing transmural vascular inflammation involving leptomeningeal or parenchymal vessels. This histopathology was granulomatous in 35 patients (60.3%), lymphocytic in 13 (22.4%), and necrotizing alone in 10 (17.2%). These histologic patterns seemed to identify subsets of disease rather than different stages of the same process because no individual patient had histologic evidence of more than 1 pattern. A favorable response to therapy including CS (prednisone) alone or in association with CYC was observed in 85% of patients. Three patients treated with biologic agents, including RTX (1 patient) and TNF-α inhibitor (2 patients) for treatment refractory disease, were also improved. Relapses were observed in 27% of patients, and 25% of patients had discontinued therapy by the time of the last follow-up visit. Although response to treatment was not associated with any histologic pattern of the biopsy specimen, treatment with CS alone was associated with more frequent relapses (odds ratio [OR], 2.90), whereas large named vessel involvement (OR, 6.14) and cerebral infarcts at the time of diagnosis (OR, 3.32) were associated with a poor response to treatment. Among the patients diagnosed exclusively by angiography alone, relapses were more frequent when there was large vessel involvement (30%) than only small vessel changes (9%), with an increased mortality because of fatal neurovascular problems caused by PCNSV. Subsets of patients with PCNSV showed equally interesting insights. Salvarani and colleagues[107] noted granulomatous vasculitis in all 8 (100%) cerebral biopsies of patients with lymphoma and PCNSV, 2 of whom had concomitant CAA. Among 131 consecutive patients with PCNSV, 11 (8.4%) had a rapidly progressive course that was resistant to immunosuppressive therapy resulting in severe disability or death. Such patients had bilateral cortical and subcortical infarction on initial brain MRI and LVV on cerebral angiography with granulomatous and necrotizing vasculitis in brain tissue biopsies. All 11 patients failed to respond to aggressive immunosuppressive therapy, only 1 of whom survived, with major fixed neurologic deficits.

In 2018, De Boysson and colleagues[105] described the treatment and long-term outcomes of an observational cohort of 112 patients with PCNSV derived from 3 main networks: the FVSG, French Neurovascular Society, and the French Internal Medicine Society. The 3 main inclusion criteria were (1) involvement of CNS vessels as shown by biopsy or based on imaging (digital subtraction angiography or magnetic resonance [MR] angiography), of intracranial arterial stenoses, occlusions, or fusiform dilations; (2) a complete work-up, including infectious and immunologic serologies (human immunodeficiency virus, HBV, HCV, syphilis, tuberculosis, antinuclear and ANCA, echocardiography, and whole-body imaging, to exclude other alternative conditions affecting CNS vessels; and (3) a follow-up at more than 6 months (unless the patient died before 6 months of a biopsy-proven PCNSV) to prevent the inclusion of other vasculopathies, such as reversible cerebral vasoconstriction syndrome in which vascular lesions reverse within the first months.[108,109] The rate of prolonged remission was defined by the absence of relapse at 12 months or longer after diagnosis, as was the functional status at last follow-up in accordance with 3 main groups of treatments administered: CS (group 1); induction treatment with CS and an immunosuppressant, but no maintenance (group 2); and combined treatment with CS and an immunosuppressant for induction followed by maintenance therapy (group 3). Good functional status was defined as a modified Rankin Scale score less than or equal to 2 at the last follow-up. Among the 112 patients reported by De Boysson and colleagues,[105] 33 (29%) patients were included with a diagnostic CNS tissue biopsy, and 68 (61%) and 11 (10%) respectively had digital subtraction angiography or MR angiography consistent with PCNSV. Remission was achieved with the initial induction treatment in 106 (95%) of the 112 patients. Prolonged remission without relapse was observed in 70 (66%) patients after a mean of 57 months (range, 12–198 months) of follow-up. A good functional status at last follow-up (ie, modified Rankin Scale score $\leq$2) was observed in 63 (56%) patients. The overall mortality was 8%. More prolonged remissions ($P = .003$) and a better functional status at the last follow-up ($P = .0004$) were observed in group 3. In multivariate analysis, the use of maintenance therapy was associated with prolonged remission (OR, 4.32 [1.67–12.19]; $P = .002$) and better functional status (OR, 8.09 [3.24–22.38]; $P<.0001$). These findings suggest that maintenance therapy with an immunosuppressant combined with CS leads to the best long-term clinical and functional outcomes in patients with PCNSV after having achieved remission with either CS alone or in combination with another immunosuppressant. In that regard, CYC in combination with CS for induction and azathioprine for maintenance, were the 2 main immunosuppressants used in this registry. Whether other combinations or sequences can achieve better results remains to be ascertained.

Childhood With a minority of positive leptomeningeal and cortical brain biopsies in established series of adult cases of PCNSV, and an estimated annual incidence rate of 2.4 cases per 1 million person-years,[8] there are no satisfactory prevalence or incidence data or evidence-based guidelines to treat cPCNSV,[110] so the results of The PedVas Initiative, a Canadian and United Kingdom collaborative study (ARChiVe Investigators Network within The PedVas Initiative [ARChiVe registry], BrainWorks, and DCVAS) of pediatric and adult cases of AAV (GPA) and PACNS (National Institutes of Health identifier, NCT02006134), are awaited. The PedVas Initiative has been prospectively collecting clinical and biobank data since January 2013 of registered cases, within 12 months of study entry, and expected completion is in December 2019. The approach to cPACNS is incorporated into the larger area of IBrainD (IBD),[23] thereby excluding angiography-positive mimics of cPACANS; and angiography-negative, brain biopsy–positive mimics of SV-cPACNS. It is difficult to reconcile the applicability of the results from The PedVas Initiative for childhood to cPACNS[98] using CS, CYC, MTX, or RTX for remission induction, and PE in conjunction with CYC and/or RTX; and AZA, MTX, RTX, MMF, and CYC for up to 12 months for remission maintenance, with the disappointing rate of remission status of 42%, and a rate of visceral organ damage of 63%.[98]

The aim of treatment in IBD has nonetheless been to rapidly control the underlying inflammatory response and stabilize the blood-brain barrier while protecting the brain from further insults. Methylprednisolone has been the first-line agent administered intravenously at a dose of 30 mg/kg/d to a maximum of 1 g/d for 3 to 5 days[111] followed by 1 to 2 mg/kg/d of oral CS to a maximum of 60 mg/d of prednisone.[101,112] After stabilization the choice of immunosuppressive treatment is directed at the inflammatory pathways involved by the primary inflammatory or vasculitic process. Induction therapy with CS and pulse CYC followed by maintenance therapy with AZA or MMF has been recommended in cPACNS.[113] Children with SV-cPACNS were treated in an open-label study[113] with CYC in doses of 500 to 750 mg/m^2 as monthly infusions for 6 months, and followed with maintenance therapy with AZA of 1 mg/kg/d and a target dose of 2 to 3 mg/kg/d, and MMF at titrated doses of 800 to 1200 mg/m^2/d followed for up to 24 months using pediatric stroke outcome measures (PSOM). Among 19 such patients, 13 completed 24 months of follow-up, of whom 9 had a good neurologic outcome by PSOM scoring, 8 experienced disease flares, and 4 achieved remission of disease. MMF was more effective than AZA. Rituximab may be appropriate therapy at doses of 375 mg/m^2 for 4 consecutive weeks or 500 mg/m^2 weekly for 2 weeks in cPACNS, as was recently reported in SV-cPACNS.[114]

Nonsystemic Vasculitic Neuropathy

The vasculitic neuropathies are heterogeneous disorders that present in the setting of systemic vasculitis or in the absence thereof, where necrotizing arteritis may remain clinically and pathologically restricted to the peripheral nerves as SOV. The Peripheral Nerve Society[115,116] established respective guidelines for the classification, diagnosis, investigation, and treatment of nonsystemic vasculitic neuropathy (NSVN) and vasculitic peripheral neuropathy. Pathologically definite vasculitic neuropathy is defined by active or chronic peripheral nerve and muscle tissue lesions that show cellular invasion of the walls of blood vessels with accompanying acute vascular damage (fibrinoid necrosis, endothelial loss/disruption, internal lamina loss/fragmentation, smooth muscle media loss/fragmentation/separation, acute thrombosis, vascular/perivascular hemorrhage, or leukocytoclasia) or chronic vascular damage (intimal hyperplasia, fibrosis of media, adventitial/periadventitial fibrosis, or chronic thrombosis chronic thrombosis with recanalization), without evidence of another primary disease process that could mimic vasculitis pathologically, such as lymphoma, lymphomatoid granulomatosis, or amyloidosis. Patients with NSVN lack symptoms, signs, or laboratory evidence of involvement of other organs (demonstrable by laboratory evidence of PR3-ANA, MPO-ANA, mixed cryoglobulins, anti-Sjögren's antibodies syndrome-related antigen A and B (SSA, SSB), Smith (Sm), ribonuclear protein (RNP), SCL-70, centromere, double-stranded DNA, or citrullinated protein (CCP) serology; erythrocyte sedimentation rate >100 mm/h, or tissue biopsy evidence of vasculitis in another organ other than muscle; serologic, polymerase chain reaction, or culture evidence of a specific infection associated with vasculitis), and no predisposing factors (other than diabetes) of a connective tissue disease, sarcoidosis, inflammatory bowel disease, active malignancy, HUV, cutaneous PAN, or exposure to drugs likely to cause vasculitis. Inflammation of microvessels less than 40 to 70 μm in diameter without vascular damage is broadly referred to as MV.

The management of NPNV has remained uncertain because the concept presumes that the vasculitic disease process is widespread within the nerves and not elsewhere in the body. This assumption has been called into question by six lines of evidence. First, the reports of equally silent lesions in medium-sized muscular arteries in patients with clinically isolated vasculitic neuropathy.[117] Patient 1 in the series of pathologically confirmed cases of PAN by Kernohan and Woltman[118] was a 54-year-old man with 5 years of progressive generalized painful peripheral neuropathy that was so severe before death that he was partially paralyzed and unable to speak or swallow. Postmortem examination showed PAN limited to the nerve trunks of the arms and legs. The brain, cranial nerves, and spinal cord were normal except for early acute changes without evidence of vasculitis. Examination of all other organs failed to reveal a single vascular lesion, except 1 small artery in the capsule of the prostate gland. Torvik and Berntzen[119] described a 76-year-old woman with diffuse fever, pain, and central scotoma of the eye that improved with CSs. A biopsy of the temporal artery and pectoralis muscle disclosed necrotizing small arteries and arterioles in small adventitial vessels of the temporal artery without frank temporal arteritis. However, postmortem examination showed evidence of healed vasculitis in numerous small arteries and arterioles of muscle and nerve tissue measuring 50 to 200 μm in diameter without vasculitis in visceral organ or the CNS.

Second, the lack of long-term follow-up in most case series ranging from 6 months to 22 years.[120]

Third, the report of only 2 proposed cases, both with foci of vasculitis outside the PNS in a visceral organ[118] or the temporal artery.[119]

Fourth, vasculitis in muscle tissue is included in the definition of NPNV,[115] making the disorder perhaps more appropriately termed PNS vasculitis or PNSV.

Fifth, finding of vasculitis in a cutaneous nerve or muscle tissue specimen aids in the diagnosis of systemic vasculitides, particularly when no other site of vasculitis can be found. An example is the FVSG database, which used nerve and muscle tissue biopsy to establish systemic vasculitis in a retrospective study cohort of PAN in the absence or presence of symptomatic peripheral neuropathy.[121] Of 129 patients who underwent nerve biopsy, including 108 with peripheral neuropathy and 21 without peripheral neuropathy, vasculitic lesions were noted respectively in 83% and 81% of patients compared with muscle biopsy, which showed vasculitis respectively in 68% and 60%.

Sixth, the exclusion of patients with diabetes according to the 2010 guidelines[115] may allow another selection bias of ascertainment. Over the years, there has been increasing support for the contribution of an autoimmune mechanism in the pathogenesis of diabetic neuropathy. Diabetes seems to be caused by autoimmune mechanisms directed at insulin-producing pancreatic beta cells, and a variety of autoantibodies have been detected in patients with type 1 diabetes or insulin-dependent diabetes mellitus, including anti–islet cell cytoplasmic antibodies, present in up to 80% of newly diagnosed patients[122]; and glutamic acid decarboxylase antibodies, also present in patients with autoimmune stiff person syndrome.[123] Younger and colleagues[10] reported the clinicopathologic and immunohistochemical findings of sural nerve biopsy tissues in a cohort of 20 patients with heterogeneous forms of diabetic neuropathy. That series was continued to a total of 107 patients,[124] 3 of whom (3%) showed MV and 3 (3%) showed necrotizing arteritis. Although diabetes has not been considered a predisposing factor in PNV, the presence or absence of diabetes became a defining feature of patients with LSRPN.[11,125] In the only postmortem case of LSRPN described by Younger,[12] sural nerve biopsy showed mononuclear inflammatory cells surrounding a small epineurial artery with extension into the vascular wall, with reactive luminal connective tissue suggesting recanalization of a thrombus. An adjacent nerve fascicle showed marked loss of myelinated nerve fibers. The patient was treated for painful diabetic lumbosacral plexopathy and PNV according to prevailing standards with 2 g/kg intravenous immunoglobulin for 5 days, followed by 750 mg of intravenous CYC and 1000 mg of methylprednisolone intravenously for 3 additional days. Acute tubular necrosis, increasing lethargy, unresponsiveness, and aspiration pneumonia supervened and the patient expired 4 weeks after admission. General autopsy showed no evidence of systemic or PNV. The brain showed diffuse loss of neurons in all sampled cortical areas, including the cerebellum, consistent with anoxia secondary to cardiac arrest. Sections of extradural lumbar plexus, sciatic, and femoral nerve tissue showed perivascular epineurial inflammation with infiltration of adjacent endoneurium. This case suggests that the restricted LSRPN may be considered a good example of true NSVN.

There are no RCTs or ongoing observational cohort studies to guide the treatment of NPNV. However, published recommendations for the treatment of NSVN[115] suggest the use of oral CS therapy at the dose of 1 mg/kg/d, with tapering over 1 year to a low dose, unless there is rapidly progressive neuropathy that warrants combination therapy with CYC, MTX, and AZA. Other agents, such as IVIg and PE, are probably effective as both initial and adjunctive therapy. Careful monitoring should be performed to observe desired therapeutic responses and to avoid potentially serious drug side effects.

REFERENCES

1. Jennette JC, Falk RJ, Bacon PA, et al. 2012 revised International Chapel Hill Consensus Conference Nomenclature of Vasculitides. Arthritis Rheum 2013; 65:1–11.

2. Younger DS, Calabrese LH, Hays AP. Granulomatous angiitis of the nervous system. Neurol Clin 1997;15:821–34.

3. Salvarani C, Brown RD Jr, Christianson TJH, et al. Adult primary central nervous system vasculitis treatment and course. Analysis of one hundred and sixty-three patients. Arthritis Rheum 2015;67(6):1637–45.

4. Cupps TR, Moore PM, Fauci AS. Isolated angiitis of the central nervous system. Prospective diagnostic and therapeutic experience. Am J Med 1983;74:97–105.

5. Lanthier S, Lortie A, Michaud J, et al. Isolated angiitis of the CNS in children. Neurology 2001;56:837–42.

6. Calabrese HL, Mallek JA. Primary angiitis of the central nervous system: report of 8 new cases, review of the literature, and proposal for diagnostic criteria. Medicine 1988;67:20–39.

7. Younger DS, Hays AP, Brust JCM, et al. Granulomatous angiitis of the brain: an inflammatory reaction of nonspecific etiology. Arch Neurol 1988;45:514–8.

8. Salvarani C, Brown RD Jr, Calamia KT, et al. Primary central nervous system vasculitis: analysis of 101 patients. Ann Neurol 2007;62:442–51.

9. Benseler SM, Silverman E, Aviv RI, et al. Primary central nervous system vasculitis in children. Arthritis Rheum 2006;54:1291–7.

10. Younger DS, Rosoklija G, Hays AP, et al. Diabetic peripheral neuropathy: a clinicopathologic and immunohistochemical analysis of sural nerve biopsies. Muscle Nerve 1996;19:722–7.

11. Dyck PJB, Windebank AJ. Diabetic and nondiabetic lumbosacral radiculoplexus neuropathies: new insights into pathophysiology and treatment. Muscle Nerve 2002;25:477–91.

12. Younger DS. Diabetic lumbosacral radiculoplexus neuropathy: a postmortem studied patient and review of the literature. J Neurol 2011;258:1364–7.

13. Gwathmey KG, Burns TM, Collins MP, et al. Vasculitic neuropathies. Lancet Neurol 2014;13:67–82.

14. Rupert N, Ozen S, Pistorio A, et al. EULAR/PINTO/PRES criteria for Henoch-Schönlein purpura, childhood polyarteritis nodosa, childhood Wegener granulomatosis and childhood Takayasu arteritis: Ankara 2008. Part I: overall methodology and clinical characterization. Ann Rheum Dis 2010;69:790–7.

15. Ozen S, Pistorio A, Iusan SM, et al. EULAR/PRINTO/PReS criteria for Henoch-Schönlein purpura, childhood polyarteritis nodosa, childhood Wegener granulomatosis and childhood Takayasu arteritis. Ankara 2008. Part II: final classification. Ann Rheum Dis 2010;69:798–806.

16. British Medical Research Council. Streptomycin treatment of pulmonary tuberculosis: a medical research council investigation. BMJ 1948;2:769–83.

17. Direskeneli H, Aydin SZ, Kermani TA, et al. Development of outcome measures for large-vessel vasculitis for use in clinical trials: opportunities, challenges, and research agenda. J Rheumatol 2011;38:1471–9.

18. Stone J, Hoffman G, Merkel P, et al. A disease-specific activity index for Wegener's granulomatosis: modification of the Birmingham vasculitis activity score. Arthritis Rheum 2001;44:912–20.

19. Hellmich B, Flossmann O, Gross W, et al. EULAR recommendations for conducting clinical studies and/or clinical trials in systemic vasculitis: focus on anti-neutrophil cytoplasm antibody-associated vasculitis. Ann Rheum Dis 2007;66:605–17.

20. Merkel P, Aydin S, Boers M, et al. Current status of outcome measure development in vasculitis. J Rheumatol 2014;41:593–8.

21. Robson JC, Dawson J, Doll H, et al. Validation of the ANCA-associated vasculitis patient-reported outcomes (AAV-PRO) questionnaire. Ann Rheum Dis 2018;77:1157–64.

22. Robson JC, Dawson J, Cronholm PF, et al. Health-related quality of life in ANCA-associated vasculitis and item generation for a disease-specific patient-reported outcome measure. Patient Relat Outcome Meas 2018;9:17–34.

23. Twilt M, Benseler SM. Childhood inflammatory brain disease: pathogenesis, diagnosis and therapy. Rheumatology (Oxford) 2014;53:1359–68.

24. Liu E, Twilt M, Tyrrell PN, et al. Health-related quality of life in children with inflammatory brain disease. Pediatr Rheumatol Online J 2018;16:73.

25. Specks U, Merkel PA, Seo P, et al, for RAVE-ITN Research Group. Efficacy of remission-induction regimens for ANCA-associated vasculitis. N Engl J Med 2013;369:417–27.

26. Guillevin L, Pagnoux C, Seror R, et al. The five-factor score revisited: assessment of prognoses of systemic necrotizing vasculitides based on the French Vasculitis Study Group (FVSG) cohort. Medicine (Baltimore) 2011;90:19–27.

27. Mukhtyar C, Guillevin L, Cid MC, et al. EULAR recommendations for the management of large vessel vasculitis. Ann Rheum Dis 2009;68:318–23.

28. Salvarani C, Cantini F, Hunder GG. Polymyalgia rheumatica and giant-cell arteritis. Lancet 2008;372:234–45.

29. Mukhtyar C, Guillevin L, Cid MC, et al. EULAR recommendations for the management of primary small and medium vessel vasculitis. Ann Rheum Dis 2009;68:310–7.

30. Jayne D, Rasmussen N, Andrassy K, et al. A randomized trial of maintenance therapy for vasculitis associated with antineutrophil cytoplasmic autoantibodies. N Engl J Med 2003;349:36–44.

31. Guillevin L, Rosser J, Cacoub P, et al. Methylprednisolone in the treatment of Wegener's granulomatosis, polyarteritis nodosa and Churg-Strauss angiitis. AP-MIS Suppl 1990;19:52–3.

32. Newburger JW, Takahashi M, Gerber MA, et al. Diagnosis, treatment, and long-term management of Kawasaki disease: a statement for health professionals from the Committee on Rheumatic Fever, Endocarditis and Kawasaki Disease, Council on Cardiovascular Disease in the Young, American Heart Association. Circulation 2004;110:2747–71.

33. Kobayashi T, Saji T, Otani T, et al. Efficacy of immunoglobulin plus prednisolone for prevention of coronary artery abnormalities in severe Kawasaki disease (RAISE study): a randomised, open-label, blinded-endpoints trial. Lancet 2012;379:1613–20.

34. Dammacco F, Sansonno D, Han JH, et al. Natural interferon-alpha versus its combination with 6-methyl-prednisolone in the therapy of type II mixed cryoglobulinemia: a long-term, randomized, controlled study. Blood 1994;84:3336–43.

35. Fauci AS, Wolff SM. Wegener's granulomatosis: studies in eighteen patients and a review of the literature. Medicine 1973;52:535–61.

36. Hoffman GS, Kerr GS, Leavitt RY, et al. Wegener granulomatosis: an analysis of 158 patients. Ann Intern Med 1992;116:488–98.

37. Guillevin L, Cordier JF, Lhote F, et al. A prospective, multicenter, randomized trial comparing steroids and pulse cyclophosphamide versus steroids and oral cyclophosphamide in the treatment of generalized Wegener's granulomatosis. Arthritis Rheum 1997;40:2187–98.

38. De Groot K, Adu D, Savage CO. The value of pulse cyclophosphamide in ANCA-associated vasculitis: meta-analysis and critical review. Nephrol Dial Transplant 2001;16:2018–27.

39. de Groot K, Harper L, Jayne DR, et al, EUVAS (European Vasculitis Study Group). Pulse versus daily oral cyclophosphamide for induction of remission in antineutrophil cytoplasmic antibody-associated vasculitis: a randomized trial. Ann Intern Med 2009;150:670–80.

40. Pillebout E, Alberti C, Guillevin L, et al. Addition of cyclophosphamide to steroids provides no benefit compared with steroids alone in treating adult patients with severe Henoch Schönlein purpura. Kidney Int 2010;78:495–502.
41. Terrier B, Semoun O, Saadoun D, et al. Prognostic factors in patients with hepatitis C virus infection and systemic vasculitis. Arthritis Rheum 2011;63:1748–57.
42. Maltzman JS, Koretzky GA. Azathioprine: old drug, new actions. J Clin Invest 2003;111:1122–4.
43. Mahr AD, Jover JA, Spiera RF, et al. Adjunctive methotrexate for treatment of giant cell arteritis: an individual patient data meta-analysis. Arthritis Rheum 2007;56:2789–97.
44. Hoffman GS, Cid MC, Hellmann DB, et al. A multicenter, randomized, double-blind, placebo-controlled trial of adjuvant methotrexate treatment for giant cell arteritis. Arthritis Rheum 2002;46:1309–18.
45. Spiera RF, Mitnick HJ, Kupersmith M, et al. A prospective, double-blind, randomized, placebo controlled trial of methotrexate in the treatment of giant cell arteritis (GCA). Clin Exp Rheumatol 2001;19:495–501.
46. Jover JA, Hernandez-Garcia C, Morado IC, et al. Combined treatment of giant-cell arteritis with methotrexate and prednisone. Ann Intern Med 2001;134:106–14.
47. Pagnoux C, Mahr A, Hamidou MA, et al, for the French Vasculitis Study Group. Azathioprine or methotrexate maintenance for ANCA-associated vasculitis. N Engl J Med 2008;359:2790–803.
48. Fulton B, Markham A. Mycophenolate mofetil. A review of its pharmacodynamic and pharmacokinetic properties and clinical efficacy in renal transplantation. Drugs 1996;51:278–98.
49. Hiemstra TF, Walsh M, Mahr A, et al, European Vasculitis Study Group (EUVAS). Mycophenolate mofetil vs azathioprine for remission maintenance in antineutrophil cytoplasmic antibody-associated vasculitis: a randomized controlled trial. JAMA 2010;304:2381–8.
50. Geetha D, Jin Q, Scott J, et al. Comparisons of guidelines and recommendations on managing antineutrophil cytoplasmic antibody-associated vasculitis. Kidney Int Rep 2018;3(5):1039–49.
51. Ntatsaki E, Carruthers D, Chakravarty K. BSR and BHPR guideline for the management of adults with ANCA-associated vasculitis. Rheumatology (Oxford) 2014;53:2306–9.
52. Yates M, Watts RA, Bajema IM. EULAR/ERA-EDTA recommendations for the management of ANCA-associated vasculitis. Ann Rheum Dis 2016;75:1583–94.
53. Dougados M, Betteridge N, Burmester GR. EULAR standardised operating procedures for the elaboration, evaluation, dissemination, and implementation of recommendations endorsed by the EULAR standing committees. Ann Rheum Dis 2004;63:1172–6.
54. De Souza AW, da Silva MD, Machado LS, et al. Short-term effect of leflunomide in patients with Takayasu arteritis: an observational study. Scand J Rheumatol 2012;41:227–30.
55. Metzler C, Miehle N, Manger K, et al. Elevated relapse rate under oral methotrexate versus leflunomide for maintenance of remission in Wegener's granulomatosis. Rheumatology 2007;46:1087–91.
56. Jayne DR, Gaskin G, Rasmussen N, et al, on behalf of the European Vasculitis Study Group. Randomized trial of plasma exchange or high-dosage methylprednisolone as adjunctive therapy for severe renal vasculitis. J Am Soc Nephrol 2007;18:2180–8.

57. Walsh M, Merkel PA, Peh CA, et al, PEXIVAS Investigators. Plasma exchange and glucocorticoid dosing in the treatment of anti-neutrophil cytoplasm antibody associated vasculitis (PEXIVAS): protocol for a randomized controlled trial. Trials 2013;14:73.

58. Levy JB, Turner AN, Rees AJ, et al. Long-term outcome of anti-glomerular basement membrane antibody disease treated with plasma exchange and immunosuppression. Ann Intern Med 2001;134:1033–42.

59. Furusho K, Kamiya T, Nakano H, et al. High-dose intravenous gammaglobulin for Kawasaki disease. Lancet 1984;2:1055–8.

60. Newburger JW, Takahashi M, Burns JC, et al. The treatment of Kawasaki syndrome with intravenous gamma globulin. N Engl J Med 1986;315:341–7.

61. Newburger JW, Takahashi M, Beiser AS, et al. A single intravenous infusion of gamma globulin as compared with four infusions in the treatment of acute Kawasaki syndrome. N Engl J Med 1991;324:1633–9.

62. Jayne DR, Davies MJ, Fox CJ, et al. Treatment of systemic vasculitis with pooled intravenous immunoglobulin. Lancet 1991;337:1137–9.

63. Jayne DR, Lockwood CM. Intravenous immunoglobulin as sole therapy for systemic vasculitis. Br J Rheumatol 1996;35:1150–3.

64. Jayne DR, Chapel H, Adu D, et al. Intravenous immunoglobulin for ANCA-associated systemic vasculitis with persistent disease activity. QJM 2000;93: 433–9.

65. Martinez V, Cohen P, Pagnoux C, et al, French Vasculitis Study Group. Intravenous immunoglobulins for relapses of systemic vasculitides associated with antineutrophil cytoplasmic autoantibodies: results of a multicenter, prospective, open-label study of twenty-two patients. Arthritis Rheum 2008;58:308–17.

66. Stone JH, Merkel PA, Spiera R, et al. Rituximab versus cyclophosphamide for ANCA-associated vasculitis. N Engl J Med 2010;363:221–32.

67. Jones RB, Tervaert JW, Hauser T, et al. Rituximab versus cyclophosphamide in ANCA-associated renal vasculitis. N Engl J Med 2010;363:211–20.

68. Guillevin L, Pagnoux C, Karras A, et al. Rituximab versus azathioprine for maintenance in ANCA-associated vasculitis. N Engl J Med 2014;371:1771–80.

69. Pugnet G, Pagnoux C, Terrier B, et al. Rituximab versus azathioprine for ANCA-associated vasculitis maintenance therapy: impact on global disability and health-related quality of life. Clin Exp Rheumatol 2016;34(3 Suppl 97):S54–9.

70. Zaja F, De Vita S, Mazzaro C, et al. Efficacy and safety of rituximab in type II mixed cryoglobulinemia. Blood 2003;101:3827–34.

71. Sansonno D, De Re V, Lauletta G, et al. Monoclonal antibody treatment of mixed cryoglobulinemia resistant to interferon alpha with an anti-CD20. Blood 2003; 101:3818–26.

72. Roccatello D, Baldovino S, Rossi D, et al. Long-term effects of anti-CD20 monoclonal antibody treatment of cryoglobulinaemic glomerulonephritis. Nephrol Dial Transplant 2004;19:3054–61.

73. Saadoun D, Resche-Rigon M, Sene D, et al. Rituximab combined with Peg-interferon-ribavirin in refractory hepatitis C virus-associated cryoglobulinaemia vasculitis. Ann Rheum Dis 2008;67:1431–6.

74. Terrier B, Saadoun D, Sene D, et al. Efficacy and tolerability of rituximab with or without PEGylated interferon alfa-2b plus ribavirin in severe hepatitis C virus-related vasculitis: a long-term followup study of thirty-two patients. Arthritis Rheum 2009;60:2531–40.

75. Ignatova TM, Kozlovskaya LV, Gordovskaya NB, et al. Hepatitis C virus-associated cryoglobulinemic vasculitis: a 20-year experience with treatment. Ter Arkh 2017;89:46–52 [in Russian].

76. Booth A, Harper L, Hammad T, et al. Prospective study of TNFα blockade with infliximab in anti-neutrophil cytoplasmic antibody-associated systemic vasculitis. J Am Soc Nephrol 2004;15:717–21.

77. Bartolucci P, Ramanoelina J, Cohen P, et al. Efficacy of the anti-TNF-alpha antibody infliximab against refractory systemic vasculitides: an open pilot study on 10 patients. Rheumatology 2002;41:1126–32.

78. Wegener's Granulomatosis Etanercept Trial (WGET) Research Group. Etanercept plus standard therapy for Wegener's granulomatosis. N Engl J Med 2005;352:351–61.

79. De Menthon M, Cohen P, Pagnoux C, et al. Infliximab or rituximab for refractory Wegener's granulomatosis: long-term follow up. A prospective randomised multicentre study on 17 patients. Clin Exp Rheumatol 2011;29:S63–71.

80. Seror R, Baron G, Hachulla E, et al. Adalimumab for steroid sparing in patients with giant-cell arteritis: results of a multicentre randomised controlled trial. Ann Rheum Dis 2014;73(12):2074–81.

81. Mekinian A, Neel A, Sibilia J, et al. Efficacy and tolerance of infliximab in refractory Takayasu arteritis: French multicentre study. Rheumatology 2012;51:882–6.

82. Frohnert PP, Sheps SG. Long-term follow-up study of periarteritis nodosa. Am J Med 1967;43:8–14.

83. Mukhtyar C, Flossmann O, Hellmich B, et al. Outcomes from studies of antineutrophil cytoplasm antibody associated vasculitis: a systematic review by the European League Against Rheumatism Systemic Vasculitis Task Force. Ann Rheum Dis 2008;67:1004–10.

84. Talar-Williams C, Hijazi YM, Walther MM, et al. Cyclophosphamide-induced cystitis and bladder cancer in patients with Wegener granulomatosis. Ann Intern Med 1996;124:477–84.

85. de Leeuw K, Kallenberg C, Bijl M. Accelerated atherosclerosis in patients with systemic autoimmune diseases. Ann N Y Acad Sci 2005;1051:362–71.

86. Little MA, Nightingale P, Verburgh CA, et al. Early mortality in systemic vasculitis: relative contribution of adverse events and active vasculitis. Ann Rheum Dis 2010;69:1036–43.

87. Xiao H, Heeringa P, Hu P, et al. Antineutrophil cytoplasmic autoantibodies specific for myeloperoxidase cause glomerulonephritis and vasculitis in mice. J Clin Invest 2002;110:955–63.

88. Little MA, Al-Ani B, Ren S, et al. Anti-proteinase 3 anti-neutrophil cytoplasm autoantibodies recapitulate systemic vasculitis in mice with a humanized immune system. PLoS One 2012;7:e28626.

89. Kain R, Exner M, Brandes R, et al. Molecular mimicry in pauci-immune focal necrotizing glomerulonephritis. Nat Med 2008;14:1088–96.

90. Popa ER, Stegeman CA, Kallenberg CG, et al. *Staphylococcus aureus* and Wegener's granulomatosis. Arthritis Res 2002;4:77–9.

91. Xing GQ, Chen M, Liu G, et al. Complement activation is involved in renal damage in human antineutrophil cytoplasmic autoantibody associated pauci-immune vasculitis. J Clin Immunol 2009;29:282–91.

92. Popa ER, Franssen CF, Limburg PC, et al. In vitro cytokine production and proliferation of T cells from patients with anti-proteinase 3- and antimyeloperoxidase-associated vasculitis, in response to proteinase 3 and myeloperoxidase. Arthritis Rheum 2002;46:1894–904.

93. Weyand CM, Goronzy JJ. Medium- and large-vessel vasculitis. N Engl J Med 2003;349:160–9.

94. Lamprecht P. Off balance: T-cells in antineutrophil cytoplasmic antibody (ANCA)-associated vasculitides. Clin Exp Immunol 2005;141:201–10.

95. De Groot K, Rasmussen N, Bacon PA, et al. Randomized trial of cyclophosphamide versus methotrexate for induction of remission in early systemic antineutrophil cytoplasmic antibody-associated vasculitis. Arthritis Rheum 2005;52:2461–9.

96. Harper L, Morgan MD, Walsh M, et al. Pulse versus daily oral cyclophosphamide for induction of remission in ANCA-associated vasculitis: long-term follow-up. Ann Rheum Dis 2012;71:955–60.

97. Faurschou M, Westman K, Rasmussen N, et al. Brief report: long-term outcome of a randomized clinical trial comparing methotrexate to cyclophosphamide for remission induction in early systemic antineutrophil cytoplasmic antibody-associated vasculitis. Arthritis Rheum 2012;64:3472–7.

98. Morishita KA, Moorthy LN, Lubieniecka JM, et al. Early outcomes in children with antineutrophil cytoplasmic antibody-associated vasculitis. Arthritis Rheum 2017; 69:1470–9.

99. Sacri AS, Chambaraud T, Ranchin B, et al. Clinical characteristics and outcomes of childhood-onset ANCA-associated vasculitis: a French nationwide study. Nephrol Dial Transplant 2015;30 Suppl 1:i104–12.

100. Ter Haar NM, Oswald M, Jeyaratnam J, et al. Recommendations for the management of autoinflammatory diseases. Ann Rheum Dis 2015;74:1636–44.

101. Golumbek P. Pharmacologic agents for pediatric neuroimmune disorders. Semin Pediatr Neurol 2010;17:245–53.

102. Graus F, Titulaer MJ, Balu R, et al. A clinical approach of autoimmune encephalitis. Lancet Neurol 2016;15:391–404.

103. Elbers J, Halliday W, Hawkins C, et al. Brain biopsy in children with primary small-vessel central nervous system vasculitis. Ann Neurol 2010;68:602–10.

104. Torres J, Loomis C, Cucchiara B, et al. Diagnostic yield and safety of brain biopsy for suspected primary central nervous system angiitis. Stroke 2016;47:2127–9.

105. De Boysson H, Arquizan C, Touze E, et al. Treatment and long-term outcomes of primary central nervous system vasculitis. Stroke 2018;49:1946–52.

106. Birnbaum J, Hellmann DB. Primary angiitis of the central nervous system. Arch Neurol 2009;66:704–9.

107. Salvarani C, Brown RD Jr, Christianson TJH, et al. Primary central nervous system vasculitis associated with lymphoma. Neurology 2018;90:e847–55.

108. Ducros A, Boukobza M, Porcher R, et al. The clinical and radiological spectrum of reversible cerebral vasoconstriction syndrome. A prospective series of 67 patients. Brain 2007;130:3091–101.

109. Singhal AB, Topcuoglu MA, Fok JW, et al. Reversible cerebral vasoconstriction syndromes and primary angiitis of the central nervous system: clinical, imaging, and angiographic comparison. Ann Neurol 2016;79:882–94.

110. Twilt M, Benseler SM. Central nervous system vasculitis in adults and children. Handb Clin Neurol 2016;133:283–300.

111. Cellucci T, Benseler SM. Central nervous system vasculitis in children. Curr Opin Rheumatol 2010;22:590–7.

112. Twilt M, Benseler SM. The spectrum of CNS vasculitis in children and adults. Nat Rev Rheumatol 2012;8:97–107.

113. Hutchinson C, Elbers J, Halliday W, et al. Treatment of small vessel primary CNS vasculitis in children: an open-label cohort study. Lancet Neurol 2010;9: 1078–84.
114. Deng J, Fang G, Wang XH, et al. Small vessel-childhood primary angiitis of the central nervous system: a case report and literature review. Zhonghua Er Ke Za Zhi 2018;56:142–7.
115. Collins MP, Dyck PJ, Gronseth GS, et al. Peripheral Nerve Society Guideline on the classification, diagnosis, investigation, and immunosuppressive therapy of non-systemic vasculitic neuropathy: executive summary. J Peripher Nerv Syst 2010;15:176–84.
116. Hadden RDM, Collins MP, Zivkovic SA, et al, the Brighton Collaboration Vasculitic Peripheral Neuropathy Working Group. Vasculitic peripheral neuropathy: case definition for collection analysis, and presentation of immunization safety data. Vaccine 2017;35:1567–78.
117. Said G, Lacroix C, Fujimura H, et al. The peripheral neuropathy of necrotizing arteritis: a clinicopathologic study. Ann Neurol 1988;23:461–5.
118. Kernohan JW, Woltman HW. A clinicopathologic study with special reference to the nervous system. Arch Neurol Psychiatry 1938;39:655–86.
119. Torvik A, Berntzen AE. Necrotizing vasculitis without visceral involvement. Postmortem examination of three cases with affection of skeletal muscles and peripheral nerves. Acta Med Scand 1968;184:69–77.
120. Dyck PJ, Benstead TJ, Conn DL, et al. Nonsystemic vasculitic neuropathy. Brain 1987;110:843–53.
121. Pagnoux C, Seror R, Henegar C, et al. Clinical features and outcomes in 348 patients with polyarteritis nodosa: a systematic retrospective study of patients diagnosed between 1963 and 2005 and entered into the French Vasculitis Study Group Database. Arthritis Rheum 2010;62:616–26.
122. Atkinson MA, Caclaren NK. The pathogenesis of insulin-dependent diabetes mellitus. N Engl J Med 1994;331:1428–36.
123. Grimaldi LME, Mertini G, Braghi S, et al. Heterogeneity of autoantibodies in stiff-man syndrome. Ann Neurol 1993;34:57–64.
124. Younger DS. Diabetic neuropathy: a clinical and neuropathological study of 107 patients. Neurol Res Int 2010;2010:140379.
125. Dyck PJ, Norell JE, Dyck PJ. Non-diabetic lumbosacral radiculoplexus neuropathy: natural history, outcome and comparison with the diabetic variety. Brain 2001;124:1197–207.

Central Nervous System Vasculitis Due to Substance Abuse

David S. Younger, MD, MPH, MS[a,b],*

KEYWORDS

- Substance abuse • Stroke • Vasculitis • Central nervous system

KEY POINTS

- Illicit drug abuse is a common differential diagnosis of acquired central nervous system vasculitis.
- There are only a handful of histopathologically confirmed cases in the literature from among the many potential classes of abused drugs traditionally implicated in this disease.
- Hemorrhagic and non-hemorrhagic stroke often preceded by vasospasm are common outcomes in confirmed cases.
- This article considers the major classes of illicit drugs in those with and without human immunodeficiency virus type-1 infection and acquired immune deficiency syndrome.

INTRODUCTION

Drug abuse is a rare cause of histopathologically verified central nervous system (CNS) vasculitis. With only a handful of confirmed patients in the literature, and rare association with progressive neurologic deficits, there is generally little justification for invasive laboratory investigation, especially given the availability of highly accurate vascular neuroimaging techniques. Management rests on avoidance of further exposure and minimizing the secondary neurotoxic effects of the abused substances and polypharmacy use. This article reviews the epidemiology, background, neuropharmacology, and histopathology of verified cases, and proposed etiopathogenic mechanisms that cause CNS vasculitis.

Disclosure Statement: The author has nothing to disclose.
[a] Department of Neurology, Division of Neuro-Epidemiology, New York University School of Medicine, New York, NY, USA; [b] School of Public Health, City University of New York, New York, NY, USA
* 333 East 34th Street, Suite 1J, New York, NY 10016.
E-mail address: youngd01@nyu.edu
Website: http://www.davidsyounger.com

Neurol Clin 37 (2019) 425–440
https://doi.org/10.1016/j.ncl.2019.01.012
0733-8619/19/© 2019 Elsevier Inc. All rights reserved.

CLASSIFICATION AND NOSOLOGY

The most widely used classification and nosology for the vasculitides is the 2012 Revised International Chapel Hill Consensus Conference Nomenclature.[1]

BLOOD BRAIN BARRIER

The past decade has witnessed extraordinary progress in our understanding of the blood brain barrier (BBB),[2] and progress in its understanding will likely afford new insights into our understanding of cerebral vasculitis and the impact of substance abuse on the nervous system. The neurovascular unit (NVU) of the BBB is composed of capillary endothelial cells, pericytes, smooth muscle cells, astrocytes, neuronal terminals, and white blood cells (in the extended NVU). Each of the components expresses a wide variety of receptors, ion channels, and transporters and resides in proximity to one another allowing for the dynamic modulation of blood flow, metabolism, and electrophysiologic regulation.[3] Many of the influx and efflux mechanisms of the BBB are present early in the developing brain, encoded by genes at much higher levels than in the adult.[4] The disruption of tight and adherens junctions, enzymatic degradation of the capillary basement membrane, or both, leads to disruption of tight junctions, altered expression and function of membrane transporters or enzymes, increased passage of inflammatory cells across the BBB from the blood to CNS, and dysfunction of astrocytes and other components. This leads to aberrant angiogenesis and neuroinflammation with concomitant vasogenic edema, accumulation of toxic substances in the brain interstitial fluid, oxidative stress, and impaired ion and water homeostasis.

AMPHETAMINES

The earliest reports of misuse of amphetamine sulfate were in late 1930 when it was used by students to avoid sleep during examination periods.[5] This was followed by reports of death by those who ingested the drug repeatedly as a stimulant for the same purpose,[6] in a suicide attempt that resulted in a fatal intracerebral hemorrhage,[7] or accidentally, when dexamphetamine and phenelzine were fatally ingested together decades later.[8] During the Second World War, amphetamine and methamphetamine were used clinically and illicitly but its abuse soared in San Francisco after 1962, wherein it was illegally produced and distributed.[9]

Amphetamine, methamphetamine, and their derivatives comprise a large spectrum of agents[10] available in powder, capsule, tablet, and injectable fluid form that can be swallowed, snorted or taken intranasally, smoked, or injected with highly variable purity and dosage equivalence. Their potent effects, which include elevation of blood pressure, pulse rate, and increased level of alertness, sometimes in association with insomnia, excitability, panic attacks, and aggressive behavior, also can be associated with seizure and stroke. Their effects distribute throughout the brain. Ecstasy refers to the different hallucinogenic amphetamine derivatives that contain 3,4-methylenedioxymethamphetamine and 3,4-methylenedioxyethylamphetamine as the main components[11] that alter brain serotonin concentrations, and postsynaptic 5-HT$_2$ receptors that play a role in the regulation of brain microvessels. The CNS toxic effects are mitigated through blocking of the reuptake of dopamine (DA) and stimulation of the release of DA and norepinephrine, as well as possible involvement on the serotonergic and endogenous opiate system. There can be DA receptor desensitization with marked reduction of DA transporters and drug levels, as well as other dopaminergic axonal markers. The neurotoxic effects of methamphetamine are believed to be mediated by multiple additional mechanisms including the generation of free radicals, nitric oxide, excitotoxicity, mitochondrial dysfunction, apoptosis, and the induction of im-mediate early inflammatory genes and transcription factors. Methamphetamine is the most potent amphetamine and the most commonly abused. All forms of amphet-amine administration increase the risk of stroke that may be ischemic, hemorrhagic and intraparenchymal,[12] which may be up to fourfold that of nonusers,[13] surpassing the rate of hemorrhagic stroke caused by cocaine use with odds ratios respectively of 4.95 versus 2.33.[14] Still, amphetamines and methamphetamine are the second commonest cause of all strokes after cocaine, occurring largely in persons younger than 45 years.

Cerebral vasculitis due to amphetamine, methamphetamine, and related agents is exceedingly rare with only 3 histopathologically studied patients in the literature.[15,16] This is surprising given the number of substances that could cause this disorder if there was a true association. Amphetamine-related multiorgan arteritis including the CNS was demonstrated by Citron and colleagues[16] in a highly publicized report of 14 Los Angeles multidrug abusers. The drug closest to a common denominator was metham-phetamine used intravenously by all but 2 patients and exclusively by 1. Acute vessel lesions of fibrinoid necrosis of the media and intima with infiltration by polymorphonu-clear cells, eosinophils, lymphocytes, and histiocytes was followed by vascular elastic and vascular smooth muscle destruction resulting in lesions considered typical for pol-yarteritis nodosa. Two patients, one abbreviated D.G. and the other E.V., who injected methamphetamine via intravenous injection had arterial lesions in cerebral and cere-bellar (D.G.) and brainstem pontine vessels (D.G. and E.V.); however, detailed histo-pathologic descriptions were not provided. Their report was followed by correspondence by Gocke and Christian[17] who contended that exposure to the Australia antigen of hepatitis B antigen was likely in their cohort[16] conceivably associ-ated with circulating immune complexes and complement activation as had recently been described.[18,19] The investigators[20] responded that no more than 30% of sera from drug abuse patients ultimately tested positive for the Australia antigen. Those with antigen-positive sera who had used drugs others than methamphetamine had no evidence of angiitis when studied angiographically. Baden[21] wrote that he had not observed a causal relation between drug abuse and necrotizing arteritis at the Of-fice of Chief Medical Examiner of New York City for the past one-half century among thousands of autopsied drug abusers. Further, 14 cases claimed documentation for angiitis was presented in only 4 patients but no substantiation for the diagnosis was given in the remainder except that 5 were asymptomatic, and 5 had a variety of nonspe-cific systemic signs and symptoms. Citron and Peters[20] responded that evidence of aneurysms so noted in 13 patients, was in their opinion ample evidence of arteritis.

Almost 2 decades later, cerebral vasculitis was demonstrated in a dubious report[15] of a 3 week postpartum woman who took her first over-the-counter Dexatrim diet pill in many months containing phenylpropanolamine, without a history of amphetamine abuse. This was followed 90 minutes later by sudden headache, nausea, vomiting, and detection of subarachnoid blood on computed tomography neuroimaging and a frontal lobe hematoma. Bilateral carotid angiography demonstrated diffuse segmental narrowing and dilatation of small, medium, and large vessels and branches of the anterior and posterior circulation. Evacuation and histopathologic analysis of the hematoma was performed showing necrotizing vasculitis of small arteries and veins with infiltration of polymorphonuclear leukocytes particularly prominent in the intima with fragmentation of the elastic lamina and areas of vessel occlusion. It was unclear whether the findings were related to primary or drug-related CNS vasculitis. However, treatment with cyclophosphamide for 6 months was associated with almost complete resolution of cerebral angiographic abnormalities.

After the report of Citron and colleagues,[16] Rumbaugh and colleagues[22] described the cerebral vascular changes due to methamphetamine abuse in 5 rhesus monkeys given amphetamine in dose ranges used by human addicts. Two of the 5 monkeys developed generalized arterial spasm during a 2-week period following intravenous injection. Three of 5 animals demonstrated decreased caliber of named cerebral artery branches and flow of the contrast agent with normalization 1 day later, whereas 2 others showed marked general decrease in small branches and large named vessels that improved in one animal and progressed in another. Histopathologic changes at postmortem examination included microaneurysmal enlargement of arteriolar segments, mononuclear perivascular cuffing of small arterioles, parenchymal necrosis, petechial hemorrhages, and swelling of brain tissue, with most of the hemorrhagic lesions centered on small-size arteriolar and capillary vessels. Although reminiscent of the clinical and histopathologic findings of Citron and colleagues,[16] necrotizing arteritis and transmural inflammation were lacking. Five years later, Rumbaugh and coworkers[23] subjected monkeys to short-duration (2 weeks; 5 animals), medium-duration (1 month; 3 monkeys), and long duration (1 year; 3 monkeys) of thrice weekly (1.5 mg/kg body weight) intravenous amphetamine and related agents including methamphetamine, secobarbital, methylphenidate, and placebo, with performance of cerebral angiography and documentation of the resulting histopathology. Their studies showed relatively severe vascular injury and brain damage from intravenous methamphetamine that included occlusions and slow blood flow in small cerebral vessels, respectively, in 2 each of the 5 monkeys in the long-term administered drug, and in 3 each of those given drug for intermediate and short durations, with some animals and controls unaffected. There was less injury caused by secobarbital and methylphenidate. Further, the possibility of vascular spasm due to subarachnoid blood was excluded by lack of blood at postmortem examination in the subarachnoid space in any of the animals.

Cocaine

Cocaine is derived from the leaves of the *Erythroxylum coca* plant and found primarily in the eastern mountains of Peru, Ecuador, and Bolivia. It is abused as cocaine hydrochloride, a water-soluble white salt in crystal, granular, and white powder that can be sniffed and "snorted" intranasally or injected parenterally. The "free-base" alkaloid form, known as "crack," derives its name from the cracking sound that occurs after dissolution of the hydrochloride salt in water, heated, and mixed with ammonia without or without baking soda. This chemical reaction converts cocaine hydrochloride to a volatile form of the drug, almost pure cocaine. Street cocaine or the noncrack form is highly variable in purity, and often cut with various agents. When smoked as freebase, it is absorbed into the pulmonary circulation and transmitted to the brain in less than 10 seconds. After appearance in the bloodstream, cocaine is rapidly hydrolyzed to benzoylecgonine, which can be accurately tested in the urine; however, levels may persist for up to 27 to 36 hours depending on the route of administration and host cholinesterase activity. In recent years, with increasing availability and purity, and a drop in the price of cocaine from the early 1970s of $85 per gram, new cohorts from all socioeconomic backgrounds and age groups have been attracted to this highly addictive drug, and use has continued to expand on a year-by-year basis.

Cocaine is a highly potent CNS stimulant that rapidly crosses the BBB due to its highly lipophilic properties and is widely distributed through the brain with its major metabolites binding at receptors with varying affinities at presynaptic sites stimulating the release of DA from synaptic vesicles and blocking DA reuptake resulting in enhanced dopaminergic neurotransmission, in addition to its local anesthetic properties. The investigation of single nucleotide polymorphisms that encode amino acid substitutions in opioid receptors and ligands implicated in drug addiction, particularly those of the mu opioid receptor (MUP-r) gene system (*OPRM1)* that releases DA from neural synapse when activated, and those of the kappa receptor (KUP-r) that instead lower extracellular dopamine levels, have contributed understanding to the variability in drug addiction among susceptible individuals.[24]

Only 10 histologically verified patients with cerebral vasculitis, including 6 men and 4 women, age 21 to 39 (mean age 28 years), occurred in the absence of other possible known causes including concomitant infection by human immunodeficiency virus type 1 infection and known causative coinfections[25–39]. In all but 1 patient,[30] who had a long-standing cocaine habit with abuse sometime in the 6 months before admission, onset of neurologic symptoms immediately followed cocaine use that was intranasal cocaine in 6 patients,[28–32] intravenous in 2,[26,27] smoked in 1,[26] and acquired via unknown modality in 1.[26] Cerebral vasculitis was associated with cerebral hemorrhage in 3 patients[29,30] and ischemia in the 7 patients[25–28,31,32] who typically presented with abrupt onset of headache and focal hemiparesis so noted in 6 patients,[25,26,29,30] confusion or agitation,[27,28,30–32] and grand mal seizures,[28] that progressed to stupor, coma, and death in 3 patients.[25,26,28] Lumbar cerebrospinal fluid (CSF) analysis showed lymphocytic pleocytosis of 10 to 65 cells/cm^3 with elevation of the protein content from 185 to 630 mg/dL,[27,32] and was completely normal in 2 other patients.[26,30] Cerebral angiography performed in 7 patients showed an avascular mass in the patient with a putaminal hemorrhage,[29] abnormal large named vessel occlusions or segmental narrowing in 3 patients,[25,26,30] poor filling and irregularities in vessel appearance in 2,[31,32] and normal in 1 patient.[27]

The pathology of cerebral vasculitis was established by brain and meningeal biopsy in 7 patients,[26–32] at postmortem examination in 2 patients,[25,28] and by both in 1 patient.[26] The underlying pathology of cerebral vasculitis was non-necrotizing with transmural mononuclear cell inflammation affecting small arteries and veins in 3 patients[26,28,29] or veins alone in 3 patients,[30–32] and perivascular cuffing of small arteries and veins in another.[27] In 2 patients there was necrosis of small cerebral vessels associated with polymorphonuclear cell inflammation of small arteries and veins[30] or large named vessels.[25] Among 3 patients so studied at postmortem examination, non-necrotizing small vessel vasculitis was noted in the brains of 2 patients without evidence of systemic involvement,[27,28] whereas necrotizing large vessel vasculitis was found in both the brain and systemic organs.[25] Treatment consisting of corticosteroid was administered to 7 patients, 5 of whom improved[26,27,30,32] and 2 who died with refractory seizures despite anticonvulsant medication[33] or as a consequence of infection, coma, and decerebration.[25] There was no mention of treatment or outcome in 3 patients,[28,29,31] including 2 patients who succumbed to coma, hypoxic-ischemic decerebration, and death.[28,29]

Although cocaine-associated cerebral vasculitis has not been rigorously studied, several independent lines of experimental evidence suggest possible etiopathogenic mechanisms in susceptible individuals. The first was the observed effects of cocaine in the induction of adhesion molecules and endothelial leukocyte migration across cerebral blood vessel endothelia walls, particularly under inflammatory conditions, which may disturb the function of the BBB. Cocaine increased the expression of the endothelial adhesion molecules intercellular adhesion molecule (ICAM)-1, vascular cell adhesion molecule-1, and endothelial leukocyte adhesion molecule-1 on brain microvascular endothelial cells (BMVEC) with a peak effect on ICAM-1 expression between 6 and 18 hours after treatment in human BMVEC cultures and increased monocyte migration in an in vitro BBB model[40–43] constructed with BMVEC and astrocytes.[44] These effects of cocaine, exerted through a cascade of augmented expression of inflammatory cytokines and endothelial adhesion molecules, may contribute to the known cerebrovascular complications of cocaine abuse.

The second is the effect of cocaine on endothelial cell permeability and apoptosis as well as the induction of chemokines and cytokines. The immunomodulatory effects of cocaine on brain microvascular endothelial cells and its proinflammatory effects on induction of proinflammatory cytokines and chemokines was investigated using a human BBB model that included human immunodeficiency virus type-1 (HIV-1) neuroinvasion.[45] Cocaine increased the in vitro permeability of endothelial cells of the BBB model and induced apoptosis of mouse thymocytes in cultures of BMVEC and monocytes using an enzyme-linked immunosorbent assay of generated accompanied by upregulation of macrophage inflammatory protein (MIP)-1, MIP-1α, inducible protein-10, and IL-8 and TNF-α expression.

A third line of investigation has been the observed synergy of cocaine in facilitating pathogenic retroviral neuroinvasion, which may confer an independent risk factor for cerebral vasculitis. Both in vitro and in vivo studies have provided valuable tools in exploring the role of cocaine in mediating HIV-associated neuropathogenesis. The importance of drug abuse in conjunction with HIV-1 has been underscored by the ability of cocaine to induce retroviral replication in mononuclear cells[46] and enhance gp120-induced neurotoxicity.[47]

Opioids

Opioids or narcotic drugs have pharmacologic properties similar to those of morphine that include the derivatives hydrocodone, oxycodone, hydromorphone, codeine, fentanyl, meperidine, methadone, and opium. The source of opioids is the exudate of seed from the poppy plant, heroin is derived from acetylation of morphine. Heroin is administered intravenously, intranasally, and subcutaneously. A higher bioavailability of heroin is present after heating on foil for inhalation compared with smoking after heating. Intravenous injection leads to extreme euphoria that peaks at 10 minutes followed by profound sedation and analgesia that lasts for up to 1 hour. Opiate overdose produces the triad of coma, respiratory depression, and miosis. The medical complications of long-term heroin exposure include endocarditis, pulmonary complications of embolism, pneumonia, and granulomatosis or fibrosis; and nephropathy, immunodepression, infection at the site of injection due to cellulitis, thrombophlebitis, and bacteremia, and hepatitis due to needle sharing.[48] It binds to endogenous opiate mu$_1$ receptors, which are responsible for most of the analgesic effects, and for the actions of the CNS and cardiovascular system leading to bradycardia, hypotension, and respiratory depression. Agonist actions at mu$_2$ receptors are responsible for respiratory depression, delayed gastrointestinal motility, miosis, and physical dependence. Agonist actions at kappa receptors lead to separate analgesia. Circulating serum morphine is transformed into morphine-3-glucuronide or morphine-6-glucuronide by the liver and the kidney. Most fatal and nonfatal overdoses occur when heroin is administered intravenously.

This author could not identify any pathologically confirmed cases of heroin-induced cerebral vasculitis reported in the literature, nor was cerebral vasculitis suggested as a likely occurrence in heroin abuse,[49] heroin addiction,[48,50] or acute overdose.[51] Moreover, detailed neuropathologic studies carried out on 134 victims of acute heroin intoxication, including 18 who survived for periods of hours or days,[52] who respectively demonstrated cerebral edema in conjunction with vascular congestion, capillary engorgement, and perivascular bleeding attributed to toxic primary respiratory failure;

and ischemic nerve cell damage resembling systemic hypoxia, showed no evidence of cerebral vasculitis, except 1 focus of lymphocytic perivascular inflammation. The brains of 10 intravenous drug abusers who died from heroin overdoses, including one due to gunshot injury,[53] likewise show no evidence of cerebral vasculitis at postmortem examination, except to a few perivascular mononuclear cells associated with pigment deposition.

The postulated mechanisms of opioid-related neuronal and CNS vascular injury include increased oxidative stress, induction of inflammatory cytokines, and increased permeability of the BBB especially in intravenous drug abuse. Ramage and colleagues[54] described increased deposition of hyperphosphorylated tau in entorhinal cortex and subiculum of the hippocampus, AT8-positive neurofibrillary tangles in entorhinal cortex, and increase in β-amyloid precursor protein (βAPP) in both the hippocampus and brainstem of drug abusers compared with controls. Several postulated causative mechanisms included repeated head injury, hypoxic-ischemic injury associated with opioid-induced respiratory depression, microglial-associated cytokine release, and drug-associated neurotoxicity.

HUMAN IMMUNODEFICIENCY VIRUS/ACQUIRED IMMUNE DEFICIENCY SYNDROME

Recognition of the propensity for cerebral vascular inflammation in association with human immunodeficiency virus type 1 infection (HIV-1)/acquired immune deficiency syndrome (AIDS) and drug abuse has provided new insights into the mechanisms of cerebral vasculitis. Early in the HIV/AIDs epidemic, it was clear that a significant proportion of infected persons engaged in intravenous drug user (IVDU). Their associated risk behavior exposed them to infection through sharing of contaminated needles, thereby increasing the risk of spread of HIV and other bloodborne infections.[55] Among 50 patients with AIDS and neurologic complication, 6 HIV-1 infected patients described by Snider and colleagues[56] were IVDUs; the others being male homosexuals and recently arrived Haitian refugees. The 2 postulated periods in the neurobiology of HIV-1 when autoimmune disease manifestations can occur that appear to be significant for the development of cerebral vasculitis are shortly after seroconversion and before the spread of productive infection[53,57] and after initiation of highly active antiretroviral therapy (HAART) in association with the immune reconstitution syndrome (IRIS).[58] The impact of IVDU in the development of cerebral vasculitis and other autoimmune sequel is not well understood; however, there is an extensive literature suggesting an independent contribution of IVDU to immune suppression, breakdown of the BBB, microglial activation, and neuronal injury,[59–65] and an additive or synergistic reinforcement of HIV-related brain damage by intravenous drug use.[66]

The timing of early HIV invasion has been difficult to ascertain based on the presence of one or more well-recognized clinicopathological HIV/AIDS syndromes. including HIV encephalitis,[67] HIV-associated dementia, and AIDS-dementia complex, all of which are indicative of symptomatic infection. HIV encephalitis is initially associated with myelin pallor and gliosis of the centrum semiovale found in more than 90% of brains from patients dying with AIDS.[68] With increasing severity of symptomatic disease, multiple glial nodules with the multinucleated cells characteristic of HIV encephalitis occur throughout the white matter, basal ganglia, cerebral and cerebellar cortex, brainstem, and spinal cord. HIV has been demonstrated in monocytes and multinucleated giant cells by electron microscopy, immunocytochemical techniques, and in situ hybridization. Vasculitides in the context of HIV infection was reviewed by Guillevin.[69]

Six patients with non-necrotizing cerebral vasculitis were described in a postmortem series of presymptomatic HIV-seropositive drug abusers by Gray and colleagues,[53] and an analogous patient was described by Yankner and coworkers[70] with rapidly fatal necrotizing granulomatous angiitis of the brain without evidence of acquired immune deficiency, circulating human T-lymphotropic virus type III (HTLV-III) or HIV-1 antibodies. Seven other patients were described by Bell and colleagues[57] with lymphocytic infiltration of the walls of leptomeningeal and subarachnoid veins, without specific reference of cerebral vasculitis. Gray and colleagues[53] studied 2 cohorts of 11 patients, one HIV-seropositive and non-AIDS, and the other HIV-seronegative heroin abusers, 10 patients of each died from heroin overdose and another of a fatal gunshot wound. Neuropathological studies showed varying degrees of vascular inflammation including "true vasculitis" exemplified by dense vascular inflammation extending through the vessel wall, associated with leptomeningitis in 6 of the 11 HIV-seropositive AIDS-negative patients. However, there was no mention as to whether inflammatory process involved arteries and vein or the vessel caliber. Vascular inflammation was comparatively mild or absent and restricted to a few perivascular mononucleated cells associated with pigment deposition, without transmural vascular inflammation or meningitis in the HIV-seronegative cohort. HIV immunocytochemistry was negative in both cohorts, and multinucleated giant cells, considered the hallmark of productive HIV infection in the brain and an essential neuropathologic feature of HIV encephalitis, were not seen. One year later, Bell and coworkers[57] described the neuropathologic findings of 23 IVDUs from the Edinburgh HIV Autopsy Cohort who died suddenly after seroconversion but while still in the presymptomatic stage of HIV infection in comparison with 10 HIV-negative IVDUs, 12 non-IVDU controls, and 9 patients with full-blown AIDS, who also died suddenly. Seven of the presymptomatic HIV-positive patients showed infiltration of T-cells in the walls of veins in association with low-grade lymphocytic meningitis; 7 others demonstrated isolated lymphocytic meningitis, and 1 patient had focal perivascular lymphocytic cuffing and macrophage collections throughout the central white matter tissue of the brain and in basal ganglia. Neither conspicuous perivascular lymphocytic infiltration nor lymphocytic meningitis was noted in HIV-negative IVDU controls, those with no drug association, or others with full-blown AIDS. Neuropathological examination in presymptomatic HIV-seropositive patients failed to reveal characteristic lesions of HIV encephalitis and none of the subjects showed immunocytochemical evidence of p24 antigen in brain tissue. Nearly a decade later, Bell and colleagues[60] reiterated that in more than 50% of pre-AIDS cases so studied, the brain was characterized by a low-grade lymphocytic meningoencephalitis in which T-cell infiltration is present in leptomeninges and the perivascular compartment, with a very occasional HIV-p24 positive lymphocyte in the lymphocytic infiltrate, but no in brain parenchyma. According to the same investigators,[60] there was conversely no clear evidence of vasculitis in IVDUs with HIV encephalitis in the Edinburgh HIV Autopsy Cohort.[33] Yankner and colleagues[70] reported the clinicopathologic findings of a homosexual man with rapidly fatal cerebral granulomatous angiitis of the brain associated with isolation of HTLV-III in CSF and brain tissue. Mononuclear cellular infiltrates were present at postmortem examination in the walls of affected large named arteries without involvement of small arteries and veins, and with rare microglial nodules and multinucleated giant cells.

The early CNS changes of HIV infection have also been investigated among patients with hemophilia examined after sudden death from intracranial hemorrhage and liver cirrhosis and in experimental animal models of simian immunodeficiency virus (SIV) syndrome and feline immunodeficiency virus infection.[34] There were comparable neuropathologic changes of gliosis, occasional microglial nodules, perivascular mononuclear infiltrates, and occasional leptomeningeal meningitis in all 3, characteristically without multinucleated giant cells or evidence of HIV in the brain.[33,34,70] HIV-infected cells were mainly perivascular, and expressed macrophage markers in the SIV model[33] suggesting transit of virus across the BBB as the main source of entry into the CNS. Moreover, the comparatively less pronounced vascular inflammation than that described in early HIV infection associated with drug abuse, suggests that IVDU contributes to vascular inflammation.

Literature of Patients with Human Immunodeficiency Virus/Acquired Immune Deficiency Syndrome–Associated Immune Reconstitution Syndrome

The introduction of HAART has changes the incidence, course, and prognosis of the neurologic complications of HIV infection concomitant with almost undetectable viral load in plasma and a rise in circulating T-lymphocytes.[35] One pathologically confirmed patient with cerebral vasculitis and IRIS was described by van der Ven and colleagues.[36] This HIV-seropositive homosexual man developed dysarthria and dysphagia after HAART with worsening and appearance of limb paresis after discontinuation of the medication. Treatment with corticosteroids preceded recommencement of HAART but there was worsening with discontinuation of corticosteroids. Biopsy of a hyperintense fronto-parietal lesion on T2-weighted MRI showed small vessel lymphocytic vasculitis, with microglial activation in the surrounding parenchyma. A severe demyelinating leukoencephalopathy in association with intense perivascular infiltration by HIV-gp41 immunoreactive monocytes/macrophages and lymphocytes was described by Langford and colleagues[37] in 7 postmortem patients. All were severely immunosuppressed and treated with HAART with presumed IRIS; however, high not low levels of HIV replication were noted and there was no consideration of cerebral vasculitis. Confirmatory neuropathology was not sought; however, Patel and coworkers[38] described an HIV-seropositive man who developed encephalitis 10 months after HAART in association with a lower thoracic dermatomal varicella zoster virus rash.

Levamisole

The anti-helminthic agent levamisole, first introduced for use in veterinary medicine, was later discovered to have potent immunomodulation properties, prompting its application in inflammatory and oncologic conditions, including rheumatoid arthritis, aphthous ulcers, and melanoma.[39] The US Food and Drug Administration approved levamisole as adjuvant therapy for the treatment of inflammatory conditions and cancer. In Asia, it has been used as an anti-helminthic and pesticide agent.

Levamisole was detected in cocaine bricks by the US Drug Enforcement Agency in 2003,[71] noting an increase from 44.1% of specimens in 2008 to 73.2% in 2009, signaling a rising public health problem. In 2011, Buchman and co-workers[72] reported a prevalence of 68% using a combination of immunoassay and gas chromatography–mass spectroscopy detection methodologies. Other drugs noted in positive urine specimens included the opioid analgesics methadone (45%), codeine (16%). heroin/6-monoacetylmorphine (6%), and morphine or oxycodone (5%). The importance of detecting levamisole in urine concomitantly with cocaine in affected cases is in being able to ascertain its separate contribution to the observed neurotoxicity in suspected cases.

Levamisole is 100-fold to 300-fold less potent than cocaine in blocking norepinephrine and dopamine uptake, and has a very low affinity for the serotonin transporter; and it does not trigger an appreciable substrate efflux. Nevertheless, the desired neuropharmacologic effects leads to its widespread contamination in cocaine production. It potentiates the euphoric effects of cocaine by inhibiting dopamine reuptake and forming amphetaminelike metabolites. Hofmaier and colleagues[73] studied the allosteric effects of levamisole and cocaine at 30 μM, a concentration at which levamisole displayed already mild effects on norepinephrine transport but without an inhibitory action on cocaine. Levamisole metabolizes to aminorex, an amphetamine-like substance that exerts strong effects on dopamine, serotonin, and norepinephrine transporters in a manner that resembled amphetamine. They concluded that although the adulterant levamisole itself had only moderate effects on neurotransmission, its metabolite, aminorex, nonetheless exerted distinct psychostimulant effects and that after the cocaine effect "fades out," the levamisole/aminorex effects "kicks in."

Exposure to levamisole-adulterated cocaine is associated with a variety of well-described hematological, skin, renal, and pulmonary pathologies,[74] often in association with positive anti-neutrophil cytoplasmic antibody (ANCA) serology. Hematologic abnormalities include agranulocytosis and neutropenia, which occur in a dose-dependent fashion, and are not commonly associated with pure cocaine-linked side or a characteristic of drug-induced vasculitis. A distinguishing feature of levamisole-adulterated cocaine exposure is small vessel vasculitis, which involves the ear lobes and the skin overlying the zygomatic arch or lower extremities, often with purpuric plaques in a retiform pattern or central necrosis. Skin biopsy shows pathologic involvement of superficial and deep dermal vessels associated with numerous neutrophils and eosinophils that surround and invade the walls of dermal vessels with extravasation of red blood cells, leukocytoclastic debris (nuclear dust), and fibrinoid necrosis on hematoxylin and eosin–stained tissue sections. Such findings are similar to children with chronic levamisole treated for nephrotic syndrome, so noted in a minority of children who developed purpuric lesions of at least the ears and biopsies revealing cutaneous vasculitis.[75] Although organ involvement has not been characteristic of levamisole-adulterated cocaine-induced autoimmune disease, there is an established association with proteinuria or hematuria, acute renal injury, and focal necrotizing and crescentic pauci-immune glomerulonephritis in some cases, and increased titers to p-ANCA. As in other drug-induced vasculitides, pulmonary involvement can complete the triad of skin, kidney, and lung pathology in the form of diffuse alveolar hemorrhages, idiopathic pulmonary hypertension, or other clinicopathologic presentations.

It has taken 25 years to recognize the causal association of levamisole-associated multifocal inflammatory leukoencephalopathy (MIL) in cocaine users. In 1992, Hook and colleagues[76] described 3 patients, ages 45 to 74 years, who developed a cerebral demyelinating disease within 3 to 5 months of beginning adjuvant therapy with 5-fluorouracil (5-FU) and levamisole. Two patients presented with progressive encephalopathy and ataxia, and a third had unexplained loss of consciousness. Brain MRI revealed multiple gadolinium-enhanced white matter lesions, predominantly in a periventricular distribution. Cerebrospinal fluid obtained in 2 patients showed oligoclonal bands (2 patients) and pleocytosis (1 patient). Pathologic studies of brain biopsy specimens from 2 patients revealed cerebral demyelination and perivascular inflammation similar to multiple sclerosis. There was clear improvement after discontinuation of chemotherapy and administration of corticosteroids. The pathogenesis was unclear, and the investigators considered the etiologic basis to be 5-FU toxicity, although the role of levamisole was not excluded.

Three years later, Kimmel and colleagues[77] described a patient age 57 years, who developed progressive confusion and ataxia over a 3-week period, 5 weeks after adjuvant therapy with levamisole for malignant melanoma. Brain MRI showed multifocal enhancing white matter lesions. CSF showed pleocytosis with an increased immunoglobulin G index. The patient improved with a 3-month tapering course of corticosteroids. The cause of the leukoencephalopathy in previously described cases[76] of 5-FU and levamisole was assigned at least in part, to levamisole.

One year later, Luppi and colleagues[78] described 2 patients, age 54 and 60 years, treated with adjuvant 5-FU and levamisole for colon cancer who, after 10 weeks and 6 weeks, respectively from onset of treatment, noted confusion, aphasia, ataxia, and progressive obtundation leading to decerebration (case 1) and nasogastric feeding (case 2). Brain MRI in both showed widespread bilaterally symmetric periventricular and hemispheric white matter hyperintensities compatible with MIL. Treatment with parenteral corticosteroids (case 2) led to clinical improvement.

A decade later, Wu and coworkers[79] described a series of 31 patients with levamisole-induced MIL, including 7 from their institution and 24 from the medical literature, treated with a combination of levamisole and 5-FU adjuvant therapy (21 patients) or levamisole alone (10 patients) for malignant cancer, most commonly colon cancer.

Onset of gait ataxia in two-thirds of cases, was delayed in those treated with combination 5-FU and levamisole compared with levamisole alone (11.7 weeks vs 2.5 weeks). Brain MRI showed enhancing periventricular or supratentorial white matter lesions. CSF showed lymphocytic pleocytosis in 47% of cases. Treatment with corticosteroids and intravenous immunoglobulin led to improved clinical status in 29 (94%) cases.

In 2009, Xu and coworkers[80] described the clinical and neuroradiological findings in 16 patients, age 8 to 52 years, treated with levamisole for recurrent aphthous ulcers or ascaris infections noting weakness (75%), aphasia (50%), neurocognitive (50%), and facial palsy (44%) as the main presenting clinical features. Brain MRI showed typical plaque and round or oval demyelinating enhancing white matter lesions and hyperintense signal on T_2/fluid-attenuated inversion recovery (FLAIR) images. Brain biopsy in 1 case showed multifocal demyelinating lesions with lymphocytic perivascular cuffs. Treatment with corticosteroids and hyperbaric oxygen was associated with full recovery.

In 2012, Blanc and colleagues[81] described a 29-year-old woman and active crack cocaine abuser with AIDS who presented with fever, malaise, and back pain and an unremarkable neurologic examination. CSF showed acellular fluid with increased protein content and oligoclonal bands. A urine drug screen showed cocaine and opiates. Brain MRI showed lesions consistent with MIL. Sera later tested for both cocaine and levamisole by gas chromatography–mass spectroscopy were negative. The investigators speculated that levamisole contamination was responsible for MIL, citing that urine testing for levamisole would have been positive if performed at the time of cocaine detection.

In 2013, Yan and colleagues[82] described the clinical and neuroradiologic features of 15 patients, age 31 to 54 years, treated with levamisole for worm expulsion for 2 weeks to 2 months before onset of fever, headache, dizziness, neurocognitive disturbance, weakness, and visual impairment. Nine patients who underwent CSF examination showed only pleocytosis. Electroencephalography in all 15 showed high-amplitude slow waves. Brain MRI showed multiple hyperintense T_2/FLAIR bilateral centrum semiovale and periventricular lesions (all patients), and two-thirds showed lesions in basal ganglia; with lesser frequency in the frontal (26%), occipital (6%), and temporal lobes (6%), or brainstem or cerebellum (6%). Treatment with "hormone therapy" was effective in all patients.

In the same year, 2013, Gonzáález-Duarte and Williams[83] described a 40-year-old woman with chronic daily use of cocaine admitted for acute confusion, aphasia, and fever. CSF showed neutrophilic pleocytosis. Brain MRI showed hyperintense signal in left parietal lobe white matter on T_2/FLAIR images. She developed sudden visual changes and hemiparesis 10 days later, and a week after, a new episode of expressive aphasia each associated with respective right and left frontal white matter lesions reminiscent of MIL. Complete recovery occurred in 2 weeks and she remained stable without further new episodes despite continued cocaine abuse. The investigators speculated a relationship to levamisole adulteration.

In 2015, Vosoughi and Schmidt[84] described MIL in 2 cocaine abusers, age 25 and 41 years, who presented respectively with unilateral progressing to bilateral sensorimotor deficits; and confusion with impaired balance. Serial brain MRI in the first patient showed increasing bilateral T_2/FLAIR enhancing white matter hyperintensities in periventricular white matter, pons and cerebellar peduncles, with similar presenting features in the second patient. Both patients improved with corticosteroids and plasma exchange. Urinary levamisole was not tested in either patient, although the investigators concluded that it was a likely cause of MIL in their cases.

Finally, Vitt and colleagues[85] described a case of MIL with positive urine testing for cocaine and levamisole in a cocaine abuser with a history of hepatitis C infection. This 63-year-old woman presented with 3 days of progressive confusion, fever, and headache. Over 2 days she developed spastic quadriparesis and stupor. Cocaine tested positive in the urine. Brain MRI revealed T2/FLAIR hyperintensities and incomplete ring-enhancement in periventricular subcortical white matter, many of which were ovoid shaped. CSF showed a lymphocytic pleocytosis and elevated protein content without oligoclonal bands. Gas chromatography–mass spectroscopy detected levamisole in the urine. High-dose intravenous methylprednisolone for 5 days followed by plasmapheresis was ineffective. The patient received intravenous cyclophosphamide with stabilization. Ten months later, the patient was minimally conscious with mutism and generalized spasticity.

The mechanisms underlying levamisole-adulterated cocaine-induced systemic pathology are not well understood, but a causal relation to ANCA-associated disease is suggested by the correlation of disease pathology, clinical relapse with detectable autoantibodies, sensitivity to immune modulatory and immunosuppressive therapy, and predictable levamisole-induced histopathology. Levamisole potentiates the production of interferon and interleukins; increases T-cell activation and proliferation, neutrophil mobility, adherence, and chemotaxis; and increases the formation of antibodies to antigens.[39] It acts as a hapten, triggering an immune response resulting in opsonization and leukocyte destruction. Levamisole may interact with neutrophil extracellular traps composed of a complex of DNA, histones, and neutrophil granules including myeloperoxidase, proteinease-3, and human neutrophil elastase. Neutrophil extracellular traps release in response to stress and provide a source of antigen that can activate the immune system.[74] There has not been a living patient or postmortem-studied case of MIL demonstrating vasculitis pathology in brain tissue.

SUMMARY

Drug abuse is a rare cause of histopathologically verified CNS vasculitis. Nonetheless, the complications of illicit substance use on the cerebral circulation can be highly lethal with secondary vasculopathy, hemorrhage, and aneurysm formation especially when the illicit substances are delivered parenterally. A likely diagnosis rests on the drug that is abused and the clinical and neuroradiologic findings of a presumptive case. Management rests on avoidance of further exposure and minimizing the secondary neurotoxic effects of the abused substances and polypharmacy use. HIV/AIDS has introduced new aspects of causation and patterns of drug use.

REFERENCES

1. Jennette JC, Falk RJ, Bacon PA, et al. 2012 revised International Chapel Hill Consensus Conference Nomenclature of Vasculitides. Arthritis Rheum 2013;65:1–11.

2. Abbott NJ, Patabendige AA, Dolman DE, et al. Structure and function of the blood-brain barrier. Neurobiol Dis 2010;37:13–25.
3. Benarroch EE. Blood-brain barrier: recent developments and clinical correlations. Neurology 2012;78:1268–76.
4. Ek CJ, Dziegielewska KM, Habgood MD, et al. Barriers in the developing brain and neurotoxicology. Neurotoxicology 2012;33:586–604.
5. Benzedrine sulfate "pep pills" [Editorial]. JAMA 1937;108:1973–4.
6. Smith L. Collapse with death following the use of amphetamine sulfate. AJAM 1939;113:1022–3.
7. Gericke O. Suicide by ingestion of amphetamine sulfate. JAMA 1945;128:1098–9.
8. Lloyd JT, Walker DR. Death after combined dexamphetamine and phenelzine. Br Med J 1965;2:168–9.
9. Anglin MD, Burke C, Perrochet B, et al. History of the methamphetamine problem. J Psychoactive Drugs 2000;32:137–41.
10. Christophersen AS. Amphetamine designer drugs - an overview and epidemiology. Toxicol Lett 2000;112-113:127–31.
11. Parrott A. Is ecstasy MDMA? A review of the proportion of ecstasy tablets containing MDMA, their dosage levels, and the changing perceptions of purity. Psychopharmacology 2004;173:234–41.
12. Fonseca AC, Ferro JM. Drug abuse and stroke. Curr Neurol Neurosci Rep 2013;13:325.
13. Petitti DB, Sidney S, Quesenberry C, et al. Stroke and cocaine or amphetamine use. Epidemiology 1998;9:596–600.
14. Westover AN, McBride S, Haley RW. Stroke in young adults who abuse amphetamines or cocaine: a population-based study of hospitalized patients. Arch Gen Psychiatry 2007;64:495–502.
15. Glick R, Hoying J, Cerullo L, et al. Phenylpropanolamine: an over-the-counter drug causing central nervous system vasculitis and intracerebral hemorrhage. Case report and review. Neurosurgery 1987;20:969–74.
16. Citron BP, Halpern M, McCarron M, et al. Necrotizing angiitis associated with drug abuse. N Engl J Med 1970;283:1003–11.
17. Gocke DC, CI. Angitiis in drug abusers [Letter]. N Engl J Med 1971;284:112.
18. Gocke DJ, Hsu K, Morgan C, et al. Polyarteritis and the Australia antigen: a new association. J Clin Invest 1970;39(35a).
19. Gocke DJ, Hsu K, Morgan C, et al. Association of polyarteritis and Australia antigen. Lancet 1970;2:1149–53.
20. Citron B, Peters R. Angiitis in drug abusers [Letter]. N Engl J Med 1971;284:111–3.
21. Baden M. Angiitis in drug abusers. N Engl J Med 1971;284:111.
22. Rumbaugh CL, Bergeron RT, Scanlan RL, et al. Cerebral vascular changes secondary to amphetamine abuse in the experimental animal. Radiology 1971;101:345–51.
23. Rumbaugh CL, Fang HC, Higgins RE, et al. Cerebral microvascular injury in experimental drug abuse. Invest Radiol 1976;11:282–94.
24. Kreek MJ, Bart G, Lilly C, et al. Pharmacogenetics and human molecular genetics of opiate and cocaine addictions and their treatments. Pharmacol Rev 2005;57:1–26.
25. Bostwick DG. Amphetamine induced cerebral vasculitis. Hum Pathol 1981;12:1031–3.

26. Krendel DA, Ditter SM, Frankel MR, et al. Biopsy-proven cerebral vasculitis associated with cocaine abuse. Neurology 1990;40:1092–4.

27. Fredericks RK, Lefkowitz DS, Challa VR, et al. Cerebral vasculitis associated with cocaine abuse. Stroke 1991;22:1437–9.

28. Morrow PL, McQuillen JB. Cerebral vasculitis associated with cocaine abuse. J Forensic Sci 1993;38:732–8.

29. Tapia JF, JM S. Case 27-1993-A 32-year-old man with the sudden onset of a right-sided headache and left hemiplegia and hemianesthesia. N Engl J Med 1993; 329:117–24.

30. Merkel PA, Koroshetz WJ, Irizarry MC, et al. Cocaine-associated cerebral vasculitis. Semin Arthritis Rheum 1995;25:172–83.

31. Martinez N, Diez-Tejedor E, Frank A. Vasospasm/thrombus in cerebral ischemia related to cocaine abuse [Letter]. Stroke 1996;27:147–8.

32. Diez-Tejedor E, Frank A, Gutierrez M, et al. Encephalopathy and biopsy-proven cerebrovascular inflammatory changes in a cocaine abuser. Eur J Neurol 1998; 5:103–7.

33. Connor MD, Lammie GA, Bell JE, et al. Cerebral infarction in adult AIDS patients: observations from the Edinburgh HIV Autopsy Cohort. Stroke 2000;31:2117–26.

34. Hurtrel M, Ganiere JP, Guelfi JF, et al. Comparison of early and late feline immunodeficiency virus encephalopathies. AIDS 1992;6:399–406.

35. Gray F, Keohane C. The neuropathology of HIV infection in the era of highly active antiretroviral therapy (HAART). Brain Pathol 2003;13:79–83.

36. van der Ven AJ, van Oostenbrugge RJ, Kubat B, et al. Cerebral vasculitis after initiation antiretroviral therapy. AIDS 2002;16:2362–4.

37. Langford TD, Letendre SL, Marcotte TD, et al. Severe, demyelinating leukoencephalopathy in AIDS patients on antiretroviral therapy. AIDS 2002;16:1019–29.

38. Patel AK, Patel KK, Shah SD, et al. Immune reconstitution syndrome presenting with cerebral varicella zoster vasculitis in HIV-1-infected patient: a case report. J Int Assoc Physicians AIDS Care 2006;5:157–60.

39. Amery WR, Bruynseels JP. Levamisole, the story and the lessons. Int J Immunopharmacol 1992;14:481–6.

40. Fiala M, Gan XH, Zhang L, et al. Cocaine enhances monocyte migration across the blood-brain barrier. Cocaine's connection to AIDS dementia and vasculitis? Adv Exp Med Biol 1998;437:199–205.

41. Fiala M, Gan X-H, Newton T, et al. Divergent effects of cocaine on cytokine production by lymphocytes and monocytes/macrophages. Adv Exp Med Biol 1996; 402:145–56.

42. Fiala M, Looney DJ, Stins M, et al. TNF- α opens a paracellular route for HIV-1 invasion across the blood-brain barrier. Mol Med 1997;3:553–64.

43. Fiala M, Rhodes RH, Shapshak P, et al. Regulation of HIV-1 in astrocytes: expression of Nef-α and IL-6 is enhanced in coculture of astrocytes and macrophages. J Neurovirol 1996;2:158–66.

44. Gan X, Zhang L, Berger O, et al. Cocaine enhances brain endothelial adhesion molecules and leukocyte migration. Clin Immunol 1999;91:68–76.

45. Zhang L, Looney D, Taub D, et al. Cocaine opens the blood-brain barrier to HIV-1 invasion. J Neurovirol 1998;4:619–26.

46. Bagasra O, Pomerantz RJ. Human immunodeficiency virus type 1 replication in peripheral blood mononuclear cells in the presence of cocaine. J Infect Dis 1993;168:1157–64.

47. Buch S, Yao H, Guo M, et al. Cocaine and HIV-1 interplay in CNS: cellular and molecular mechanisms. Curr HIV Res 2012;10:425–8.

48. Louria DB, Hensle T, Rose T. The major medical complications of heroin addiction. Ann Intern Med 1967;67:1–22.
49. Caplan LR, Hier DB, Banks G. Current concepts of cerebrovascular disease–stroke: stroke and drug abuse. Stroke 1982;13:869–72.
50. Richter RW, Pearson J, Bruun B, et al. Neurological complications of addictions to heroin. Bull N Y Acad Med 1973;49:3–21.
51. Sporer KA. Acute heroin overdose. Ann Intern Med 1999;130:584–90.
52. Oehmichen M, Meissner C, Reiter A, et al. Neuropathology in non-human immunodeficiency virus-infected drug addicts: hypoxic brain damage after chronic intravenous drug abuse. Acta Neuropathol 1996;91:642–6.
53. Gray F, Lescs MC, Keohane C, et al. Early brain changes in HIV infection: neuropathological study of 11 HIV seropositive, non-AIDS cases. J Neuropathol Exp Neurol 1992;51:177–85.
54. Ramage SN, Anthony IC, Carnie FW, et al. Hyperphosphorylated tau and amyloid precursor protein deposition is increased in the brains of young drug abusers. Neuropathol Appl Neurobiol 2005;31:439–48.
55. UNAIDS/WHO. AIDS epidemic update 2005. 2005. Available at: http://data.unaids.org/publications/irc-pub06/epi_update2005_en.pdf.
56. Snider WD, Simpson DM, Nielsen S, et al. Neurological complications of acquired immune deficiency syndrome: analysis of 50 patients. Ann Neurol 1983;14:403–18.
57. Bell JE, Busuttil A, Ironside JW, et al. Human immunodeficiency virus and the brain: investigation of virus load and neuropathologic changes in pre-AIDS subjects. J Infect Dis 1993;168:818–24.
58. Nachega JB, Morroni C, Chaisson RE, et al. Impact of immune reconstitution inflammatory syndrome on antiretroviral therapy adherence. Patient Prefer Adherence 2012;6:887–91.
59. Kumar A. HIV and substance abuse. Curr HIV Res 2012;10:365.
60. Bell JE, Arango JC, Robertson R, et al. HIV and drug misuse in the Edinburgh cohort. J Acquir Immune Defic Syndr 2002;31(Suppl 2):S35–42.
61. Bell JE, Arango JC, Anthony IC. Neurobiology of multiple insults: HIV-1-associated brain disorders in those who use illicit drugs. J Neuroimmune Pharmacol 2006;1:182–91.
62. Donahoe RM, Vlahov D. Opiates as potential cofactors in progression of HIV-1 infections to AIDS. J Neuroimmunol 1998;83:77–87.
63. Bane A, Annessley-Williams D, Sweeney E, et al. Cerebral vasculitis and haemorrhage in a HIV positive intravenous drug abuser. Ir Med J 1999;92:340.
64. Tomlinson GS, Simmonds P, Busuttil A, et al. Upregulation of microglia in drug users with and without pre-symptomatic HIV infection. Neuropathol Appl Neurobiol 1999;25:369–79.
65. Gosztonyi G, Schmidt V, Nickel R, et al. Neuropathologic analysis of postmortal brain samples of HIV-seropositive and -seronegative i.v. drug addicts. Forensic Sci Int 1993;62:101–5.
66. Bell JE, Donaldson YK, Lowrie S, et al. Influence of risk group and zidovudine therapy on the development of HIV encephalitis and cognitive impairment in AIDS patients. AIDS 1996;10:493–9.
67. Sharer LR, Kapila R. Neuropathologic observations in acquired immunodeficiency syndrome (AIDS). Acta Neuropathol 1985;66:188–98.
68. Petito CK. Review of central nervous system pathology in human immunodeficiency virus infection. Ann Neurol 1988;23(Suppl):S54–7.

69. Guillevin L. Vasculitis in the context of HIV infection. AIDS 2008;22(Suppl3): S27–33.
70. Yankner BA, Skolnik PR, Shoukimas GM, et al. Cerebral granulomatous angiitis associated with isolation of human T-lymphotropic virus type III from the central nervous system. Ann Neurol 1986;20:362–4.
71. Valentino AM, Fuentecilla K. Levamisole: an analytical profile. Microgram J 2005; 3:134–7.
72. Buchman JA, Heard K, Burbach C, et al. Prevalence of levamisole in urine toxicology screens positive for cocaine in an inner-city hospital. JAMA 2011;305: 16571658.
73. Hofmaier T, Luf A, Seddik A, et al. Aminorex, a metabolite of the cocaine adulterant levamisole, exerts amphetamine like actions at monoamine transporters. Neurochem Int 2014;73:32–41.
74. Nolan AI, Kuang-Yu J. Pathologic manifestations of levamisole-adulterated cocaine exposure. Diagn Pathol 2015;10:48.
75. Rongioletti F, Chio L, Ginevi F, et al. Purpura of the ears: a distinctive vasculopathy with circulating autoantibodies complicating long-term treatment with levamisole in children. Br J Dermatol 1999;140:948–51.
76. Hook CC, Kimmel DW, Kvols LK, et al. Multifocal inflammatory leukoencephalopathy with 5-fluorouracil and levamisole. Ann Neurol 1992;31:262–7.
77. Kimmel DW, Wijdicks FM, Rodriguez M. Multifocal inflammatory leukoencephalopathy associated with levamisole therapy. Neurology 1995;45:374–6.
78. Luppi G, Zoboli A, Barbieri F, et al. Multifocal leukoencephalopathy associated with 5-fluorouracil and levamisole adjuvant therapy for colon cancer. A report of two cases and review of the literature. Ann Oncol 1996;7:412–5.
79. Wu V-C, Huang J-W, Lien H-C, et al. Levamisole-induced multifocal inflammatory leukoencephalopathy. Clinical characteristics, outcome, and impact of treatment in 31 patients. Medicine 2006;85:203–13.
80. Zu N, Zhou W, Shuyu LI, et al. Clinical and MRI characteristics of levamisole-induced leukoencephalopathy in 16 patients. J Neuroimaging 2009;19:326–31.
81. Blanc PD, Chin C, Lynch KL. Multifocal inflammatory leukoencephalopathy associated with cocaine abuse: Is levamisole responsible? Clin Toxicol 2012;50: 534–5.
82. Yan R, Wu Q, Ren J, et al. Clinical features and magnetic image analysis of 15 cases of demyelinating leukoencephalopathy induced by levamisole. Exp Ther Med 2013;6:71–4.
83. Gonzáález-Duarte A, Williams R. Cocaine-induced recurrent leukoencephalopathy. Neuroradiol J 2013;26:511–3.
84. Vosoughi R, Schmidt BJ. Multifocal leukoencephalopathy in cocaine users: a report of two cases and review of the literature. BMC Neurol 2015;15:208.
85. Vitt JR, Brown EG, Chow DS, et al. Confirmed case of levamisole-associated multifocal inflammatory leukoencephalopathy in a cocaine user. J Immunol 2017;305:128–30.

Central Nervous System Vasculitis due to Infection

David S. Younger, MD, MPH, MS[a,b,*], Patricia K. Coyle, MD[c]

KEYWORDS

- Infection • Central nervous system • Vasculitis

KEY POINTS

- Several pathogens have a propensity to involve blood vessels during central nervous system infection, which can lead to cerebrovascular complications.
- Infection is a recognized cause of secondary central nervous system vasculitis.
- It is very important not to miss the diagnosis of infection-related central nervous system vasculitis because specific antimicrobial therapy may be necessary.
- This article reviews the major implicated organisms and the etiopathogenic mechanism of central nervous system vasculitis.

INTRODUCTION

Vasculitis or angiitis is defined as inflammation of blood vessels. Vasculitic involvement of large-, medium-, and small-caliber vessels, respectively, leads to arteritis, venulitis, and capillaritis alone or in combination. Central nervous system (CNS) vasculitis typically affects blood vessels within the brain and rarely the spinal cord. It can also lead to a range of complications, including ischemic infarction (stroke), intracerebral or subarachnoid hemorrhage, mycotic aneurysms, venous thrombosis, and transient ischemic attacks (TIA). Three suggestive clinical patterns are shown in **Box 1**.[1] The diagnosis of CNS can be challenging based on the current options for classifying definite case using neuroradiologic and histopathologic studies, which are used to categorize cases of granulomatous angiitis of the brain (GAB) or nervous system,[2] the prototypical, albeit least common and most lethal subtype of primary CNS vasculitis (PCNSV).[3] Vessel narrowing, beading, multiple dilatations, aneurysms, avascular mass lesions, and normal studies, and granulomatous angiitis with epithelioid cells, giant cells, and vascular necrosis, can be encountered in GAB and angiitis of other

Disclosure Statement: The authors have nothing to disclose.
[a] Department of Neurology, Division of Neuro-Epidemiology, New York University School of Medicine, New York, NY, USA; [b] School of Public Health, City University of New York, New York, NY, USA; [c] Department of Neurology, Clinical Affairs, MS Comprehensive Care Center, Stony Brook University Medical Center, HSC T12, Room 020, Stony Brook, NY, USA
* Corresponding author. 333 East 34th Street, Suite 1J, New York, NY 10016.
E-mail address: youngd01@nyu.edu

Box 1
Clinical neurologic presentations of central nervous system vasculitis

- Encephalopathy with headache
- Intracranial mass lesion with headache and other abnormalities
- Atypical relapsing multiple sclerosis picture (with headache, seizures, encephalopathy, and strokelike features)

Adapted from Coyle PK. Central nervous system vasculitis due to infection. Chapter 27. In: Younger DS, editor. The vasculitides, volume 2. Nervous system vasculitis and treatment. New York: Nova Biomedical; 2015. p. 127–50; with permission.

---

origins, including diverse infections.[2] However, the management of PCNSV and infectious-mediated vasculitis will differ.[4]

Infection can injure blood vessels in different ways. The pathogen may bind to or actually infect endothelium, or may trigger an adjacent immune or toxic response that indirectly affects vasculature. Blood vessel injury may reflect the sequela of direct infection, compressive inflammatory exudate, septic emboli, or formation of mycotic aneurysms. The infectious agents associated with CNS blood vessel disease are shown in **Box 2**.

Box 2
Infectious agents associated with central nervous system blood vessel disease

Bacterial pathogens:
- Agents of acute bacterial meningitis (*S pneumoniae, N meningitidis*)
- *M tuberculosis*
- Spirochetal infections (*T pallidum, B burgdorferi*, and Leptospira)
- *Mycoplasma pneumoniae*
- *Bartonella*
- *T whippelii*

Viral pathogens:
- Herpes pathogens (VZV, CMV, HSV 1 and 2; EBV)
- Retroviruses (HIV, HTLV-1)
- Hepatitis agents (HBV, HCV)
- Parvovirus B19
- West Nile virus

Fungal pathogens:
- Aspergillus
- Candida
- Coccidioides
- Cryptococcus
- *E rostratum*
- *H capsulatum*
- Mucormycosis

Parasitic pathogens:
- *T solium*
- *P falciparum*
- *S mansoni*
- *T gondii*

Rickettsial pathogens:
- *R rickettsia*
- Scrub typhus

BACTERIA

Acute septic bacterial meningitis is associated with vascular complications in up to 20% of patients.[5] Vascular complications typically occur early, including days to weeks following initiation of antibiotic therapy. Invasive pneumococcal disease is defined as a proven isolation of *Streptococcus pneumoniae* bacteria from normally sterile sites, such as blood or cerebrospinal fluid (CSF). It remains a major cause of morbidity and mortality worldwide despite the availability of antibiotic therapy and vaccines. Host as well as bacterial factors contribute to its pathogenicity. Ethnicity, extremes of age, comorbidities, and alcoholism are well-known host risk factors associated with increased susceptibility and higher mortality. Pneumococcal meningitis remains a potentially devastating disease with high mortality and neurologic damage among those who survive. Focal neurologic findings may be present during the acute phase of bacterial meningitis, but more often occur after a few days as immunologic complication of meningitis. Case death rates and risk of sequelae following meningitis are higher for *S pneumoniae* than *Neisseria meningitidis* or *Haemophilus influenzae* infection.

The proinflammatory cascade triggered by *S pneumoniae* and self-perpetuated by a dysregulated host inflammatory response triggers mediators with vascular toxicity resulting in seizures, diffuse brain swelling, hydrocephalus, hearing loss, and ischemic or hemorrhagic stroke. Arteries are involved more often than veins and show narrowing on ultrasonography.[5] Ischemic complications result from vasculitis, vasospasm, associated endocarditis, or intra-arterial thrombosis.[5]

Among 87 consecutive adult patients with pneumococcal meningitis, mortality was 24.1%.[6] Cerebrovascular arterial complications were seen in 21.8%, and venous complications were seen in 10.3% of cases. Bacterial meningitis produces a subarachnoid inflammatory exudate that worsens over time, encasing large vessels at the base of the brain. Invasion of blood vessel walls by inflammatory cells leads to edema, focal stenosis and dilation, and intimal thickening. Large and medium vessels are typically involved in the circle of Willis and along the terminal internal carotid artery (ICA), but the process can spread to involve smaller vessels as well. Although vasculitis and vasospasm lead to cerebral ischemia and infarction however, disseminated intravascular coagulation may also supervene in the setting of septic meningitis and hypercoagulability, with activation of antifibrinolytic, proinflammatory, and procoagulant pathways. Pneumococcal meningitis was associated with cerebral venous thrombosis and carotid and vertebral artery dissection in one reported patient.[7] There are reports of late stroke with pneumococcal meningitis involving small penetrating arterioles.[8]

There can be delayed or chronic vasculopathy and progressive arterial stenosis consistent with late immune-mediated mechanisms, the hypercoagulable state, or rebound inflammatory effects.[4,8,9] Such patients are exceptional but may respond to corticosteroid therapy.

Infection of the endocardial inner lining of the heart can involve heart valves, mural endocardium, and septal defects[10]; valvular heart disease is a predisposing factor for infective endocarditis. The commonest site of valvular infection is the mitral followed by the aortic valve; the pulmonic valve is the least frequently involved. Mitral valve carries the highest risk for CNS emboli, as noted in **Box 2**. Both sterile and infected emboli may occur because of endocarditis.[11]

Endocarditis is generally due to bacterial infection, although fungi, *Rickettsiae*, and viruses are occasional agents. The microorganisms most commonly implicated are *Staphylococcus aureus*, followed by *Streptococcus viridans*, coagulase-negative

Staphylococci, other streptococci, and gram-negative rod organisms[12]; S aureus in particular infects endothelial cells. Streptococcus bovis is a rare cause of infective endocarditis in association with occult gastrointestinal tumors in up to 56% of cases.[10] Bacteremia associated with gingivitis due to HACEK (Haemophilus, Actinobacillus, Cardiobacterium, Eikenella, and Kingella) organism with pneumonia or pyelonephritis can infect sterile fibrin-platelet vegetation. Infection occurs with trivial everyday activities, such as brushing of teeth, bowel movements, and invasive procedures, such as dental extraction, prostate removal, endoscopy or colonoscopy, barium enema, and transesophageal echocardiography. Intravenous (IV) drug use is a risk factor for infectious-related endocarditis. Indwelling lines can be a source of bacteremia. Internal jugular lines are more likely to become infected than subclavian lines. Not only is subacute endocarditis associated with embolism but also it promotes the formation circulating immune complexes, cryoglobulins, and agglutinating and complement-fixing bactericidal antibodies.

CNS complications occur in 20% to 40% of patients with infective endocarditis, the commonest of which is stroke due to septic embolism.[11,13,14] Clinically diagnosed intracranial mycotic aneurysms complicate 2% to 3% of infective endocarditis cases, although the postmortem rate is in the range of 5% to 10%. About 2% to 6% of all intracranial aneurysms are due to infection, tending to affect distal portions of secondary and tertiary branches of the middle cerebral artery (MCA).

The clinical features of neurologic involvement in endocarditis may initially be very subtle with nonspecific fever; headache, fatigue, and malaise are common. Abnormalities on physical examination suggestive of embolism include Janeway lesions, splinter hemorrhages, and Roth spots; multiple ischemic strokes may also be present. Rupture of resultant mycotic aneurysm can lead to acute catastrophic hemorrhage, the symptoms of which depend on the location. Multiple microscopic emboli can lead to nonfocal encephalopathy.

A recent analysis of neurologically asymptomatic patients with infective endocarditis[13] found that 71.5% of cases manifested occult brain MRI abnormalities consisting mainly of multiple small infarcts in a watershed distribution, and cerebral microscopic hemorrhages within cortical regions.

Most affected patients demonstrate leukocytosis, elevated acute phase reactants, and positive blood cultures. Diffusion-weighted and gradient-echo MRI sequences are recommended to image the commonest findings in affected patients that include ischemia and hemorrhage. Although brain computed tomographic angiography (CTA) and MR angiography (MRA) detect mycotic aneurysms measuring 3 mm to 4 mm or larger in size, digital subtraction angiography (DSA) remains the gold standard, but can be associated with serious complications.

The differentiation of infective endocarditis and primary cerebral vasculitis is extremely important.[15] Therapy for infective endocarditis includes both supportive care and medical interventions, whereas cerebral vasculitis requires immunosuppression. Failure to accurately distinguish the 2 can result treatment failures and heightened morbidity and mortality. A comparison of the findings of 6 patients with biopsy-proven CNS vasculitis with the data of 6 patients with infective endocarditis showed that the former was generally younger (27–62 years) and presented with multiple strokes (n = 4), intracerebral hemorrhage (n = 1), epileptic seizures (n = 2), or encephalopathy (n = 1). All had pathologic CSF findings, including pleocytosis (n = 5), protein elevation (n = 4), and angiography that revealed multilocular stenosis in 2 cases, whereas DSA was normal in 4. Those with infective endocarditis were generally older (32–77 years) and presented with multiple (n = 3) or single ischemic strokes (n = 2) or encephalopathy and headache (n = 2). Although all patients showed inflammatory serum findings (C-reactive protein, n = 6; leukocytosis, n = 4), CSF-pleocytosis was present in 2 cases only. Angiography revealed a vasculitic pattern in 2 patients. The diagnosis of bacterial endocarditis was established based on trans-esophageal echocardiography and blood cultures. Leptomeningeal and brain bi-opsies performed in 2 cases were normal. Patients with either cerebral vasculitis or infective endocarditis may present with multiple strokes and encephalopathy. The frequency of a vasculitic pattern in angiography is similar in both conditions. Although inflammatory serum findings are the rule in infective endocarditis, pathologic CSF findings were present in all of those with cerebral vasculitis. Transesophageal echocardiography and blood cultures should be performed in order to diagnose or exclude infective endocarditis in those at higher risk. Notwithstanding, immunosuppressive therapy may be dangerous in suspected cases of cerebral vasculitis without confirmatory brain and leptomeningeal biopsy.

Mycobacteria

Mycobacterium tuberculosis (TB) meningitis was the first type of meningitis to be described clinically as *dropsy* of the brain in 1768 and subsequently shown to be inflammatory when meningeal tubercles and visceral tubercles were found to be identical in 1830. The tuberculoma, once the commonest intracranial tumor, is now exceptionally rare. The chief neurologic signs and symptoms of tuberculous meningitis reflecting meningeal irritation are neck stiffness and positive Kernig sign, and raised intracranial pressure notably headache and vomiting with mental changes, seizures, and focal neurologic signs. Arteritis is the rule in the vicinity of tuberculous lesions, wherein vessel walls are invaded by mononuclear cells, with the adventitia more heavily involved than the media.[16] The subintimal and intimal regions form a layer of homogenous fibrinoid material that later involves the media, and the vessel lumen is reduced by inflammatory cell exudation beneath the fibrinoid material, the end results of which are reduction or complete obliteration of the lumen, proliferative endarteritis, and cerebral infarction. The vessels most heavily involved are those at the base of the brain and others in the Sylvian fissure. CNS involvement, which occurs in only 1% of TB infections, has the greatest mortality of any organ involvement, with fatality or severe residual mortality noted in up to one-half of cases of resultant TB meningitis.[17] Children and human immunodeficiency virus (HIV)-infected individuals are at special risk for developing CNS involvement. Polymorphisms in genes involved in the innate immune response, such as the toll-like receptor 2 gene, may influence dissemination and development of TB meningitis.[17] The pathogenesis of infection is usually due to rupture of a previously seeded meningeal, subpial, or subependymal focus. Chronic meningitis produces a thick, gelatinous inflammatory exudate that results in intimal thickening with obliterative vasculitis involving vessels at the base of the brain. Stroke occurs in 15% to 60% of affected patients and may be more common in HIV-infected individuals.[4,18,19] Cerebral infarction can be clinically silent, overshadowed by the meningeal features, or insidious in development. TB-related strokes show a prediction for the anterior rather than posterior circulation. A basal exudate produces inflammatory vascular changes within the circle of Willis. Distal ICA, proximal MCA, and its perforating branches are particularly affected.[17] More severe meningitis carries a greater risk for vascular involvement. Vasospasm affects strokes in the early period, whereas proliferative intimal disease is a factor in later outcome. The immune reconstitution inflammatory syndrome (IRIS) can supervene during treatment of extraneural TB, unmasking latent TB meningitis and presenting with neurologic features, including stroke. Hydrocephalus is a common sequela with often-associated meningeal enhancement, particularly along basal brain regions. Contrast-enhanced MRA is more sensitive in the detection of small-vessel involvement. Pathologically proven TB-associated CNS vasculitis has been described in 5 heterogeneous patients to date.[16]

The diagnosis is confirmed by detection of TB bacilli in CSF using a Ziehl-Neelsen stain and culture as well as a positive polymerase chain reaction (PCR). A positive yield is increased with large sample volumes, and ventricular CSF demonstrating an even higher yield than lumbar CSF. Interferon (IFN)-γ releasing assays and TB antigen analysis can be studied in CSF.[20] Neuroimaging features of basilar exudate and hydrocephalus are suggestive.

Treatment involves induction therapy for 2 months with isoniazid, rifampin, pyrazinamide, and a fourth drug, either streptomycin or ethambutol, followed by maintenance therapy with 2 drugs for an additional 7 to 10 months, typically isoniazid and rifampin. Fluoroquinolones are used in multidrug-resistant cases. Adjunctive corticosteroids may be warranted in the first 6 to 8 weeks. Aspirin is potentially useful in reducing stroke and mortality.[20]

Spirochetes

Syphilis

Syphilis is a spirochetal infection due to *Treponema pallidum*. Infection is acquired or congenital, with an estimated worldwide annual incidence of 12 million new adult cases.[21] About 4% to 10% of untreated patients develop CNS involvement. Symptomatic neurosyphilis presents with meningitis and meningovascular syndromes. Meningitis occurs in the first year of infection, producing basilar meningitis often culminating in stroke and vasculitis.

Meningovascular syphilis comprises 39% to 61% of all symptomatic cases of neurosyphilis. It is characterized by obliterative endarteritis that affects blood vessels of the brain, spinal cord, and leptomeninges, precipitating substantial ischemic injury. Often referred to as Heubner arteritis, it involves medium-sized to large arteries with lymphoplasmacytic intimal inflammation and fibrosis; however, there is a variant form termed Nissl-Alzheimer arteritis that characteristically affects small vessels and produces both adventitial and intimal thickening. Both types can lead to vascular thrombotic occlusions and cerebral infarction, with preferential involvement of the MCA.

Meningovascular syphilis occurs months to years later and is associated with perivascular inflammatory endarteritis that leads to luminal narrowing and rarely dilatation. It typically involves large and medium-sized intracranial vessels, in particular the MCA, as many small intracranial vessels, altogether comprising 15% to 23% of cases.[4]

Patients may experience prodromal symptoms of headache, vertigo, insomnia, and behavioral changes. Stroke symptoms developed in a subacute progressive pattern in one-quarter of patients. A recent Australian series[21] noted a prevalence of 4% for stroke or TIA among those with seropositive meningovascular syphilis.

The affected supraclinoid ICA and proximal vessels of the circle of Willis show smooth or beaded segmental narrowing on neuroimaging, without common or cavernous ICA involvement atypical for atherosclerotic disease. Amorphous proteinaceous firm masses with a necrotic center surrounded by inflammatory tissue termed gumma are noted in the brain of patients with tertiary syphilis and meningovascular disease.

The fluorescent *Treponemal* antibody, which detects specific *T pallidum* antibodies later in the course of the disease, can be used to confirm the results of plasma reagin (RPR) and Venereal Disease Research Laboratory (VDRL) tests, which register reactivity to cardiolipin-lecithin-cholesterol antigen elaborated early in the course of syphilis exposure. The CSF in affected patients with neurosyphilis demonstrates pleocytosis, reactive VDRL, and increased intrathecal *T pallidum* antibody index. All patients should be checked for HIV infection. Treatment of neurosyphilis is IV penicillin for 10 to 14 days with CSF monitoring in HIV-positive individuals to document normalization. Aspirin 81 mg daily can be added for stroke prophylaxis.

The search for the cause of stroke in young adults should include meningovascular syphilis as a potential cause. Sudden acute severe headache heralded onset of occlusion of bilateral vertebral and proximal basilar artery documented by MRA and was noted in an African man who responded to thrombectomy with restoration of blood flow but succumbed to fatal pontine and subarachnoid hemorrhages.[22] Postmortem examination revealed RPR and a positive VDRL test in CSF with CNS vasculitis characterized by mural thrombi along the vertebrobasilar arteries with well-defined lines of Zahn of alternating layers of fibrin, platelet, and red blood cell aggregates, and inflammatory cell infiltration of the arterial walls particularly in the adventitia. Another patient with abrupt onset of confusion, aphasia, and hemiparesis had carotid angiography that documented normal named cerebral vessels except for smaller than average caliber, with an abnormal complement fixation test of the blood and CSF, positive colloidal gold curve test, and leptomeningeal biopsy that showed lymphocytic infiltration, focal fibrosis, and chronic perivasculitis consistent with meningovascular syphilis.[23]

Lyme neuroborreliosis

Veenendaal-Hilbers and colleagues[24] introduced the term Lyme neuroborreliosis in 1988 to emphasize CNS involvement due to Lyme disease. *Borrelia burgdorferi sensu lato* is the spirochete responsible for Lyme disease. *B burgdorferi sensu stricto*, hereafter referred to a *B burgdorferi*, is the species agent that causes Lyme disease and its neurologic complications in North America; *Borrelia garinii* and *Borrelia afzelii* species predominate outside of North America. Virtually all cases result from an infected *Ixodes* tick bite. Lyme disease is a systemic infection with most patients manifesting the prototypical expanding skin lesion at the bite site termed erythema migrans. Both the CNS and the peripheral nervous system (PNS) are targeted body organs. CNS vasculitis, although exceedingly uncommon, probably accounted for less than 1% of all Lyme disease cases in endemic areas. Patients with Lyme neuroborreliosis may present with cerebral infarction, intracerebral or subarachnoid hemorrhage, and TIA.[25–30]

Only 3 patients reported in the literature with neurovascular clinical syndromes ascribed to CNS vasculitis in which detailed information was available, including documentation of positive CSF Lyme serology, were ultimately found to have verified vasculitis.[28–30] Two patients,[28] who presented with headache, were ultimately noted to have histopathologically confirmed vasculitis on brain biopsy. Patient 3 of Oksi and colleagues[28] was an 11-year-old boy with headache and hyperactivity syndrome who developed gait difficulty concomitantly with a stroke visualized on brain MRI. Subsequent craniotomy and biopsy of the area of enhancement disclosed lymphocytic vasculitis of small vessels without fibrinoid necrosis, and CSF *B burgdorferi* serology was positive. Headache and the MRI improved with IV antimicrobial therapy. Patient 2 of Topakian and coworkers[29] presented with headache, fatigue, malaise, nausea, and vomiting first considered migrainous and then psychosomatic until subsequent MRI disclosed ischemic brain infarctions. MRA was compatible with diffuse vasculitis, and CSF showed lymphocytic pleocytosis with positive oligoclonal bands, and diagnostic CSF and serum *B burgdorferi* serology. Brain biopsy showed vasculitis-involving leptomeningeal arteries comprising lymphoplasmacytic vessel wall infiltration with focal necrosis. Epithelioid cells were beaded in multiple granuloma-like formations in the leptomeninges. There was symptomatic improvement after a course of IV antimicrobial therapy. The third patient reported by Miklossy and colleagues,[30] a 50-year-old man with leg spasticity and CSF pleocytosis for 15 months who progressed to hemiparesis and ventilatory support, was later found to have diagnostic *B burgdorferi* serology in serum and CSF. Postmortem examination showed perivascular lymphocytic inflammation of leptomeningeal vessels, some of which displayed infiltration of the vessel walls, duplication of the elastic lamina, narrowing of lumina, and complete obstruction of some leptomeningeal vessels by organized thrombi.

There are rare instances of cerebral venous sinus thrombosis. *B burgdorferi* infection in the CNS may be associated with lymphocytic cerebral vasculitis[28] preceding clues of which include headache, arthralgia, myalgia, peripheral facial nerve palsy, and flulike illness during the summer months. Laboratory evaluation may demonstrate meningeal enhancement on brain MRI, although there appears to be a propensity of vasculitis to involve the posterior circulation. Lumbar CSF analysis typically reveals pleocytosis, increased protein, and intrathecal Lyme antibody production. CNS vasculitis due to Lyme neuroborreliosis should be treated with IV ceftriaxone 2 g daily for 4 weeks via midline or PIC (permanent intravenous catheter) line with daily acidophilus to lower risk of *Clostridium difficile* colitis.

Leptospira

Leptospirosis is a worldwide zoonotic infection due to a spirochete from the genus *Leptospira*. It is transmitted by the urine of infected animals to people exposed to the pathogenic organism through contact with contaminated water, blood, or soil. Infection is biphasic, with flulike symptoms, followed by a second immune phase that can involve meningitis, jaundice with liver injury, and renal failure. Infection can be asymptomatic. About 90% of symptomatic infections manifest a benign biphasic febrile illness with 10% involving icteric Weil disease, and a fatality rate of 10%. Spirochetes are found in blood and CSF early in the course of the illness, and in the urine later in the disease. Leptospirosis more commonly causes meningitis or meningoencephalitis. Clinically apparent CNS vascular involvement is unusual but can result in stroke, hemorrhage, and venous sinus thrombosis.[31–33] Diagnostic tests include screening serology via enzyme-linked immunosorbent assay, microscopic agglutination test, and PCR. Vasculitis is a recognized feature of this infection involving capillaries, with consequent edema, necrosis, and lymphocytic infiltration. Therapy involves primarily doxycycline; however, other effective antibiotics include cefotaxime, penicillin, ampicillin, and amoxicillin.

Relapsing fever

Relapsing fever is spread by tick or lice bites. Louse-borne relapsing fever is due to *Borrelia recurrentis*. Tick-borne relapsing fever is due to at least 15 different *Borrelia* species. Clinical illness is characterized by febrile episodes accompanied by prominent headache and myalgia. Neurologic involvement is characterized by meningitis, facial palsy, myelitis, radiculitis, and focal or diffuse CNS dysfunction.[34] Neuropathologic changes involve edema, subarachnoid, and parenchymal hemorrhage, with perivascular mononuclear infiltrates. Spirochetes can be found in the cerebral microvasculature and interstitial spaces. Diagnosis is based on culture and stain. Treatment includes administration of doxycycline, oxytetracycline, or cephalosporin.

Other Bacteria

Mycoplasma

Mycoplasmas are very small bacteria that have a plasma membrane boundary, but lack a cell wall. The nervous system is a major extrapulmonary target, and neurologic disease can occur after primary atypical pneumonia or de novo.[35] Mycoplasma encephalitis reflects direct brain invasion or an immune-mediated syndrome. There is evidence for vascular injury and microthrombi, with endothelial cell infection.[35,36] Stroke occurs in both children and adults.[37] Diagnosis is based on serology and PCR when positive. Therapy involves a course of macrolide antibiotics, although neurologic involvement may be postinfectious and immune mediated. Anticoagulation can be considered for thrombotic disease.

Rosales and colleagues[37] described isolation of *Mycoplasma gallisepticum* and *Mycoplasma synoviae* from the brains of poultry showing meningeal vasculitis and encephalitis, postulating a role for invasive mycoplasma species in human across the blood-brain barrier.

Bartonella

Bartonella are facultative gram-negative intracellular bacteria that cause human and zoonotic disease. *Bartonella henselae* causes cat scratch disease. Several *Bartonella* species are associated with neuroretinitis, a retinal vasculitis. Immunocompromised hosts are vulnerable to more severe infections. *Bartonella* species can produce cutaneous and systemic vasoproliferative lesions.[38] *B henselae* is known to invade and colonize vascular endothelial cells, among others. Among a broad neurologic spectrum, there are rare cases of ischemic stroke and cerebral arteritis. Diagnosis is based on serology and PCR. Therapy involves doxycycline or azithromycin.

Balakrishnan and colleagues[39] described isolation of *B henselae* DNA by PCR from a 12-year-old with headaches, visual and auditory hallucinations, anxiety, vision loss, bouts of paralysis, facial palsy, chronic insomnia, seizures, dizziness, cognitive dysfunction, and memory loss, resulting in cerebral infarction. However, frank vasculitis lesions were not observed.

Whipple disease

Tropheryma whippelii, a member of gram-positive Actinobacteria family, is the etiologic agent of Whipple disease, which is the soil-borne gram-positive bacillus. CNS involvement, which occurs in up to 43% of cases, may be the initial presentation of infection in 5% of cases.[40] CNS involvement occurs in the setting of active Whipple disease as well as in those relapsing previously treated disease and isolated CNS involvement.[41] Stroke presentation, although very rare, has been described[42] and should be in the differential diagnosis of CNS vasculitis. Stroke also occurs with leptomeningeal arterial fibrosis and thrombosis, or associated with endocarditis.[40] Clues to diagnosis are extraneural disease, including weight loss, fever, polyarthritis, diarrhea, and uveitis. Oculomasticatory myorhythmia and supranuclear gaze palsy are characteristic neurologic features. The diagnosis can be confirmed with PCR and tissue biopsy that reveal macrophages that stain positive for glycogen with the periodic acid Schiff assay, or the identification of the causative organism by immunoreactive antigen. Effective treatment includes administration of third-generation cephalosporins followed by long-term, on average 2 years of ,trimethoprim-sulfamethoxazole and doxycycline.

Famularo and colleagues[43] identified arterial and arteriolar fibrosis, thrombosis, and thickening associated with inflammation of adjacent brain parenchyma and leptomeninges and cerebral vasculitis in a patient with cerebral Whipple disease and stroke syndrome of without gastrointestinal involvement due to hematogenous spread of *T whippelii*.

VIRUSES
Herpesviruses

Herpesviruses are a large family of enveloped DNA viruses. Several distinct agents affect humans, and all result in lifelong latent infection. Varicella zoster virus (VZV) is the cause of childhood chickenpox, and most children manifest only mild neurologic sequelae, and an important infectious agent of associated blood vessel disease. After the infection resolves, the virus becomes latent in neurons of cranial and spinal ganglia of nearly all individuals and has the propensity to reactivate in elderly adults and immunocompromised individuals to produce shingles. An uncommon but serious complication of virus reactivation is ischemic and hemorrhagic stroke. VZV vasculopathy affects both immunocompetent and immunocompromised individuals, typically presenting with headache and mental status changes with or without focal neurologic deficits and a spectrum of vascular damage from vasculopathy to vasculitis with stroke. Both large and small vessels can be involved, and MRI shows multifocal ischemic lesions, commonly at gray-white matter junctions. The diagnosis of VZV can be missed when symptoms and signs occur months after zoster, or in the absence of a typical zoster rash.

It is the only virus documented to replicate in human arteries and is a recognized risk factor for ischemic stroke in children, and stroke and TIA in adults under age 40.[44,45] It is latent in cranial nerve, dorsal root, and autonomic nervous system ganglia. VZV, when reactivated, spreads to arteries of the brain and spinal cord to produce a large- and small-vessel vasculopathy. Cerebral blood vessels show multinucleated giant cells, Cowdry type A inclusion bodies with viral particles, and detectable VZV antigens and DNA, consistent with direct infection. In one series of 30 patients,[7] 50% had both large- and small-vessel involvement; 37% showed small artery involvement, and 13% manifested large-artery invasion.[46] Clinical sequelae include infarction, aneurysm, hemorrhage, and ICA dissection.[47] Recently, VZV vasculopathy was recognized as an etiologic agent in patients presenting with giant cell arteritis despite noninformative temporal artery biopsy. Vascular involvement can be unifocal or multifocal. Both immunocompetent and immunocompromised hosts are affected, although more commonly it is the immunocompromised patient. Infarctions can be superficial or deep. Gray-white matter junction lesions are suggestive. With regard to primary infection, there are unusual cases of cerebral infarction or hemorrhage in children. With regard to reactivated infection, vasculopathy can occur up to 6 months after a zoster outbreak. Herpes zoster ophthalmicus (HZO) can be followed weeks later by delayed contralateral hemiparesis, with segmental carotid siphon arteritis, typically in immunocompetent individuals.

Small-vessel involvement may lead to central retinal or posterior ciliary artery involvement, with monocular vision loss. Neuroimaging in these VZV cases is typically abnormal. CSF is often abnormal with an increase in white and red blood cells, raised CSF protein content, and present oligoclonal bands. The CSF VZV immunoglobulin G (IgG) antibody should be measured along with a sample for PCR analysis; however, the former is more likely to be informative in true cases. CNS VZV vasculopathy often presents with headache and progressive neurologic deficits without a history of zoster rash; rarely is VZV associated with spinal cord infarction. Treatment involves antiviral therapy with IV acyclovir; however, oral valacyclovir can be used to extend the length of treatment in more profoundly affected or refractory cases due to concomitant HIV infection.

Thirteen patients with VZV-related vasculopathy with detailed clinicopathologic data including histologic findings of vasculitis have been described in the literature. VZV DNA and VZV-specific antigen were found in 3 of 5 cerebral arteries examined with histologically confirmed CNS vasculitis involving the circle of Willis. Patient 1 of Eidelberg and colleagues[48] who presented with headache and HZO rash was deemed to have CNS vasculitis based on complete occlusion of the MCA and so treated; however, postmortem examination showed no evidence of vasculitis. One patient with contralateral hemiplegia 1 month after HZO was found at postmortem examination to have endarteritis of unilateral anterior cerebral artery (ACA), MCA, and posterior cerebral artery (PCA)[49] with VZV DNA from the involved vessels.

Cytomegalovirus (CMV) replicates in leukocytes and vascular endothelial cells during primary infection with single patient reports of CMV associated with vasculitis. Venous involvement can be found in addition to occlusive arteritis. Affected individuals are usually HIV-positive or an immunocompromised host.[50] Diagnosis involves serologic studies, PCR, culture, and histopathologic tissue analysis for the causative organism. Therapy includes IV ganciclovir, foscarnet, or a combination of both. One recently described elderly woman with CMV encephalitis[51] later developed a postinfectious PCNSV. Koeppen and coworkers[52] described rapidly progressive CNS and PNS deterioration 2 years after chemotherapy for small cell undifferentiated lymphoma in whom postmortem examination demonstrated occlusive arteritis in gray and white matter with involvement of veins indicative of vasculitis, in addition to Cowdry A inclusions and chorioretinitis.

Herpes simplex virus (HSV), types 1 and 2, and Epstein-Barr virus (EBV) have been associated with CNS vasculitis[53,54]; however, vessel wall contrast enhancement may be a clue in suspected patients,[54] and a positive findings in CSF PCR is adequate to justify antiviral therapy. However, in contrast to VZV, where reactivation is the mechanism of causation, CNS vasculitis may be problematic due to latency of infection. Kano and colleagues[55] described EBV-associated CNS vasculitis in brain biopsy tissue of a patient with rapid CNS deterioration and positive EBV DNA in CSF.

RETROVIRUSES
Human Immunodeficiency Virus

Approximately 1% to 5% of individuals infected with HIV are at risk of developing a stroke due to opportunistic infections, coagulopathy, cardioembolism, HIV-associated vasculopathy, and frank vasculitis.[56] Moreover, HIV-associated arterial vasculitis is thought to account for 13% to 28% of ischemic strokes. CNS vasculitis, which is estimated to occur in less than 1% of cases of HIV infection, is a diagnosis of exclusion. Typically, patients are in an advanced stage of the infection. HIV can be associated with a granulomatous inflammation involving small arteries and veins within the brain and leptomeninges. HIV patients with vasculitis should be assessed for cryoglobulins and accompanying infection, especially TB, syphilis, CMV, VZV, hepatitis B and C virus (HBV and HCV), or a drug-induced vasculitis. Therapy typically involves highly active antiretroviral therapy (HAART), with corticosteroids reserved for refractory cases due to vasculitis.

Early in the HIV and the AIDS epidemic, it was clear that a significant proportion of infected persons were IV drug users. Their associated risk behavior exposed them to infection through sharing of contaminated needles, thereby increasing the risk of spread of HIV and other blood-borne infections. The 2 postulated periods in the neurobiology of HIV when autoimmune disease manifestations and cerebral vasculitis can occur are shortly after seroconversion and before the spread of productive infection, and after initiation of HAART in association with the IRIS. The timing of early HIV invasion has been difficult to ascertain based on the presence of one or more well-recognized clinicopathologic HIV/AIDS syndromes, including HIV encephalitis, HIV-associated dementia, and AIDS-dementia complex, all of which are indicative of symptomatic infection. Six presymptomatic HIV-seropositive drug abusers by Gray and colleagues[57] had nonnecrotizing cerebral vasculitis at postmortem examination.

Human T-cell lymphotropic virus-type 1

Human T-cell lymphotropic virus-type 1 (HTLV-1) was the first described human retrovirus. It causes adult T-cell leukemia and lymphoma as well as a progressive myelopathy referred to as tropical spastic paraparesis–HTLV-1–associated myelopathy in less than 1% of infections. Neurologic syndromes associated with HTLV-1 infection appear to be due to active and selective expansion of retrovirus-infected T cells that harbor provirus that selectively expresses HTLV-1 proteins, such as Tax. In particular, activated cytotoxic CD8$^+$ T cells are increased. Perivascular inflammation is a frequent histopathologic feature. The laboratory diagnosis of HTLV-1 infection is based on serologic and PCR studies. There is no proven antiviral therapy. Ma and co-workers[58] reported vasculitis in brain biopsy tissue of a patient with HTLV-1 infection.

Hepatitis Virus Agents

Hepatitis C is estimated to affect 170 million people worldwide with extrahepatic involvement that occurs in 38% to 74% of cases. Hepatitis C is associated with cryoglobulinemia, arthritis, and palpable purpura. There is an immune response to the Fc portion of immunoglobulin, characterized by the Wa idiotype. The resulting immune complex, which contains virus, idiotypic antibody, and antibody, precipitates in the cold and produces a small-vessel vasculitis. HCV can cause CNS vasculitis independent of cryoglobulinemia, and CNS vasculitis may be the first clinical manifestation of hepatitis C infection.

Affected patients present with progressive headache, multiple strokes, and typical angiographic patterns. Therapy includes the antiviral agent interferon (IFN), ribavirin, sofosbuvir, protease inhibitors, and corticosteroids. Both HBV and HCV have been associated with polyarteritis nodosa[59] that typically involves the PNS, but unusual cases may involve the CNS. In such cases, antiviral therapy is added to corticosteroids, and cyclophosphamide, in more severe cases. The resultant choice of therapy might involve the virostatic agent lamivudine or IFN-α for HBV and ribavirin for HCV.[60] Plasma exchange and rituximab can be added in specific cases as needed.

Parvovirus B19

Parvovirus B19 is a small nonenveloped DNA virus that only infects humans. It causes erythema infectiosum, also known as fifth disease, a benign childhood condition characterized by a classic slapped-cheek appearance. It can cause anemia with preexisting disease as well as arthritis. The cellular receptor for parvovirus B19 is an antigen of the P blood group present on endothelial cells and erythroid progenitor cells. Rare patients with CNS vasculitis have been reported in association with parvovirus B19 infection.[61] The diagnosis is based on serologic studies and PCR testing. There is no specific antiviral therapy for parvovirus B19 infection; however, both intravenous immune globulin (IVIG) and corticosteroids have been used therapeutically.

West Nile Virus

West Nile virus is a flavivirus typically transmitted by the bite of infected culex mosquitoes. Less than 1% of patients develop invasive neurologic disease that includes meningitis, encephalitis, and resultant flaccid paralysis, with rarely reported cases of ischemic infarction and CNS vasculitis[62–64] and occlusive retinal artery vasculitis. Patients with a history of diabetes and alcohol abuse, and older individuals are at increased risk for ischemic complications. Diagnosis is based on IgM antibody and viral RNA detection as well as virus isolation. There is no antiviral therapy, but IVIG has been beneficial in individual patients.

Zika Virus

Zika virus is an arbovirus belonging to the Flaviviridae family. Younger[65] has reviewed the epidemiology of Zika virus. Originally isolated in Uganda, Zika virus is known to cause mild clinical symptoms similar to those of dengue and chikungunya. Zika is transmitted by different species of *Aedes* mosquitoes. Nonhuman primates and possibly rodents play a role as reservoir. Direct interhuman transmission has been reported to occur perinatal, through blood transfusion, and sexually. The first human cases were reported in Africa, but recent outbreaks have been seen in several regions of the world, including Brazil, highlighted the needs of the scientific and public health community to consider it an emerging global threat.

Its clinical profile is that of a dengue-like febrile illness, but recently, associated Guillain-Barré syndrome and microcephaly have appeared. There is neither a vaccine nor prophylactic medications available to prevent Zika virus infection, so current public health recommendation advises pregnant women to postpone travel to areas where Zika viral infection is epidemic, and if not, to follow steps to avoid mosquito bites to avert fetal brain injury associated with intrauterine infection. Viral RNA indicating Zika virus, Chikungunya virus, and Dengue infection can be pathogenically isolated from the CSF of adults with neurologic symptoms with meningitis or encephalitis, Guillain-Barré syndrome, and CNS vasculitis.

FUNGI
Aspergillus

Aspergillosis is the most common invasive mold infection worldwide. It typically causes disease in immunocompromised hosts, although CNS vasculitis and stroke occur in immunocompetent patients.[66,67] The major human pathogens are from the *Aspergillus fumigatus*, *Aspergillus niger*, and *Aspergillus flavus* species. Patients with hematologic malignancies and a history of bone marrow transplantation can have fulminant CNS courses with mortalities of 85% to 99%.[4]

The *Aspergillus* organisms invade blood vessels with resultant production of proteases that weaken the vessel wall leading to aneurysm formation.[68] The course can be more chronic and insidious in those with lesser degrees of immune compromise, such as due to diabetes mellitus. Spread to the CNS occurs via hematogenous routes from the lung or by direct extension through the paranasal sinuses and orbits. CNS involvement, which occurs in 10% to 50% of systemic infections, includes meningoencephalitis and intracerebral hemorrhage as well as vasculopathy, and mycotic aneurysm formation leading, respectively, to stroke and potentially fatal subarachnoid hemorrhage with greater involvement of penetrating than larger named vessels.

Aspergillus infection should be considered in immunocompromised hosts with pulmonary disease and either ischemic or hemorrhagic stroke. The diagnosis can be difficult because CSF cultures are positive in less than 50% of cases, and PCR is investigational. Two antigen assays, each for biomarkers including galactomannan and beta-D-glucan, have not been standardized in the CSF. Tissue biopsy can be confirmatory. Brain neuroimaging may demonstrate ring-enhancing lesions, meningeal enhancement, and ischemic or hemorrhagic stroke. Therapy involves oral voriconazole and surgical resection of focal cerebral and extraneural sites of involvement.

Candida

Candida species are part of normal human flora and thus typically are not pathogenic unless there is mitigating systemic immune compromise. Neutropenia is a major risk factor for invasive disease. *Candida* is considered a yeast infection with *Candida albicans* the most common agent in humans. It invades small blood vessels and can be associated with thrombosis and infarction. Neurologic involvement most often takes the form of meningitis that may predispose to basilar artery thrombosis.[69] One affected patient with HIV/AIDS and subacute meningitis who was treated empirically for tuberculosis and initiated on HAART therapy developed fatal worsening due to postmortem-proven basilar *Candida* meningitis and cerebral vasculitis characterized by CD8[+] T-cell infiltration and microinfarcts, consistent with IRIS.[70] The diagnosis of Candida infection is based on a positive culture and informative PCR, and suggestive findings on antigen assays to mannan and beta-D-glucan are not routinely performed. Effective treatment depends on the age and severity of infection with lipid formulations of amphotericin, fluconazole, or echinocandin.

Lipton and colleagues[71] described CNS vasculitis at postmortem examination in 48% of 29 patients with systemic candidiasis, only 21% of whom had suspected antemortem involvement, noting that immunosuppression represents a risk factor for both systemic and cerebral mycoses.

Coccidioides immitis

Coccidioides immitis is a soil-based fungus endemic to the arid southwest and Latin America. Infection may be asymptomatic or the cause of mild pulmonary issues, such as occurs in valley fever. About one-half of disseminating cases involve the CNS, resulting in basilar meningitis with a local vasculitis of small and medium arteries, and occasionally, larger ones that are more likely to occur in immunocompromised hosts.[72] Cerebral infarction complicates about 40% of patients with *coccidioides* meningitis, leading to alteration of mental status and emergency of focal deficits.[4] Stroke can occur years later following the initial infection.[72] In general, acute infectious-related injury can predispose to vasculitic changes that include transmural inflammation with thrombosis and fibrinoid necrosis, whereas chronic injury leads to intimal thickening, proliferation, and narrowing of the lumen with little or no inflammation.

CSF culture is positive in 33% of cases, often in association with eosinophilic pleocytosis. Complement fixation is positive in about 40% of serum and CSF specimens, but seroconversion can take up to 12 weeks. Treatment involves high-dose fluconazole followed by maintenance therapy. Voriconazole is a second-line agent. A self-limited course of corticosteroids can be given in the setting of cerebral infarction to reduce inflammation.

Eron and colleagues[72] described vasculitis and encephalitis as complications of *C immitis* infection of the CNS in 6 cases of apparent and 4 cases of histologically proven vasculitis, including one with vasculitis and encephalitis associated with coccidioidal meningitis. Vasculitic complications include mental status changes, aphasia, hemianopsia, and hemiparesis.

Cryptococcus neoformans

The yeast form, *Cryptococcus neoformans*, is the commonest cause of fungal meningitis.[4] Vessels of the circle of Willis are most affected by the resultant basilar exudate. Vascular involvement occurs early or late in 4% to 32% of cases. Diagnosis is made by the presence of CSF cryptococcal antigen, India ink stain, and culture. Treatment involves induction therapy with IV amphotericin and flucytosine for 2 weeks followed by consolidation with fluconazole once CSF cultures are negative. Corticosteroids may offer a benefit in the setting of stroke.[73]

Exserohilum rostratum

Exserohilum rostratum is a dematiaceous fungus and black mold that does not typically cause human disease. It is a major contaminant in iatrogenic infections due to mold contamination of methylprednisolone acetate. There was one fatal case of meningitis and CNS vasculitis in an immunocompetent host who received a cervical epidural steroid injection for chronic neck pain.[74] The diagnosis is based on culture and PCR of CSF. Recommended therapy is liposomal amphotericin B and voriconazole, with monitoring of drug levels.[75]

Lyons and colleagues[76] described angioinvasive septate fungal hyphae associated with diffuse vasculitis at postmortem examination in the brainstem of a patient with fatal *Exserohilum* meningitis following cervical epidural methylprednisolone injection for new occipital headaches.

Histoplasma capsulatum

Histoplasma capsulatum is a dimorphic fungus that is endemic in the Ohio and Mississippi River Valley as well as parts of Latin America, Asia, and Africa.[4,70] Although infection in immunocompetent hosts may remain asymptomatic or lead to mild lower respiratory tract illness, others can experience disseminated infection with CNS involvement in up to 20% of cases. The latter most commonly manifests meningitis; however, strokes may accompany associated infective *histoplasma* endocarditis or associated meningovascular disease with ensuing mortality of 11% to 100%. Antihistoplasma antibodies can support CSF culture and antigen studies, which show evidence of CNS infection. Treatment includes liposomal amphotericin followed by itraconazole or fluconazole for at least 1 year.

Mucormycosis

Mucormycosis is due to infection by filamentous fungi of the order Mucorales and class Zygomycetes. They are ubiquitous organisms in bread mold, soil, manure, and decaying vegetation, and the second commonest invasive mold infection.[77,78] *Rhizopus*, *Mucer*, and *Lichtheimia* are the most common genera to cause mucormycosis. Immunocompromised hosts are at particular risk. Underlying conditions include diabetes mellitus, hematologic malignancy, trauma, solid cancers, and solid organ transplants.

Sites of infection include lung, skin, gastrointestinal tract, and the rhino-orbito-cerebral region. Iron is an important component in this infection. These fungi contain spore coat homolog proteins that are unique and required for angioinvasion. The result of this blood vessel invasion is vessel thrombosis and tissue necrosis. The rhino-orbito-cerebral form may produce suggestive necrotic nasal or sinus eschars. Patients may experience carotid or basilar artery thrombosis, cavernous sinus thrombosis, or intracerebral hemorrhage.[74,79]

Diagnosis is based on clinical suspicion confirmed by biopsy, scraping, or culture. PCR is being evaluated. Treatment involves a combination of surgery and systemic therapy. Liposomal amphotericin B is favored therapy; however, thiazoles and posaconazole antibiotics have been used in selected individuals.

PARASITES
Taenia solium

Cysticercosis due to infection with the larval stage of the pork cestode tapeworm *Taenia solium* is the commonest CNS parasite, accounting for 10% of stroke cases in endemic areas, and a major cause of headache and seizures. Lenticulostriate lacunar infarcts are more common than large artery stroke; however, TIA and intracranial hemorrhages also occur.[4,80–82] Among 28 patients with subarachnoid cysticercosis, 15 (53%) had angiographic evidence of cerebral arteritis, 12 (80%) of whom had a stroke syndrome ($P = .02$). Eight of the 15 patients (53%) with cerebral arteritis had evidence of cerebral infarction on MRI, whereas only one patient without cerebral arteritis had cerebral infarction ($P = .05$). The most commonly involved vessels were the MCA and PCA. Small vessels are preferentially affected, with superficial cortical vessel thrombosis, occlusive endarteritis, and focal arteritis. Larger circle of Willis vessels are involved when severe arachnoiditis is present. Diagnosis involves antibody testing and suggestive findings on neuroimaging; however, antigen testing is not routinely used. Antihelminthic therapies include the benzimidazole drug albendazole and the antihelminthic drug praziquantel with corticosteroids.

Plasmodium falciparum

Plasmodium falciparum is a unicellular parasitic protozoan that infects humans, causing more severe forms of malaria. The disease is typically transmitted by the bite of an infected female *Anopheles* mosquito. Inoculated sporozoites infect and multiply in liver cells and then differentiate into merozoites that are released and invade red blood cells. Infection leads to expression of adhesive surface proteins that cause the red cells to stick to the walls of small blood vessels. Intercellular adhesion molecule-1 is a major host binding site.

Falciparum malaria is a leading cause of morbidity and mortality in tropical countries. Cerebral malaria is the most severe neurologic manifestation. It is defined by coma that is not due to seizures, hypoglycemia, or any other identifiable cause, and that is associated with a positive blood smear for parasitized red blood cells.

Pathophysiology is thought to be due to parasitic sequestration in cerebral microvessels. As infected red cells adhere to the endothelium, they cause further erythrocyte agglutination along with platelet clumping. There is endothelial activation, and direct cytotoxic injury. Perfusion is abnormal, and tissue oxygenation is compromised. There may also be injury mediated by soluble factors, including various chemokines, cytokines, nitric oxide, and quinolinic acid. Diagnosis is based on blood smear and antigen-based rapid diagnostic tests. Patients diagnosed with uncomplicated malaria can be effectively treated with the oral antimalarial drug chloroquine phosphate (Aralen) or hydroxychloroquine (Plaquenil). Patients who are considered to have severe disease should be treated aggressively with parenteral antimalarial therapy. Treatment of severe malaria involves parenteral quinidine gluconate given by continuous infusion for at least 24 hours in an intensive care setting plus one of the following: doxycycline, tetracycline, or clindamycin orally or IV followed by oral administration for a full course of 7 days.

There is an investigational new drug protocol that can be obtained by contacting the Centers for Disease Control and Prevention that uses artesunate followed by one of the following: atovaquone-proguanil (Malarone), doxycycline (clindamycin in pregnant women), or mefloquine (Lariam).

Schistosoma mansoni

This Trematode infection, which involves a flatworm, is endemic to sub-Saharan Africa and South America. There is percutaneous penetration of cercariae in the invasive stage followed by mating worms that inhabit the inferior mesenteric veins where they excrete eggs in the adult stage. Neurologic involvement occurs in later stages of infection wherein adult worms can be found in spinal meningeal veins and the intracranial venous system. Ectopic eggs migrate to the brain provoking granuloma formation. Cerebrovascular lesions are found in 20% of patients from postmortem series.

CNS vasculitis occurs in both early and later stages of *Schistosoma* infection[83,84] associated with multiple infarctions, marked eosinophilia, and a corticosteroid response reflective of eosinophil-mediated injury. Presumptive diagnosis is suggested by a known travel history and compatible clinical presentation combined with serologic testing and documentation of eggs in the stool. Treatment involves praziquantel.

Toxoplasma gondii

Toxoplasma gondii is an obligate intracellular protozoan that causes toxoplasmosis. During the initial acute phase of the infection, rapidly dividing tachyzoites spread throughout the host. The development of an effective cellular immune response suppresses the replication of tachyzoites and eradicates most of them, ending the acute phase of the infection. In the brain, the parasites undergo conversion to bradyzoites, which remain viable in the form of cysts because of the low levels of class I major histocompatibility complex and, in addition, the parasites within the cyst are surrounded by the parasitophorous vacuole that is enclosed by a cyst wall; thus, a small amount of antigen escapes into the cytoplasm of the cyst-containing host cell. The organisms reproduce slowly throughout the life of the host and can remain viable within intact nerve cells. Cyst rupture occurs rarely and, in immunocompetent individuals, a rapid immune response leading eventually to microglial nodule formation limits the damage to small inflammatory foci. However, in immunocompromised hosts, cyst rupture may reactivate the infection, leading to the conversion of bradyzoites to the active and rapidly replicating tachyzoites and development of severe tissue injury. Therefore, the CNS may be affected in congenital toxoplasmosis, as a primary infection in immunocompetent individuals or as an opportunistic infection in immunosuppressed individuals. Thus, most CNS infections represent reactivation of old lesions and hematogenous spread from prior infections instead of primary infection.

The resulting disease is widely distributed worldwide among domestic animals and humans. The oocyst form is excreted in cat feces and can be the source of infection. Eating infected raw or undercooked meat is another source of infection. Most infections are asymptomatic; however, immunocompromised hosts are particularly vulnerable to clinical disease. Toxoplasmosis is the leading cause of focal CNS disease in patients with HIV/AIDS and low $CD4^+$ T-cell counts.

Congenital toxoplasmosis causes the characteristic eye lesion termed chorioretinitis, cerebral calcifications, hydrocephalus, and CSF pleocytosis. The pathologic features include periventricular microglial nodules surrounded by lymphocytic vasculitis and necrotic foci. Toxoplasma encephalitis shows well-circumscribed areas of hemorrhage and necrosis, with vascular thrombosis and present tachyzoites. The resulting clinical presentation is usually headache with constitutional symptoms that progress to encephalopathy and focal neurologic deficits.

Pittella[85] has reviewed toxoplasmosis as an opportunistic infection in immunosuppressed individuals. In HIV-infected patients, the disorder presents as a mass lesion, usually multiple, with the basal ganglia, thalamus, and the cerebral gray and white matter junctions being the preferred sites. The lesions consist of well-defined areas of coagulative necrosis, with or without hemorrhage, containing karyorrhectic debris. Blood vessel changes are common, characterized by necrosis, vasculitis, and thrombosis. Mononuclear inflammatory cells and reactive astrocytes in variable numbers are seen surrounding the necrosis. Bradyzoites and tachyzoites are present in large numbers, the former at the periphery of the lesion and the latter within the necrosis. The immunohistochemical identification of tachyzoites is especially useful when bradyzoites are not seen. In more chronic lesions, macrophages may surround the necrosis associated or not with calcification, and parasites are reduced in number. In treated patients, the lesions undergo cystic change and are surrounded by macrophages, scanty inflammatory infiltrate, and astrocytosis.

Serologic testing is generally positive, but may not be so in immunocompromised patients. Parasites can sometimes be observed in biopsy-stained tissues and CSF; however, a positive CSF PCR is helpful. Culture is typically too time-consuming to perform. Compatible features of the disorder on brain MRI include single or multiple lesions in the basal ganglia and white matter, with mass effect and homogeneous or ring-enhancing lesions. However, brain neuroimaging may also be normal when there is diffuse CNS involvement.

Treatment includes pyrimethamine, sulfadiazine, and folinic acid administered for 6 weeks and treatment of any underlying immunocompromised condition. Alternative therapy includes trimethoprim-sulfamethoxazole and clindamycin for patients allergic to sulfa medication.

Rickettsial Pathogens

Rickettsiae are obligate intracellular gram-negative coccobacillary agents that multiply in eukaryotic cells. Phylogenetically, they fall between bacteria and viruses. Both mammals and arthropods are natural hosts. Within the genus *rickettsia*, there are 3 biogroups that cause illness: the spotted fever group, the typhus group, and the scrub typhus biogroup. *Rickettsiae* adhere to and invade endothelium with increased vascular permeability, leakage, edema, and hypotension. They are capable of eliciting a generalized vasculitic response in the CNS.

Rickettsia rickettsia

Rrickettsia causes Rocky Mountain spotted fever. More than 90% of infections in the United States occur from April through September via tick bite. The tick vectors are larger soft ticks, including *Dermacentor andersoni* and *Dermacentor variabilis* and *Amblyomma americanum*. Within the CNS, the vasculitis provokes a damaging immune response that is predominantly cell mediated. The overall associated mortality is about 4%.

Symptomatic infection involves severe headache, abdominal pain, persistent fever, peripheral macular centripetal rash, confusion, and myalgia. The classic triad is fever, headache, and rash. Conjunctivitis may also be noted. Neurologic involvement includes meningoencephalitis, focal deficits, and coma. Suggestive laboratory abnormalities are thrombocytopenia, hyponatremia, and elevated liver enzymes. A deficiency of glucose-6-phosphate dehydrogenase enzyme is associated with more severe infection.

Diagnosis is made on clinical grounds, confirmed by positive serology. Therapy involves doxycycline for 7 to 14 days. Kumar and Pramod[86] described a young male Indian with high fever and severe acute headache followed by mental change who developed facial weakness, hyperreflexia, and right posterior cerebral and bilateral thalamopeducular infarcts on computerized tomography of the brain, with filling defects in the origin in the P1 segment of the right PCA on CTA. CSF showed lymphocytic pleocytosis and a positive Weil-Felix test for the proteus antigen OX19. The patient was diagnosed with cerebral vasculitis; however, confirmatory histopathology was not obtained.

Scrub typhus

Scrub typhus (Tsutsugamushi disease) involves infection with different species of *Orientia tsutsugamushi*. Most cases occur in the southwest Pacific and Southeast Asia. Infection occurs with the bite of the larval form of trombiculid mites or chiggers, resulting in small-vessel perivasculitis. The ensuing illness is typically mild and self-limited, but can progress to life-threatening neurologic illness,[87–89] including meningoencephalitis.

Suggestive features of the disorder include necrotic eschar at the site of the mite bite so noted in 50% of case; generalized lymphadenopathy, and mild truncal rash. CSF shows a pattern of aseptic meningitis. Serologic testing is available, and therapy involves doxycycline or another tetracycline.

SUMMARY

Underlying infections are important to consider in patients with CNS vasculitis, and when seriously suspected, warrant prompt and thorough investigation. Selected antimicrobial therapy combined with supportive care can be lifesaving; however, a self-limited course of corticosteroids can lead to prompt reduction in associated inflammation and preservation of neurologic integrity.

REFERENCES

1. Coyle PK. Central nervous system vasculitis due to infection [Chapter 27]. In: Younger DS, editor. The vasculitides, volume 2. Nervous system vasculitis and treatment. New York: Nova Biomedical; 2015. p. 127–50.
2. Younger DS, Hays AP, Brust JCM, et al. Granulomatous angiitis of the brain. An inflammatory reaction of diverse etiology. Arch Neurol 1988;45:514–8.
3. Salvarani C, Brown RD Jr, Christianson TJH, et al. Adult primary central nervous system vasculitis: treatment and course. Arthritis Rheum 2015;67:1637–45.
4. Younger DS. Overview of primary and secondary vasculitides [Chapter 2]. In: Younger DS, editor. The vasculitides, vol. 1, 2nd edition. New York: Nova Biomedical; 2019. [Epub ahead of print].
5. Klein M, Koedel U, Pfefferkorn T, et al. Arterial cerebrovascular complications in 94 adults with acute bacterial meningitis. Crit Care 2011;15:R281.
6. Kastenbauer S, Pfister HW. Pneumococcal meningitis in adults: spectrum of complications and prognostic factors in series of 87 cases. Brain 2003;126:1015–25.
7. Panicio M, Foresto R, Mateus L, et al. Pneumococcal meningitis, cerebral venous thrombosis, and cervical arterial dissection: a run of bad luck? Neurohospitalist 2013;3:20–3.
8. Schut E, Brouwer M, de Gans J, et al. Delayed cerebral thrombosis after initial good recovery from pneumococcal meningitis. Neurology 2009;73:1988–95.
9. Kato Y, Takeda H, Dembo T, et al. Delayed recurrent ischemic stroke after initial good recovery from pneumococcal meningitis. Intern Med 2012;51:647–50.
10. Choucair J. Infectious causes of vasculitis. In: Sakhas LI, Katsiori C, editors. Updates in the diagnosis and treatment of vasculitis. 2013. https://doi.org/10.5772/55189.
11. Chaudhary G, Lee J. Neurologic complications of infective endocarditis. Curr Neurol Neurosci Rep 2013;13:380.
12. Bor D, Woolhandler S, Nardin R, et al. Infective endocarditis in the US, 1998-2009: a nationwide study. PLoS One 2013;3(8):e60033.
13. Hess A, Klein I, Lavallee P, et al. Brain MRI findings in neurologically asymptomatic patients with infective endocarditis. AJNR Am J Neuroradiol 2013;4:1579–84.
14. Ruttmann E, Willeit J, Ulmer H, et al. Neurological outcome of septic cardioembolic stroke after infective endocarditis. Stroke 2006;37:2094–9.
15. Berit P. Isolated angiits of the CNS and bacterial endocarditis: similarities and differences. J Neurol 2009;256:792–5.
16. Smith HV, Daniel P. Some clinical and pathological aspects of tuberculosis of the central nervous system. Tuberculosis 1947;28:64–80.

17. Thwaites G, Van Toorn R, Schoeman J. Tuberculous meningitis: more questions, still too few answers. Lancet Neurol 2013;12:999–1010.

18. Pasticci MB, Paciaroni M, Floridi P, et al. Stroke in patients with tuberculous meningitis in a low TB endemic country: an increasing medical emergency? New Microbiol 2013;36:193–8.

19. Lammie G, Hewlett R, Schoeman J, et al. Tuberculous cerebrovascular disease: a review. J Infect 2009;59:156–66.

20. Thwaites G. Advances in the diagnosis and treatment of tuberculous meningitis. Curr Opin Neurol 2013;26:295–300.

21. Cordato D, Djekic S, Taneja S, et al. Prevalence of positive syphilis serology and meningovascular neurosyphilis in patients admitted with stroke and TIA from a culturally diverse population. J Clin Neurosci 2013;20:943–7.

22. Feng W, Caplan M, Matheus M, et al. Meningovascular syphilis with fatal vertebrobasilar occlusion. Am J Med Sci 2009;338:169–71.

23. Rabinov KR. Angiographic findings in a case of brain syphilis. Radiology 1963; 80:622–4.

24. Veenendaal-Hilbers JA, Perquin WVM, Hoogland PH, et al. Basal meningovasculitis and occlusion of the basilar artery in two cases of *Borrelia burgdorferi* infection. Neurology 1988;38:1317–9.

25. Romi F, Kråkenes J, Aarli J, et al. Neuroborreliosis with vasculitis causing stroke-like manifestations. Eur Neurol 2004;51:49–50.

26. Schmiedel J, Gahn G, von Kummer R, et al. Cerebral vasculitis with multiple infarcts caused by Lyme disease. Cerebrovasc Dis 2004;17:79–80.

27. Jacobi C, Schwark C, Kress B, et al. Subarachnoid hemorrhage due to *Borrelia burgdorferi*-associated vasculitis. Eur J Neurol 2006;13:536–8.

28. Oksi J, Kalimo H, Marttila RJ, et al. Inflammatory brain changes in Lyme borreliosis: a report on three patients and review of literature. Brain 1996;119:2143–54.

29. Topakian R, Stieglbauer K, Nussbaumer K, et al. Cerebral vasculitis and stroke in Lyme neuroborreliosis. Two case reports and review of current knowledge. Cerebrovasc Dis 2008;26:455–61.

30. Miklossy J, Kuntzer T, Bogousslavsky J, et al. Meningovascular form of neuroborreliosis: similarities between neuropathological findings in a case of Lyme disease and those occurring in tertiary neurosyphilis. Acta Neuropathol 1990;80: 568–72.

31. Watt G, Manaloto C, Hayes C. Central nervous system leptospirosis in the Philippines. Southeast Asian J Trop Med Public Health 1989;20:265–9.

32. George P. Two uncommon manifestations of leptospirosis: Sweet's syndrome and central nervous system vasculitis. Asian Pac J Trop Med 2001;4:83–4.

33. Turhan V, Senol M, Sonmez G, et al. Cerebral venous thrombosis as a complication of leptospirosis. J Infect 2006;53:e247–9.

34. Cadavid D. Lyme disease and relapsing fever [Chapter 38]. In: Sheld WM, Whitley RJ, Marra CM, editors. Infections of the central nervous system. 3rd edition. Philadelphia: Lippincott Williams and Wilkins; 2004. p. 659–90.

35. Rhodes R, Monastersky B, Tyagi R, et al. Mycoplasma cerebral vasculopathy in a lymphoma patient: presumptive evidence of *Mycoplasma pneumonia* microvascular endothelial cell invasion in a brain biopsy. J Neurol Sci 2011;309:18–25.

36. Koskiniemi M. CNS manifestations associated with *Mycoplasma pneumoniae* infections: Summary of cases at the University of Helsinski and review. Clin Infect Dis 1993;17(Suppl. 1):S52–7.

37. Rosales RS, Puleio R, Loria GR, et al. Mycoplasmas: brain invaders? Res Vet Sci 2017;113:56–61.

38. Spinella A, Lumetti F, Sandri G, et al. Beyond cat scratch disease: a case report of *Bartonella* infection mimicking vasculitic disorder. Case Rep Infect Dis 2012. https://doi.org/10.1155/2012/334625.

39. Balakrishnan N, Ericson M, Maggi R, et al. Vasculitis, cerebral infarction and persistent Bartonella henselae infection in a child. Parasit Vectors 2016;9:254.

40. Peters G, du Plessis D, Humphrey P. Cerebral Whipple's disease with a stroke-like presentation and cerebrovascular pathology. J Neurol Neurosurg Psychiatry 2002;73:336–9.

41. Compain C, Sacre K, Puéchal X, et al. Central nervous system involvement in Whipple disease: clinical study of 18 patients and long-term follow-up. Medicine 2013;92:324–30.

42. El-Helou J, Saliba G, Kolev I, et al. Neuro-Whipple confirmed five years after a presumptive diagnosis of a primitive CNS vasculitis. J Neurol 2008;255:925–6.

43. Famularo G, Minisola G, De Simone C. A patient with cerebral Whipple's disease and a stroke-like syndrome. Scand J Gstroenterol 2005;40:607–9.

44. Baskin H, Hedlund G. Neuroimaging of herpesvirus infections in children. Pediatr Radiol 2007;7:949–63.

45. Breuer J, Pacou M, Gauthier A, et al. Herpes zoster as a risk factor for stroke and TIA. Neurology 2014;82:206–12.

46. Nagel M, Cohrs R, Mahalingam R, et al. The varicella zoster virus vasculopathies. Clinical, CSF, imaging, and virologic features. Neurology 2008;70:853–60.

47. Gilden D, Cohrs R, Mahalingam R, et al. Varicella zoster virus vasculopathies: diverse clinical manifestations, laboratory features, pathogenesis, and treatment. Lancet Neurol 2009;8:731–40.

48. Eidelberg D, Sotrel A, Horoupian S, et al. Thrombotic cerebral vasculopathy associated with herpes zoster. Ann Neurol 1985;19:7–14.

49. Melanson M, Chalk C, Georgevich L, et al. Varciella-zoster virus DNA in CSF and arteries in delayed contralateral hemiplegia: evidence for viral invasion of cerebral arteries. Neurology 1996;47:569–70.

50. Anderson A, Fountain J, Green S, et al. Human immunodeficiency virus-associated cytomegalovirus infection with multiple small vessel cerebral infarcts in the setting of early immune reconstitution. J Neurovirol 2010;16:179–84.

51. Rosales D, Garcia-Garcia C, Salgado E, et al. Primary central nervous system vasculitis triggered by cytomegalovirus encephalitis. Neurology 2013;80. POI.231.

52. Koeppen A, Lansing L, Peng S, et al. Central nervous system vasculitis in cytomegalovirus infection. J Neurol Sci 1981;51:395–410.

53. Naides S. Known infectious causes of vasculitis in man. Cleve Clin J Med 2002; 69:SII15–9.

54. Guerrero W, Dababneh H, Hedna S, et al. Vessel wall enhancement in herpes simplex virus central nervous system vasculitis. J Clin Neurosci 2013;20:1318–9.

55. Kano K, Katayama T, Takeguchi S, et al. Biopsy-proven case of Epstein-Barr virus (EBV)-associated vasculitis of the central nervous system. Neuropathology 2017; 37:259–64.

56. Benjamin L, Bryer A, Emsley H, et al. HIV infection and stroke: current perspectives and future directions. Lancet Neurol 2012;11:878–90.

57. Gray F, Marie-Claude L, Keohane C, et al. Early brain changes in HIV infection: Neuropathological study of 11 HIV seropositive, non-AIDS cases. J Neuropathol Exp Neurol 1992;51:177–85.

58. Ma WL, Li CC, Yu SC, et al. Adult T-cell lymphoma/leukemia presenting as isolated central nervous system T-cell lymphoma. Case Rep Hematol 2014;2014: 917369.

59. Semmo AN, Baumert TF, Kreisel W. Severe cerebral vasculitis as primary manifestation of hepatitis B-associated polyarteritis nodosa. J Hepatol 2002;37:414–6.

60. Broussalis E, Trinka E, Kraus J, et al. Treatment strategies for vasculitis that affects the nervous system. Drug Discov Today 2013;18:818–35.

61. Bilge I, Sadikoğlu B, Sevinç E, et al. Central nervous system vasculitis secondary to parvovirus B19 infection in a pediatric renal transplant patient. Pediatr Nephrol 2005;20:529–33.

62. Kulsta A, Wichter M. West Nile encephalitis presenting as a stroke. Ann Emerg Med 2003;4:283.

63. Alexander J, Lasky A, Graf W. Stroke associated with central nervous system vasculitis after West Nile virus infection. J Child Neurol 2006;21:623–5.

64. Zafar S, Dash D, Chachere M, et al. West Nile virus infection associated with central nervous system vasculitis and strokes. Neurology 2012;78. P03. 264. [abstract].

65. Younger DS. Epidemiology of Zika virus. Neurol Clin 2016;34:1049–56.

66. Abenza-Abildua M, Fuentes-Gimeno B, Morales-Bastos C, et al. Stroke due to septic embolism resulting from *Aspergillus* aortitis in an immunocompetent patient. J Neurol Sci 2009;284:209–10.

67. Martins H, Rodrigo da Silva T, Scalabrini-Neto A, et al. Cerebral vasculitis caused by *aspergillus* simulating ischemic stroke in an immunocompetent patient. J Emerg Med 2010;38:597–600.

68. Laurencikas E, Sandstedt B, Söderman M. Intrathecal aspergillosis and fusiform arterial aneurysms in an immunocompromised child: a clinic-pathological case report. Childs Nerv Syst 2006;22:1497–501.

69. Grimes D, Lach B, Bourque P. Vasculitic basilar artery thrombosis in chronic Candida albicans meningitis. Can J Neurol Sci 1998;25:76–8.

70. Trofa D, Nosanchuk J. Histoplasmosis of the central nervous system. J Neuroparasitology 2012;3:1–7.

71. Lipton SA, Hickey WF, Morris JH, et al. Candidal infection in the central nervous system. Am J Med 1984;76:101–8.

72. Williams P, Johnson R, Pappagianis D, et al. Vasculitic and encephalitic complications associated with *Coccidioides immitis* infection of the central nervous system in human: report of 10 cases and review. Clin Infect Dis 1992;14:673–82.

73. Lane M, McBride J, Archer J. Steroid responsive late deterioration in *Cryptococcus neoformans variety gattii* meningitis. Neurology 2004;63:713–4.

74. Takahashi S, Horiguchi T, Mikami S, et al. Subcortical intracerebral hemorrhage caused by mucormycosis in a patient with a history of bone-marrow transplantation. J Stroke Cerebrovasc Dis 2009;18:405–6.

75. Bell W, Dalton J, McCall C, et al. Iatrogenic *Exserohilum* infection of the central nervous system: mycological identification and histopathological findings. Mod Pathol 2013;26:166–70.

76. Lyons JL, Gireesh ED, Trivedi JB, et al. Fatal Exserohilum meningitis and central nervous system vasculitis after cervical epidural methylprednisolone injection. Ann Intern Med 2012;157:835–6.

77. Hong H, Lee Y, Kim T, et al. Risk factors for mortality in patients with invasive mucormycosis. Infect Chemother 2013;45:292–8.

78. Katragkou A, Walsh T, Roilides E. Why is Mucormycosis more difficult to cure than more common mycoses? Clin Microbiol Infect 2013. https://doi.org/10.1111/1469-0691. 12466.

79. Maffini F, Cocorocchio E, Pruneri G, et al. Locked-in syndrome after basilary artery thrombosis by Mucormycosis masquerading as meningoencephalitis in a lymphoma patient. Ecancermedicalscience 2013;7:382.

80. Alarcón F, Hidalgo F, Moncayo J, et al. Cerebral cysticercosis and stroke. Stroke 1992;23:224–8.

81. Marquez J, Arauz A. Cerebrovascular complications of neurocysticercosis. Neurologist 2012;18:17–22.

82. Barinagarrementeria F, Cantú C. Frequency of cerebral arteritis in subarachnoid cysticercosis: an angiographic study. Stroke 1998;29:123–5.

83. Camuset G, Wolff V, Marescaux C, et al. Cerebral vasculitis associated with *Schistosoma mansoni* infection. BMC Infect Dis 2012;12:220.

84. Jauréguiberry S, Ansart S, Perez L, et al. Acute neuroschistosomiasis: two cases associated with cerebral vasculitis. Am J Trop Med Hyg 2007;76:964–6.

85. Pittella JEH. Pathology of CNS parasitic infections. Handb Clin Neurol 2013;114:65–88.

86. Kumar P, Pramod K. Neurorickettsioses: a rare presentation with stroke in a young adult. J Clin Diagn Res 2014;8:MD03–4.

87. Kim D, Chung J, Yun N, et al. Scrub typhus meningitis or meningoencephalitis. Am J Trop Med Hyg 2013;89:1206–11.

88. Boorugu H, Chrispal A, Gopinath K, et al. Central nervous system involvement in scrub typhus. Trop Doct 2014;44:36–7.

89. Pai H, Sohn S, Seong Y, et al. Central nervous system involvement in patients with scrub typhus. Clin Infect Dis 1997;24:436–40.

Dermatologic Aspects of Systemic Vasculitis

David S. Younger, MD, MPH, MS[a,b,]*, Andrew Carlson[c]

KEYWORDS

- Infection • Dermatology • Vasculitis

KEY POINTS

- Systemic and localized vasculitis affects the skin and subcutis, due to their large vascular beds as well.
- Initial cutaneous manifestations of vasculitides include discoloration, swelling, hemorrhage, and necrosis.
- Affected patients present with localized, self-limited disease to the skin without any known trigger or associated systemic disease.
- Cutaneous vasculitis manifests as urticaria, erythema, petechiae, purpura, purpuric papules, hemorrhagic vesicles and bullae, nodules, livedo racemosa, deep punched-out ulcers, and digital gangrene.
- Skin biopsy and dermatopathology contribute relevant information.

INTRODUCTION

Systemic and localized vasculitis affects the skin and subcutis, due to their large vascular beds as well as hemodynamic factors, such as stasis in lower extremities, and environmental influences, as occur in cold exposure. The initial cutaneous manifestations of vasculitis includes diverse and dynamic patterns of discoloration, swelling, hemorrhage, and necrosis. One-half of affected patients present with localized, self-limited disease to the skin without any trigger or associated systemic disease, known as idiopathic cutaneous leukocytoclastic vasculitis (LCV).[1] Cutaneous vasculitis manifests as urticaria, erythema, petechiae, purpura, purpuric papules, hemorrhagic vesicles and bullae, nodules, livedo racemosa, deep punched-out ul-

Author Disclosure Statement: The authors have nothing to disclose.
[a] Department of Neurology, Division of Neuro-Epidemiology, New York University School of Medicine, New York, NY 10016, USA; [b] School of Public Health, City University of New York, New York, NY, USA; [c] Department of Pathology, Division of Dermatology and Dermatopathology, Albany Medical College, 43 New Scotland Avenue, MC-81, Albany, NY 12208, USA
* Corresponding author. 333 East 34th Street, 1J, New York, NY 10016.
E-mail address: youngd01@nyu.edu
Website: http://www.davidsyounger.com

Neurol Clin 37 (2019) 465–473
https://doi.org/10.1016/j.ncl.2019.01.017
0733-8619/19/© 2019 Elsevier Inc. All rights reserved.

cers, and digital gangrene.[2] Skin biopsy and dermatopathology contribute relevant information; however, they require correlation with the clinical history, physical examination, and laboratory findings to reach an accurate diagnosis in a given affected patient. This article reviews the dermatologic aspects of primary and secondary vasculitides.

GENERAL CONCEPTS AND NOSOLOGY

The skin receives its blood supply from penetrating vessels from within the underlying subcutaneous fat, which contains medium-sized vessels.[3] Branches of medium-sized vessels give rise to 2 vascular plexuses that intercommunicate, the deep vascular plexus lying at the interface between the dermis and subcutaneous fat and the superficial plexus located in the superficial aspects of the reticular dermis. Further distally, the papillary dermis forms by capillary loops.

The type of cutaneous lesions closely correlates with the size of vessel affected by vasculitis. For example, in cutaneous LCV, immune complexes deposition and inflammation targeting postcapillary venules result in small palpable purpura (**Fig. 1**).

Inflammation that targets arterioles and arteries results in large purpuric lesions with irregular borders (**Fig. 2**). Ulcers, nodules, pitted scars, and livedo reticularis are

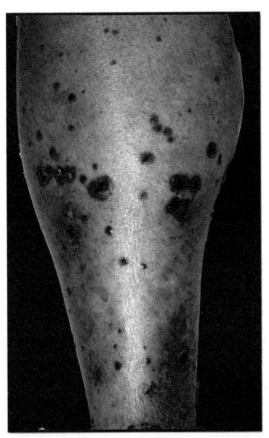

Fig. 1. Typical palpable purpura, some with central necrosis in a patient with idiopathic cutaneous vasculitis of the legs.

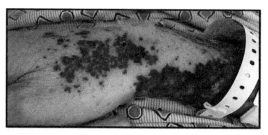

Fig. 2. Large purpuric lesions with irregular borders affecting the left wrist of a patient with idiopathic systemic vasculitis.

associated with arterial muscular vessel involvement localized to the dermal-subcutis interface or within the subcutis.[4]

EPIDEMIOLOGY

The incidence of cutaneous vasculitis ranges from 15.4 to 29.7 cases per million per year, affecting adults more than children of all ages, with slight female predominance, and up to 90% of children diagnosed with Henoch-Schönlein purpura (HSP)/IgA vasculitis (IgAV).[1] Approximately one-half of patients presenting with cutaneous vasculitis have idiopathic LCV skin lesions, whereas the remainder are attributed to recent infection and drug ingestion. LCV that results from drugs or infection is termed, *hypersensitivity* or *allergic vasculitis*. The antinuclear cytoplasmic antibody (ANCA)-associated vasculitides (AAV) include eosinophilic granulomatosis with polyangiitis (previously known as Churg-Strauss syndrome), microscopic polyangiitis, and granulomatosis with polyangiitis (GPA) (previously known as Wegener granulomatosis) which may present with cutaneous vasculitis.[3] The onset of cutaneous vasculitis may be an indication of secondary vasculitis in association with connective tissue disease (CTD), such as systemic lupus erythematosus vasculitis (LV),[5] and rheumatoid arthritis (RA)-related vasculitis (RAV).[6]

The evolution of cutaneous vasculitis occurs in 3 phases. The first is a single acute, self-limited episode that resolves in less than or equal to 6 months in association with drug exposure or an infectious trigger, so noted in 60% of patients. The second is relapsing disease with symptom-free periods, usually found in patients with HSP/IgAV and cryoglobulinemic vasculitis (CV), so noted in 20% of patients. The third is chronic, unremitting disease most often associated with primary systemic and secondary vasculitides in association with CTD, CV, or malignancy, altogether in approximately 20% of patients. The duration of vasculitis ranges from 1 week to 318 months, with mean and median durations of 28 months and 3.7 months, respectively. Fewer than 20% of cutaneous vasculitis cases have extracutaneous or visceral vasculitis. Fatal disease occurs in fewer than 7% of patients.[4]

CLINICAL PRESENTATION

Systemic symptoms of fever, malaise, weight loss, arthritis, and arthralgia most often accompany cutaneous vasculitides. The resulting lesions affect dependent sites of the legs, especially under tight fitting clothes, less so along the arms, trunk, head, and neck, signifying more severe disease or coexisting systemic vasculitis.[7] Cutaneous vasculitis commonly manifests as palpable purpura and infiltrated erythema, indicating dermal small vessel vasculitis (SVV), and less frequently as nodular erythema, livedo racemosa, punched-out ulcers, or digital gangrene due to muscular-vessel vasculitis. The type of cutaneous lesions closely correlates with the size of vessel affected by vasculitis. Sparse superficial perivascular neutrophilic infiltrates associated with nuclear debris and extravasated red blood cells result in urticarial papules and plaques, which last greater than 24 hours, burn rather than itch, and resolve with residual pigmentation. A predominant SVV results in purpuric macules and infiltrated erythema, whereas deeper dermal SVV correlate with palpable purpura and vesiculobullous lesions. Ulcers, nodules, pitted scars, and livedo reticularis are associated with arterial muscular vessel involvement located at the dermal-subcutis interface or within the subcutis.[8]

LABORATORY EVALUATION
Histopathologic Studies

A diagnosis of cutaneous vasculitis of small and medium-sized muscular vessels is established by biopsy and examination of hematoxylin-eosin–stained sections followed by direct immunofluorescent (DIF) studies. Fibrinoid necrosis is composed of fibrin deposition within and around the vessel wall and is a feature of nearly all early vasculitic lesions. Inflammatory infiltrates within and around the walls of vessels accompanied by fibrin deposition (**Fig. 3**) may be accompanied by endothelial damage in the form of endothelial swelling and shrinkage due to apoptosis and sloughing. The finding of inflammatory cells infiltrating the adventitia and media and disrupting the endothelium or endothelialitis is a de facto sign of vasculitis (**Fig. 4**). Secondary changes that suggest underlying vasculitis include extravasation of red blood cells causing purpura, necrosis leading to infarction, and ulceration secondary to the ischemia and vessel obstruction. Circumstantial evidence of vessel wall damage includes lamination of the adventitia, media, and/or intima of vessels or so-called onion skinning; perivascular nuclear dust or leukocytoclasia without fibrin deposits, such as in early evolving LCV; sharply defined loss of the elastic lamina associated with acellular scar tissue in the healed stage of muscular vessel vasculitis; and subendothelial, intramuscular, and adventitial inflammatory cells. Neovascularization of the adventitia and the formation of small capillaries are prominent features of mature and older lesions in chronic

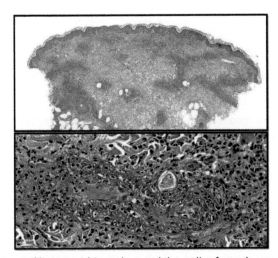

Fig. 3. Inflammatory infiltrates within and around the walls of vessels accompanied by fibrin deposition indicative of vasculitis, seen in low magnification (*upper panel*) and higher magnification (*lower panel*).

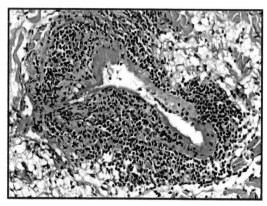

Fig. 4. Lymphocytes infiltrate the adventitia and media of a small vein and the intima shows extensive fibrin deposits.

localized SVV, such as erythema elevatum dinutum; medium vessel vasculitides, such as polyarteritis nodosa; and large vessel vasculitides, such as giant cell arteritis. Immunofluorescence analysis of a tissue biopsy of involved skin lesions is indispensable. The most common immunoreaction found in vessels by DIF is C3, followed by IgM, IgA, and IgG and fibrin deposits.[1,8] The type of immunoglobulin and pattern of deposits in DIF are of additional diagnostic value. For example, predominance of IgA in HSP/IgAV directs attention to renal involvement. Basement membrane zone or keratinocyte nuclear or in vivo ANA and IgG immunoreactions found in vasculitides associate with CTD, such as LV. The finding of basement membrane zone immunoreactions occur especially in those with CTDs. IgM deposition in blood vessels, circulating RF, and monoclonal production of IgM occur in CV and RA-related vasculitis.

Drug-Induced Cutaneous Vasculitis

Hypersensitivity vasculitis due to adverse drug reactions manifests as superficial dermal neutrophilic or lymphocytic SVV on skin biopsy and represents approximately 20% of cases of cutaneous vasculitis.[1,8–10] Tissue eosinophilia is a useful indicator of drug-induced cutaneous SVV.

Tumor necrosis factor α

Tumor necrosis factor (TNF)-α inhibitors used in the treatment of autoimmune and rheumatic diseases were the reported cause of cutaneous vasculitis in 8 patients so treated for 2 months to 72 months,[11] 4 patients with RA, 3 patients with ulcerative colitis, and 1 patient with Crohn disease. The most common presenting manifestation of the patients was palpable purpura, followed by ulcerated lesions, erythematous macules, and blisters. After discontinuation of anti–TNF-α, none had recurrent vasculitis. Appearance of ANCA titers in patients under anti–TNF-α therapy should prompt excluding AAV overlap, for which anti–TNF-α is not efficacious and that requires switching to disease-specific therapy.

Levamisole

Levamisole was originally introduced as an anthelmintic agent and later used in Behçet disease and RA for immunosuppression. It has been used in colon cancer, enhancing the immunity by potentiating the T-cell–mediated immune response. More recently levamisole was added to cocaine to potentiate the stimulant effects because it has a dopamine agonistic effects provoking a synergistic effect with cocaine.[5] Affected patients have constitutional symptoms, arthralgia, leukopenia, agranulocytosis, and cutaneous vasculitis with purpuric lesions of the ears, nose, cheeks, and extremities. The lesions have bright-red borders with central necrosis (**Fig. 5**). Despite the severe and dramatic clinical appearance of these lesions, they usually resolve spontaneously within a few weeks of drug discontinuation but can recur with subsequent contaminated cocaine abuse. Subsequently, clinicians need to differentiate this presentation from other forms of vasculitis, particularly with GPA, because the degree of immune suppression differs between both. The degree of skin necrosis has been as severe and large as to require skin grafting and removing the offender combined with a short course of corticosteroids suffice to control the disease, contrasting with the management for GPA, which requires more aggressive immune suppression. One-half of affected patients demonstrated positive anti-MPO or positive anti-PR3 antibodies.[6] In addition, cocaine contaminated with levamisole by unclear mechanisms is the mediator of ANCA-mediated vasculitis. The target, differing from AAV, was found the neutrophil elastase within the granules, eliciting an atypical ANCA-positive antibody response. Furthermore, elastase, a constituent of neutrophil extracellular traps (NETs), is a target of patients exposed to cocaine/levamisole. It has been suggested that the programmed cell death of neutrophils by NETs release, which is the extrusion of nuclear (chromosomal material) and mitochondrial DNA containing proinflammatory and thrombogenic peptides, is potentiated by cocaine/levamisole. This combination of drugs induces the release of highly immunogenic NETs, containing high concentrations of elastase.[12]

TNF receptor–associated periodic syndrome (TRAPS) is an autosomal dominant disorder consisting of periodic fever episodes lasting from 3 days to 21 days and in which manifestations show pleuritic chest pain, abdominal pain, conjunctivitis, periorbital edema, monoarthritis, testicular pain, myalgia, and papulomacular and urticarial rash. A report revealed SVV and panniculitis in a 66-year-old patient diagnosed with TRAPS with migratory macular erythematous rash and with positive ANCA against elastase, successfully treated with etanercept.

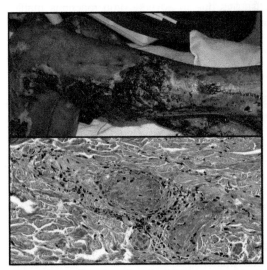

Fig. 5. Levamisole-induced vasculitis shows histologic signs of a vaso-occlusive disorder and vasculitis. The *upper panel* shows the site of clinical vasculitis and the *lower panel* shows the associated histopathology.

SYSTEMIC MALIGNANCY

Lymphoproliferative, myeloproliferative, and carcinomatous tumors comprise less than 5% of cases of paraneoplastic cutaneous vasculitis (**Fig. 6**), a diagnosis that may be considered in patients with recurrent purpura; hematologic abnormalities, including cytopenia, monoclonal gammopathy, and immature blood cells; hematuria, abnormal tissue, or nodal masses on imaging studies; and refractory responses to immune therapies. There are 3 such categories of patients, including those with true paraneoplastic vasculitic syndromes wherein the vasculitis improves with extirpation or treatment of the tumor; vasculitis masquerading as malignancy, such as lung masses in GPA; and malignancy masquerading as vasculitides, as in emboli from an atrial myxoma and superficial migratory thrombophlebitis with pancreatic cancer. Most paraneoplastic cutaneous vasculitic syndromes are the result of a paraproteinemia secondary to lymphoproliferative disorders, including cryoglobulinemia in association with lymphocytic lymphoma and Waldenström macroglobulinemia.

PROGNOSIS

The distinction between localized cutaneous vasculitis and systemic vasculitis is important because the former carries a relatively favorable outcome, whereas the latter conveys the likelihood of permanent organ damage and increased morbidity and mortality. Approximately 20% to 40% of patients with cutaneous vasculitis

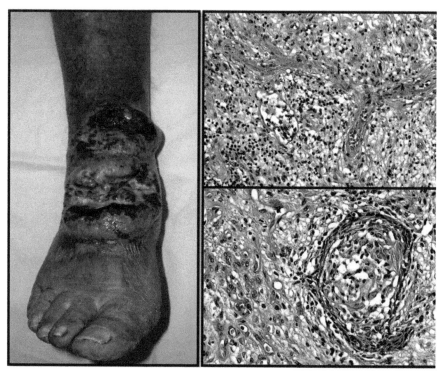

Fig. 6. Myelodysplastic syndrome presenting as erythema elevatum diutinum. A large ulcerative tumor shows localized fibrosing leukocytoclastic vasculitis. The *left panel* shows the site of clinical vasculitis. The *upper and lower right panel* shows the associated histopathology. (*Courtesy of* Juan Carlos Graces, MD, Guayaquil, Ecuador.)

have concomitant limited systemic vasculitis, notably in the kidney, such as renal-dermal vasculitis, whereas the likelihood of chronicity and systemic progression is enhanced when there is coexisting CTD, cryoglobulinemia, frank ulceration, arthralgia, more than 1 form of cutaneous vasculitic lesion such as ulceration and palpable pur-pura, putative muscular vessel vasculitis and SVV, normal serum IgA levels, pares-thesia, fever, painless lesions, and cutaneous necrosis.[12] Histologically, the severity of vessel injury in cutaneous vasculitis correlates with the clinical severity and course.[13,14] Up to 60% of patients presenting with cutaneous vasculitis on skin biopsy have SVV restricted to the dermis whereas the remainder have deep dermal and pan-nicular SVV and muscular vessel involvement.[15]

THERAPY

Therapy depends on the nature and severity of the vasculitis. Mild hypersensitivity due to drug reactions should be treated with discontinuation of the offending agents, an-tihistamines for urticaria-associated pruritus, and a short course of corticosteroids in more severe cases. Simple observation may be adequate for mild cases and transient lesions of HSP/IgAV-related purpura. Nonsteroidal anti-inflammatory agents, colchi-cine, antihistamines, and dapsone may be used in chronic cutaneous vasculitis without recognizable cause and in selected patients prior to administration of cortico-steroids and cytotoxic drugs. Rituximab has remission-induction efficacy equivalent to cyclophosphamide in AAV, each in conjunction with corticosteroids.[15] Morphologic alternations of the vessel wall lumina and perivascular areas may be useful in treat-ment strategy. Healed arteritis with intimal thickening due to luminal occlusion should suggest the need for anticoagulation and vascular dilating agents, whereas patholog-ically confirmed acute and subacute arteritis generally warrants combination immuno-suppressive therapy to suppress ongoing vascular inflammation and tissue damage.

REFERENCES

1. Carlson JA, Ng BT, Chen KR. Cutaneous vasculitis update: diagnostic criteria, classification, epidemiology, etiology, pathogenesis, evaluation and prognosis. Am J Dermatopathol 2005;27:504–28.
2. Carlson JA. The histological assessment of cutaneous vasculitis. Histopathology 2010;56:3–23.
3. Lane SE, Watts R, Scott DG. Epidemiology of systemic vasculitis. Curr Rheumatol Rep 2005;7:270–5.
4. Tai YJ, Chong AH, Williams RA, et al. Retrospective analysis of adult patients with cutaneous leukocytoclastic vasculitis. Aust J Dermatol 2006;47:92–6.
5. Chang A, Osterloh J, Thomas J. Levamisole: a dangerous new cocaine adul-terant. Clin Pharmacol Ther 2010;88:408–11.
6. McGrath MM, Isakova T, Rennke HG, et al. Contaminated cocaine and antineu-trophil cytoplasmic antibody-associated disease. Clin J Am Soc Nephrol 2011; 6:2799–805.
7. Ioannidou DJ, Krasagakis K, Daphnis EK, et al. Cutaneous small vessel vascu-litis: an entity with frequent renal involvement. Arch Dermatol 2002;138:412–4.
8. Chen KR, Carlson JA. Clinical approach to cutaneous vasculitis. Am J Clin Der-matol 2008;9:71–92.
9. Carlson JA, Chen KR. Cutaneous vasculitis update: neutrophilic muscular vessel and eosinophilic, granulomatous, and lymphocytic vasculitis syndromes. Am J Dermatopathol 2007;29:32–43.

10. Lee JS, Loh TH, Seow SC, et al. Prolonged urticaria with purpura: the spectrum of clinical and histopathologic features in a prospective series of 22 patients exhibiting the clinical features of urticarial vasculitis. J Am Acad Dermatol 2007;56: 994–1005.
11. Sokumbi O, Wetter DA, Makol A, et al. Vasculitis associated with tumor necrosis factor-alpha inhibitors. Mayo Clin Proc 2012;87:739–45.
12. Lood C, Hughes GC. Neutrophil extracellular traps as a potential source of auto-antigen in cocaine-associated autoimmunity. Rheumatology (Oxford) 2017;56: 638–43.
13. Ratnam KV, Boon YH, Pang BK. Idiopathic hypersensitivity vasculitis: clinicopath-ologic correlation of 61 cases. Int J Dermatol 1995;34:786–9.
14. Hodge SJ, Callen JP, Ekenstam E. Cutaneous leukocytoclastic vasculitis: correlation of histopathological changes with clinical severity and course. J Cutan Pathol 1987;14:279–84.
15. Geetha D, Kallenberg C, Stone JH, et al. Current therapy of granulomatosis with polyangiitis and microscopic polyangiitis: the role of rituximab. J Nephrol 2015; 28:17–27.

Moving?

Make sure your subscription moves with you!

To notify us of your new address, find your **Clinics Account Number** (located on your mailing label above your name), and contact customer service at:

Email: journalscustomerservice-usa@elsevier.com

800-654-2452 (subscribers in the U.S. & Canada)
314-447-8871 (subscribers outside of the U.S. & Canada)

Fax number: 314-447-8029

Elsevier Health Sciences Division
Subscription Customer Service
3251 Riverport Lane
Maryland Heights, MO 63043

*To ensure uninterrupted delivery of your subscription, please notify us at least 4 weeks in advance of move.

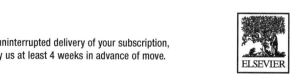

Printed and bound by CPI Group (UK) Ltd, Croydon, CR0 4YY

03/10/2024

01040405-0008